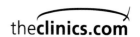

# NEUROLOGIC CLINICS

Brain Tumors in Adults

GUEST EDITORS
Patrick Y. Wen, MD
David Schiff, MD

CONSULTING EDITOR
Randolph W. Evans, MD

November 2007 • Volume 25 • Number 4

**SAUNDERS**

An Imprint of Elsevier, Inc.
PHILADELPHIA   LONDON   TORONTO   MONTREAL   SYDNEY   TOKYO

**W.B. SAUNDERS COMPANY**
*A Division of Elsevier Inc.*

1600 John F. Kennedy Blvd., Suite 1800, Philadelphia, PA 19103-2899

http://www.theclinics.com

**NEUROLOGIC CLINICS**
November 2007
Editor: Donald Mumford

Volume 25, Number 4
ISSN 0733-8619
ISBN-13: 978-1-4160-5195-4
ISBN-10: 1-4160-5195-3

The ideas and opinions expressed in *Neurologic Clinics* do not necessarily reflect those of the Publisher. The Publisher does not assume any responsibility for any injury and/or damage to persons or property arising out of or related to any use of the material contained in this periodical. The reader is advised to check the appropriate medical literature and the product information currently provided by the manufacturer of each drug to be administered to verify the dosage, the method and duration of administration, or contraindications. It is the responsibility of the treating physician or other health care professional, relying on independent experience and knowledge of the patient, to determine drug dosages and the best treatment for the patient. Mention of any product in this issue should not be construed as endorsement by the contributors, editors, or the Publisher of the product or manufacturers' claims.

*Neurologic Clinics* (ISSN 0733-8619) is published quarterly by Elsevier Inc., 360 Park Avenue South, New York, NY 10010–171. Months of issue are February, May, August, and November. Business and editorial offices: 1600 John F. Kennedy Blvd., Suite 1800, Philadelphia, PA 19103-2899. Customer Service Office: 6277 Sea Harbor Drive, Orlando, FL 32887–4800. Accounting and circulation offices: 6277 Sea Harbor Drive, Orlando, FL 32887-4800. Periodicals postage paid at New York, NY, and additional mailing offices. Subscription prices are $218.00 per year for US individuals, $344.00 per year for US institutions, $109.00 per year for US students, $273.00 per year for Canadian individuals, $404.00 per year for Canadian institutions, $285.00 per year for international individuals, $404.00 per year for international institutions, and $145.00 for Canadian and foreign students/residents. To receive student/resident rate, orders must be accompanied by name of affiliated institution, date of term, and the *signature* of program/residency coordinator on institution letterhead. Orders will be billed at individual rate until proof of status is received. Foreign air speed delivery is included in all *Clinics* subscription prices. All prices are subject to change without notice. POSTMASTER: Send address changes to *Neurologic Clinics*, Elsevier Periodicals Customer Service, 6277 Sea Harbor Drive, Orlando, FL 32887-4800. **Customer Service: 1-800-654-2452 (US). From outside of the US, call 1-407-345-4000.**

*Neurologic Clinics* is also published in Spanish by Nueva Editorial Interamericana S.A., Mexico City, Mexico.

*Neurologic Clinics* is covered in *Current Contents/Clinical Medicine, Index Medicus, EMBASE/Excerpta Medica*, and *PsycINFO*, and *ISI/BIOMED*.

Printed in the United States of America.

# CONSULTING EDITOR

**RANDOLPH W. EVANS, MD,** Clinical Professor of Neurology, Department of Neurology and Neuroscience, Weill Medical College of Cornell University, New York, New York; Department of Neurology, The Methodist Hospital; and Clinical Associate Professor of Neurology, Baylor College of Medicine, Houston, Texas

# GUEST EDITORS

**PATRICK Y. WEN, MD,** Associate Professor in Neurology, Harvard Medical School; Director, Division of Neuro-Oncology, Department of Neurology, Brigham and Women's Hospital; and Clinical Director, Center for Neuro-Oncology, Dana-Farber/Brigham and Women's Cancer Center, Boston, Massachusetts

**DAVID SCHIFF, MD,** Professor of Neurology, Neurological Surgery and Medicine (Hematology/Oncology), University of Virginia, Charlottesville, Virgina

# CONTRIBUTORS

**LAUREN E. ABREY, MD,** Associate Attending Neurologist, Department of Neurology, Memorial Sloan-Kettering Cancer Center, New York, New York

**GALAL AHMED, MD,** Department of Neurological Surgery, University of Virginia, Charlottesville, Virginia

**ASHOK R. ASTHAGIRI, MD,** Staff Neurosurgeon, National Institutes of Health/NINDS, Bethesda, Maryland

**ROBERT CAVALIERE, MD,** Assistant Professor of Neurology, Division of Neuro-Oncology, Ohio State University, Columbus, Ohio

**LISA M. DeANGELIS, MD,** Chair, Department of Neurology, Memorial Sloan-Kettering Cancer Center, New York, New York

**JAN DRAPPATZ, MD,** Instructor in Neurology, Harvard Medical School; Division of Neuro-Oncology, Department of Neurology, Brigham and Women's Hospital; and Center for Neuro-Oncology, Dana-Farber/Brigham and Women's Cancer Center, Boston, Massachusetts

**CHRISTOPHER J. FARRELL, MD,** Department of Neurosurgery, Massachusetts General Hospital and Harvard Medical School, Boston, Massachusetts

**JAMES L. FISHER, PhD,** Research Scientist, The Arthur G. James Cancer Hospital and Richard J. Solove Research Institute and Comprehensive Cancer Center at The Ohio State University, Columbus, Ohio

**MARK R. GILBERT, MD,** Professor and Deputy Chair, Department of Neuro-Oncology, University of Texas M.D. Anderson Cancer Center, Houston, Texas

**GREGORY A. HELM, MD, PhD,** Associate Professor, Department of Neurological Surgery, University of Virginia Health Sciences Center, Charlottesville, Virginia

**JAY JAGANNATHAN, MD,** Department of Neurological Surgery, University of Virginia Health System, Charlottesville, Virginia

**JOHN A. JANE, Jr, MD,** Department of Neurological Surgery, University of Virginia Health System, Charlottesville, Virginia

**ADAM S. KANTER, MD,** Department of Neurosurgery, University of California San Francisco, San Francisco, California

**SANTOSH KESARI, MD, PhD,** Assistant Professor of Neurology, Harvard Medical School; Department of Cancer Biology, Dana-Farber Cancer Institute; Division of Neuro-Oncology, Department of Neurology, Brigham and Women's Hospital; and Center for Neuro-Oncology, Dana-Farber/Brigham and Women's Cancer Center, Boston, Massachusetts

**FREDERICK F. LANG, MD,** Professor, Department of Neurosurgery, University of Texas M.D. Anderson Cancer Center, Houston, Texas

**EDWARD R. LAWS, Jr, MD, FACS,** Department of Neurosurgery, Stanford University, Palo Alto, California

**MINESH P. MEHTA, MD,** Professor and Chair, Department of Human Oncology, University of Wisconsin, Madison, Wisconsin

**NIMISH A. MOHILE, MD,** Fellow, Department of Neurology, Memorial Sloan-Kettering Cancer Center, New York, New York

**TERI D. NGUYEN, MD,** Fellow, Department of Neurology, Memorial Sloan-Kettering Cancer Center, New York, New York

**ANDREW D. NORDEN, MD,** Instructor in Neurology, Harvard Medical School, Division of Neuro-Oncology, Department of Neurology, Brigham and Women's Hospital; and Center for Neuro-Oncology, Dana-Farber/Brigham and Women's Cancer Center, Boston, Massachusetts

**SCOTT R. PLOTKIN, MD, PhD,** Department of Neurology, Massachusetts General Hospital and Harvard Medical School, Boston, Massachusetts

**NADER POURATIAN, MD, PhD,** Department of Neurological Surgery, University of Virginia, Charlottesville, Virginia

**DAVID A. REARDON, MD,** Associate Professor, Department of Surgery; Department of Pediatrics; and Associate Deputy Director, The Preston Robert Tisch Brain Tumor Center, Duke University Medical Center, Durham, North Carolina

**JEREMY N. RICH, MD,** Associate Professor, Department of Medicine; Department of Surgery; Department of Neurobiology; Department of Pharmacology; and Department of Cancer Biology, The Preston Robert Tisch Brain Tumor Center, Duke University Medical Center, Durham, North Carolina

**SITH SATHORNSUMETEE, MD,** Division of Neurology; and Division of Neurosurgery, The Preston Robert Tisch Brain Tumor Center, Duke University Medical Center, Durham, North Carolina; Division of Neurology, Department of Medicine, Faculty of Medicine at Siriraj Hospital, Mahidol University, Bangkok, Thailand

**CLAIRE M. SAUVAGEOT, PhD,** Instructor in Neurology, Department of Cancer Biology, Dana-Farber Cancer Institute; Department of Neurology, Brigham and Women's Hospital; and Harvard Medical School, Boston, Massachusetts

**DAVID SCHIFF, MD,** Professor of Neurology, Neurological Surgery and Medicine (Hematology/Oncology), University of Virginia, Charlottesville, Virgina

**JUDITH A. SCHWARTZBAUM, PhD,** Associate Professor, Comprehensive Cancer Center at The Ohio State University and Division of Epidemiology, College of Public Health, The Ohio State University, Columbus, Ohio; Institute of Environmental Medicine, Karolinksa Institute, Stockholm, Sweden

**MARK E. SHAFFREY, MD,** Professor and Chairman, Department of Neurological Surgery, University of Virginia, Charlottesville, Virginia

**JASON P. SHEEHAN, MD, PhD,** Assistant Professor, Department of Neurological Surgery, University of Virginia Health Sciences Center, Charlottesville, Virginia

**JONATHAN SHERMAN, MD,** Department of Neurological Surgery, University of Virginia, Charlottesville, Virginia

**VOLKER W. STIEBER, MD,** Assistant Professor, Department of Radiation Oncology, Wake Forest University School of Medicine, Winston-Salem, North Carolina

**CHARLES D. STILES, PhD,** Professor of Microbiology and Molecular Genetics, Department of Cancer Biology, Dana-Farber Cancer Institute; and Harvard Medical School, Boston, Massachusetts

**MARTIN J. VAN DEN BENT, MD,** Neuro-Oncology Unit, Daniel den Hoed Cancer Clinic/Erasmus University Medical Center, Rotterdam, the Netherlands

**PATRICK Y. WEN, MD,** Associate Professor in Neurology, Harvard Medical School; Director, Division of Neuro-Oncology, Department of Neurology, Brigham and Women's Hospital; and Clinical Director, Center for Neuro-Oncology, Dana-Farber/Brigham and Women's Cancer Center, Boston, Massachusetts

**JOSEPH L. WIEMELS, PhD,** Associate Professor, Division of Cancer Epidemiology, Department of Epidemiology and Biostatistics, University of California, San Francisco, California

**MARGARET WRENSCH, PhD,** Professor, Departments of Neurological Surgery and Epidemiology and Biostatistics, University of California, San Francisco, California

**GEOFFREY S. YOUNG, MD,** Director of MRI Neuroimaging, Department of Radiology, Brigham and Women's Hospital; and Instructor in Radiology, Harvard Medical School, Boston, Massachusetts

# CONTENTS

that will eventually allows us to manage this primary cause of treatment failure.

## Advances in Radiation Therapy for Brain Tumors

Volker W. Stieber and Minesh P. Mehta

Radiation therapy is used postoperatively as adjunctive therapy to decrease local failure; to delay tumor progression and prolong survival; as a curative treatment; as a therapy that halts further tumor growth; to alter function; and for palliation. Registration of MRI scan data sets with the treatment-planning CT scan is essential for accurate definition of the tumor and surrounding organs at risk. Integrating additional imaging studies that reflect the biologic characteristics of central nervous system tumors is an area of active research. Conformal treatment delivery is used to spare adjacent normal tissue from receiving unnecessary dose. In the dose range used when treating these tumors, the probability of causing serious late toxicity is relatively low and secondary malignancies are rare.

## Medical Management of Brain Tumor Patients

Jan Drappatz, David Schiff, Santosh Kesari, Andrew D. Norden, and Patrick Y. Wen

Brain tumors can present challenging medical problems. Seizures, peritumoral edema, venous thromboembolism, fatigue, and cognitive dysfunction can complicate the treatment of patients who have primary or metastatic brain tumors. Effective medical management results in decreased morbidity and mortality and improved quality of life for affected patients.

## Management of Patients with Low-Grade Gliomas

Mark R. Gilbert and Frederick F. Lang

The accurate diagnosis and management of patients who have infiltrating low-grade gliomas is increasing in importance. Recent advances in molecular characterization, imaging, and treatment of these tumors underscore this current focus of investigations.

## Anaplastic Oligodendroglioma and Oligoastrocytoma

Martin J. van den Bent

Until approximately 15 years ago, the diagnosis of an oligodendroglioma (OD) was merely as a pathologic entity. The only clinical relevant meaning of this histologic diagnosis was the observation that the prognosis of OD was in general better than that of astrocytic tumors of similar grade. This changed with the recognition of the marked sensitivity to PCV chemotherapy of these tumors, although the best timing of chemotherapy still is unclear. Observations have led to the current tendency to consider 1p/19q loss low-grade and anaplastic oligodendroglioma a separate biologic entity, at least within clinical trials, since they have a much better outcome.

## Diagnosis and Treatment of High-Grade Astrocytoma

Sith Sathornsumetee, Jeremy N. Rich, and David A. Reardon

High-grade astrocytomas include the most common adult central nervous system (CNS) tumor, glioblastoma multiforme, and anaplastic astrocytoma—a highly aggressive cancer with short median survival despite maximal multimodality therapy. Diagnosis is by clinical and radiographic findings confirmed by histopathology. Standard-of-care therapy includes surgical resection, radiotherapy, and temozolomide. Nearly all patients who have high-grade astrocytomas develop tumor recurrence or progression after this multimodality treatment. Two treatment challenges are molecular/genetic heterogeneity of tumors and limited CNS tumor delivery. It is probable that targeted therapies will be most effective in combination with one another or with cytotoxic therapies. This article discusses diagnosis and current treatment of high-grade astrocytomas.

## Novel Therapies for Malignant Gliomas

Robert Cavaliere, Patrick Y. Wen, and David Schiff

The impact of cytotoxic therapies on the outcome of glioblastoma has been modest thus far. Yet it is clear that subsets of high-grade gliomas exist that are sensitive to treatment. Patients deemed resistant to the current standard approach may be selected for alternative therapies, thereby avoiding treatment toxicity from an ineffective treatment. The future of novel therapies lies in our understanding of the molecular biology of gliomas and their stem cells. Not only will this drive the development of new agents, it will also lead to tailored therapies for specific tumors. Yet much research is still needed at all levels, from the identification of molecular markers to the development and application of novel therapeutics.

## Brain Metastases

Teri D. Nguyen and Lisa M. DeAngelis

Brain metastases are a common complication of cancer and alter patient management more than metastases at any other site of distant progression. Supportive therapies include steroids and antiseizure medications. Definitive treatments include radiation therapy, surgery, and chemotherapy. The optimal choice of treatment and overall prognosis largely depend on patient characteristics and the extent and distribution of disease. Delaying or decreasing neurologic cause of death and disability are important therapeutic goals for this population. While better definitive strategies are investigated, physicians must remember to optimize the use of supportive therapies to ameliorate symptoms and maintain quality of life.

# FORTHCOMING ISSUES

# RECENT ISSUES

NEUROLOGIC
CLINICS

ELSEVIER
SAUNDERS

Neurol Clin 25 (2007) xiii–xv

# Preface

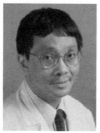 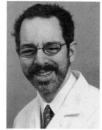

Patrick Y. Wen, MD    David Schiff, MD
*Guest Editors*

Each year in the United States there are approximately 40,000 new cases of primary brain tumors and 150,000 to 200,000 new cases of brain metastases in adults. These tumors tend to occur between the 4th and 7th decades of life, and they produce a disproportionately significant impact in terms of morbidity and mortality compared to other neoplasms. Since the last issue of *Neurologic Clinics* that was devoted to brain tumors in adults was published more than 10 years ago, there has been substantial progress in understanding the molecular pathogenesis of these tumors, especially in the critical role of tumor stem cells. In addition, there have been important technologic advances in surgery and radiation therapy that have significantly improved the safety of these therapies, and these advances have allowed the widespread application of techniques, such as stereotactic radiosurgery, to treat brain metastases and some primary brain tumors that cannot be removed surgically. Most excitingly, improved understanding of the biology of brain tumors finally is being translated into novel therapies using targeted molecular agents, inhibitors of angiogenesis, and immunotherapies. The preliminary results with these therapies are encouraging, but there remains significant work ahead before the promise of these treatments are fulfilled.

This issue of *Neurologic Clinics* attempts to summarize the recent progress made in the diagnosis and treatment of brain tumors in adults. The focus of the majority of articles in this volume is on patient management. However, the scientific and technologic underpinnings of current

0733-8619/07/$ - see front matter © 2007 Elsevier Inc. All rights reserved.
doi:10.1016/j.ncl.2007.08.001                                    *neurologic.theclinics.com*

practice also are reviewed and referenced to allow readers to investigate particular areas in more detail as their interest or clinical needs demand.

This issue is divided into three parts. The first part reviews, in dedicated articles, the epidemiology of brain tumors, the molecular pathogenesis of brain tumors and the role of stem cells, and the genetic syndromes that give rise to brain tumors and the important insights they have contributed to our understanding of the pathogenesis of these tumors.

The second set of articles summarizes the advances in technologies that diagnose and treat brain tumors. The first article in this set discusses the important advances in magnetic resonance imaging that have significantly improved brain tumor diagnosis and potentially may allow better monitoring of therapies and prediction of responses in the future. Other articles discuss the advances in neurosurgery and radiation therapy that have been responsible for much of the progress in the treatment of brain tumors over the past decade.

The third set of articles focuses upon the management of the most common forms of brain tumors in adults. The first article in this third set reviews the optimal medical management of brain tumors. This important topic includes the optimal use of antiepileptic drugs and the treatment of peritumoral edema, venous thromboembolism, fatigue, and cognitive deficits. Succeeding articles cover the diagnosis and treatment of specific types of brain tumors, including low grade gliomas, anaplastic oligodendrogliomas and oligoastrocytomas, anaplastic astrocytomas and glioblastomas, primary central nervous system lymphomas, brain metastases, and benign brain tumors, such as meningiomas, schwannomas, and pituitary tumors. Novel therapies for malignant gliomas also are discussed.

As this issue demonstrates, there has been much progress in understanding the pathogenesis of brain tumors and in the development of more effective therapies over the past decade. Nonetheless, for many patients who have brain tumors, the prognosis remains poor. There remains an urgent need to develop more effective therapies for these patients.

We thank all of the authors for their outstanding contributions and the editor, Donald Mumford, and his colleagues at WB Saunders/Elsevier for their help with this issue. We especially thank our patients and their families. Their courage and strength in the face of terrible adversity provide the inspiration for all of us to work toward the day when we will have cures for these devastating tumors.

Patrick Y. Wen, MD
*Center for Neuro-Oncology*
*Dana Farber/Brigham and Women's Cancer Center*
*SW430*
*44 Binney Street*
*Boston, MA 02115, USA*

*E-mail address:* pwen@partners.org

David Schiff, MD
*Departments of Neurology, Neurological Surgery, and*
*Medicine (Hematology/Oncology)*
*University of Virginia*
*Box 800342*
*Charlottesville, VA 22908, USA*

*E-mail address:* ds4jd@virginia.edu

ELSEVIER
SAUNDERS

NEUROLOGIC
CLINICS

Neurol Clin 25 (2007) 867–890

# Epidemiology of Brain Tumors

James L. Fisher, PhD[a,b,*],
Judith A. Schwartzbaum, PhD[b,c,d],
Margaret Wrensch, PhD[e], Joseph L. Wiemels, PhD[f]

[a]*The Arthur G. James Cancer Hospital and Richard J. Solove Research Institute,
2050 Kenny Road, Suite 940, Columbus, Ohio 43221, USA*
[b]*Comprehensive Cancer Center at The Ohio State University, Columbus, Ohio, USA*
[c]*Division of Epidemiology, College of Public Health, The Ohio State University,
300 West 10th Avenue, B-121 Starling Loving Hall, Columbus, Ohio 43210, USA*
[d]*Institute of Environmental Medicine, Karolinksa Institute, Stockholm, Sweden*
[e]*Departments of Neurological Surgery and Epidemiology and Biostatistics,
University of California, San Francisco, UCSF Box 1215, 44 Page Street 503,
San Francisco, California 94143-1215, USA*
[f]*Division of Cancer Epidemiology, Department of Epidemiology and Biostatistics,
University of California, San Francisco, UCSF Box 0441, 1 Irving Street,
AC34, San Francisco, California 94143-0441, USA*

Brain tumors are classified on the basis of histopathology into the following major histologic groupings: tumors of neuroepithelial tissue (hereafter referred to as glioma, including astrocytoma [grade II], anaplastic astrocytoma [grade III], glioblastoma [grade IV], oligodendroglioma, and ependymoma), tumors of meninges (including meningioma and hemangioblastoma), germ cell tumors, and tumors of sellar region (including pituitary tumors and craniopharyngioma). This article reviews the incidence of brain tumors in terms of temporal, demographic, and geographic variation. The incidence and survival probability of brain tumors are summarized using information from the Central Brain Tumor Registry of the United States (CBTRUS) [1] and the Surveillance, Epidemiology and End Results (SEER) program of the National Cancer Institute [2] and literature is reviewed pertaining to risk and prognostic factors, focusing on compelling and promising lines of research that have emerged from the brain tumor literature and from descriptive comparisons. Because only recent research has considered variation in risk factors according to histologic subtypes,

* Corresponding author. The Arthur G. James Cancer Hospital and Richard J. Solove Research Institute, 2050 Kenny Road, Suite 940 Columbus, Ohio 43221, USA.
*E-mail address:* Jay.Fisher@osumc.edu (J.L. Fisher).

0733-8619/07/$ - see front matter © 2007 Elsevier Inc. All rights reserved.
doi:10.1016/j.ncl.2007.07.002 *neurologic.theclinics.com*

we are not always able to report findings in refined histologic categories. Approximately 75% of all primary brain tumors are classified as glioma or meningioma; therefore, this article focuses primarily on these more common brain tumors.

## Descriptive epidemiology

During the years 1998 to 2002, the average annual rate of occurrence of incident (newly diagnosed) primary brain tumors in the United States was 14.4 per 100,000 persons [1]. The incidence of brain tumors has increased over time and differs according to gender, age, race and ethnicity, and geography.

Based on nine geographic areas surveyed by the United States SEER program since 1973, the age-adjusted incidence rate for malignant brain tumors has increased among men (from 5.9 per 100,000 men in 1973 to 7.0 per 100,000 men in 2003) and women (from 4.1 per 100,000 women in 1973 to 5.2 per 100,000 women in 2003) [2]. Most, if not all, of this increase probably is attributable to improvements in diagnostic imaging (eg, use of CT and MRI), increased availability of medical care and neurosurgeons, changing approaches in the treatment of older patients, and changes in classifications of specific histologies of brain tumors [3–5].

For all central nervous system (CNS) tumors, of which brain tumors are the majority, the age-adjusted average annual (1998 to 2002) incidence rate for women (15.1 per 100,000 person years) is slightly greater than that for men (14.5 per 100,000 person years) [1]. Table 1 shows average annual (1997 to 2001) age-adjusted incidence rates and median ages at diagnosis for the major histologic groupings and selected common histologic subtypes of brain tumors. As shown in Table 1, glioma and germ cell tumors are more common in men, whereas meningioma is approximately twice as common in women. This gender difference is greater, approximately fourfold, among Polynesians [6].

In the United States, the median age at diagnosis among all patients diagnosed with a primary brain tumor between 1998 and 2002 was 57 years [1]. Average annual incidence rates of the major histologic groupings according to age at diagnosis are shown in Fig. 1. Average annual incidence rates, according to age at diagnosis, for selected histologies common among adults and children/adolescents (ages 0 to 19), respectively, are shown in Figs. 2 and 3. Among adults (see Fig. 2), incidence rates of meningioma and glioblastoma increase with advancing age, except for a decline in the incidence rate of glioblastoma in people ages 85 years and older. (A logarithmic scale is used in Fig. 2, so that variation by histology can be displayed.) Among children/adolescents (see Fig. 3), incidence rates of all non–germ cell histologies decrease through childhood and adolescence, whereas the incidence of germ cell tumors reaches a peak during the adolescent years. Variation in incidence according to histologic type may reflect diagnostic

Table 1
Number of cases, median ages at diagnosis, and age-adjusted average annual (1998–2002) incidence rates of primary brain tumors (major histologic groupings and selected histologic subtypes), according to gender

| Histologic group | Number of cases | Median age at diagnosis (years) | Rate | Male rate | Female rate |
|---|---|---|---|---|---|
| Tumors of neuroepithelial tissue/glioma | 27,776 | 53 | 6.42 | 7.67 | 5.35 |
| Pilocytic astrocytoma | 1465 | 12 | 0.33 | 0.34 | 0.32 |
| Diffuse astrocytoma | 428 | 46 | 0.10 | 0.11 | 0.08 |
| Anaplastic astrocytoma | 2029 | 51 | 0.47 | 0.56 | 0.38 |
| Glioblastoma | 12,943 | 64 | 3.05 | 3.86 | 2.39 |
| Oligodendroglioma | 1559 | 41 | 0.35 | 0.38 | 0.33 |
| Anaplastic oligodendroglioma | 781 | 48 | 0.18 | 0.20 | 0.16 |
| Ependymoma/anaplastic ependymoma | 1126 | 39 | 0.26 | 0.29 | 0.22 |
| Mixed glioma | 722 | 42 | 0.16 | 0.19 | 0.14 |
| Malignant glioma, not otherwise specified | 1668 | 43 | 0.38 | 0.42 | 0.35 |
| Benign and malignant neuronal/glial, neuronal and mixed | 944 | 26 | 0.21 | 0.23 | 0.19 |
| Embryonal/primitrive/ medulloblastoma | 1094 | 9 | 0.24 | 0.29 | 0.19 |
| Tumors of meninges | 19,980 | 63 | 4.70 | 2.95 | 6.18 |
| Meningioma | 19,190 | 64 | 4.52 | 2.75 | 6.01 |
| Germ cell tumors | 397 | 17 | 0.09 | 0.12 | 0.06 |
| Tumors of sellar region | 4496 | 48 | 1.03 | 1.05 | 1.03 |

Rates are per 100,000 population, age-adjusted to the 2000 United States (19 age groups) standard and based on cancer incidence data from the following registries: Arizona, Colorado, Connecticut, Delaware, Idaho, Maine, Massachusetts, Minnesota, Montana, New Mexico, New York, North Carolina, Texas, Utah, and Virginia.
*From* CBTRUS statistical report: Primary Brain Tumors in the United States, 1998–2002.

practices and access to diagnoses in different age groups in addition to actual biologic variations of brain tumors with age.

Gliomas are approximately twice as common among whites as compared with blacks, as are germ cell tumors. From 1998 to 2002, the incidence rate of glioma among whites was 6.8 per 100,000 persons and 3.5 per 100,000 persons among blacks. During this same time, the incidence of glioma among non-Hispanics (6.7 per 100,000 persons) was greater than that of Hispanics (4.9 per 100,000 persons). There are no well-described explanations for the observed race and ethnicity differences; however, genetic differences (as described later) may contribute to race-related incidence differences.

Brain tumor incidence rates vary moderately by geographic region in areas that report to CBTRUS [1]. The lowest age-adjusted average annual (1998 to 2002) incidence of all CNS tumors is found in Virginia (9.6 per

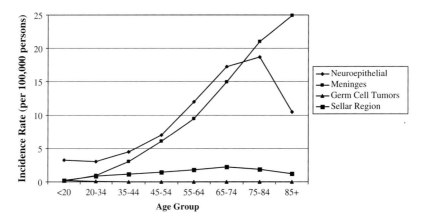

Fig. 1. Age-specific incidence rates of primary CNS tumors, 1998–2002, according to major histologic groupings, CBTRUS. (*Reported in tabular form in* CBTRUS (2005) statistical report: Primary Brain Tumors in the United States, 1998–2002.)

100,000 person years), and the highest is located in Colorado (21.9 per 100,000 person years) [1]. For malignant brain tumors, a similar degree of variation is reported in the geographic SEER regions [2]. There also is worldwide geographic variation in the incidence of brain tumors; for example, malignant brain tumors occur in Japan with less than half the frequency of that in Northern Europe. Countries reporting a high incidence of malignant brain tumors include Australia, Canada, Denmark, Finland, Sweden, New Zealand, and the United States, whereas areas of the world with a lower

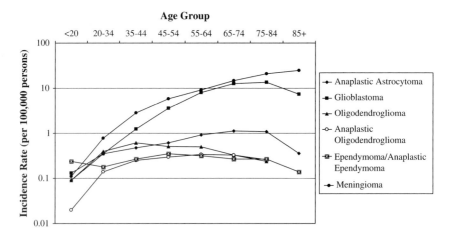

Fig. 2. Age-specific incidence rates of primary neuroepithelial brain tumors and meningioma, 1998–2002, CBTRUS. (*Reported in tabular form in* CBTRUS (2005) statistical report: Primary Brain Tumors in the United States, 1998–2002.)

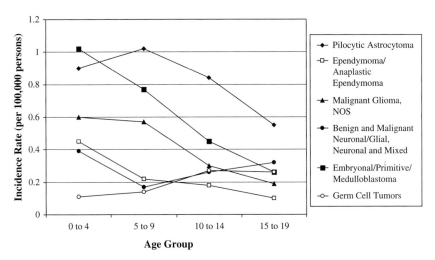

Fig. 3. Age-specific incidence rates of primary CNS histologies more common among children, 1998–2002, CBTRUS. (*Reported in tabular form in* CBTRUS (2005) statistical report: Primary Brain Tumors in the United States, 1998–2002.)

incidence—such as Rizal, Philippines, and Bombay, India—have an incidence approximately one fourth that of the high-incidence countries [5,7]. Differences in diagnostic practices and completeness of brain tumor reporting make all geographic, especially international, comparisons difficult [5]. In addition, higher incidence rates appear in countries (and within the United States—in some states) with greater access to health care and better medical care [5,7]. In one study, although American immigrants had a lower risk for death from all causes, their risk for death from brain tumors was greater than that for their American-born counterparts. This suggests that country of birth alters risk, that exposures occurring early in life may afford protection to the American born, or that potential early exposures in non-American countries increase brain tumor risk [8].

## Survival probability and prognostic factors

### Glioma and glioma subtypes, including glioblastoma

Survival time after brain tumor diagnosis varies greatly by histologic type and age at diagnosis, as shown in Fig. 4 [1]. For each age group, relative survival probability is lowest for patients who have glioblastoma. In general, survival probability is lower for those in older age groups. The relative 2-year and 5-year survival probabilities associated with primary malignant brain tumors diagnosed between 1998 and 2003 are 37.7% and 30.2%, respectively [2]. For the period 1973 to 2003, the 2-year relative probability of surviving a malignant brain tumor for men (35.2%) was slightly less than

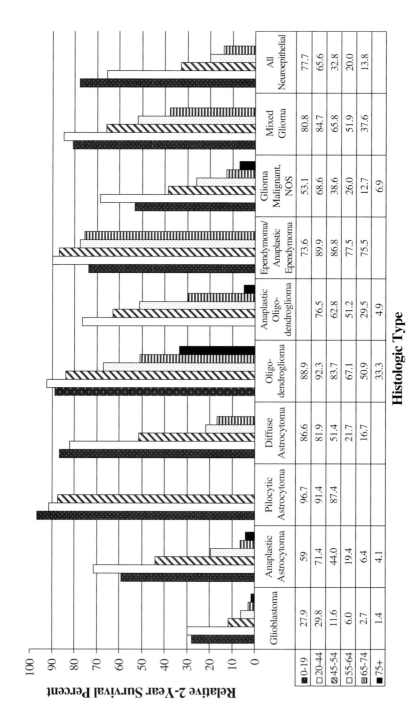

**Histologic Type**

Fig. 4. Two-year relative survival probabilities of primary malignant CNS tumors according to age at diagnosis and histologic type, based on the follow-up of individuals diagnosed between 1973 and 2002, SEER, compiled by CBTRUS. (*Reported in tabular form in* CBTRUS (2005) statistical report: Primary Brain Tumors in the United States, 1998–2002.)

that for women (35.6%) [2]. Although the prognosis is poor for many patients who have malignant brain tumors, 2-year survival probability for patients who have malignant brain tumors has increased from 28.5% in 1975 to 38.7% in 2002 [2]. Much of this increase occurred in patients younger than 65 years of age who were diagnosed with tumors other than anaplastic astrocytoma and glioblastoma. This increase in survival may be an artifact of improved ascertainment of indolent brain tumor subtypes rather than improved clinical management. There has been little change in the survival probability for patients diagnosed with glioblastoma.

Because of the poor prognosis for patients who have glioblastoma—less than one third survive longer than 1 year [2]—investigators have sought to determine factors associated with survival probability and survival time from glioblastoma. Based on previous findings, the following are known to be related to glioblastoma prognosis: age, Karnofsky Performance Status score, extent of resection, capacity for complete resection, degree of necrosis, enhancement on preoperative MRI studies, volume of residual disease, therapeutic approach, pre- and postoperative tumor size, noncentral tumor location (defined as infiltration of splenium, basal ganglia, thalamus, or midbrain), patient deterioration, patient condition before radiation therapy, and presurgical serum albumin level [9–12]. Recent efforts to identify prognostic factors for glioblastoma and other glioma subtypes have focused on genetic factors and molecular markers. For oligodendroglioma, it is now well established that the combined loss of 1p and 19q confers a more favorable prognosis [13]. Although results are inconsistent, and effects may be modified by other factors, such as age, there is some evidence that the following are prognostic indicators for glioblastoma and other glioma subtypes: p53 mutation and expression [14–23], overexpression or amplification of epidermal growth factor receptor (EGFR) [15,17,18,20–22], CDKN2A alterations and deletions [15,17,20], and MDM2 amplifications [14,17,20,22,24]. Simmons and colleagues [25] demonstrated the complex relationship of survival with age at diagnosis, p53, and EGFR in patients who have glioblastoma. They found that in patients younger than the median age, there was a shorter survival time in patients whose tumors overexpressed EFGR but had normal p53 immunohistochemistry [25]. In interpreting their findings, it should be remembered that post-hoc subgroup analysis increases the risk for false-positive findings [26]. Age-dependent associations between glioblastoma survival and 1p and CDKN2A also have been demonstrated [15]. p53 protein expression probably decreases with advancing age [15,25], and the association between p53 expression and survival from glioblastoma may be hidden when confounding by age is adjusted statistically. Loss of heterozygosity (LOH) on chromosome 10q is associated with shorter duration of survival from glioblastoma [23,27], and the combined LOH on 1p and 19q may afford a more favorable prognosis to patients who have glioblastoma [23]. There may be a strong association between different genotypes of human telomerase MNS16A and glioblastoma survival time (24.7 months median survival time for the SS genotype, compared with 14.0 months and 13.1 months for the SL and LL genotypes, respectively) [28]. These results are promising because human telomerase MNS16A may be exploitable as a biomarker of treatment success.

Recently, Wrensch and colleagues [22] reported that glutathione S-transferases (GST) theta (T)1 deletion afforded a less favorable glioma prognosis, whereas higher glioma survival probability was afforded to patients who had glioma and who had the ERCC1 (a DNA excision repair gene) C8092A polymorphism. EGFR expression in patients who had anaplastic astrocytoma was associated with nearly threefold poorer survival [22]. Patients who had glioblastoma and who had elevated IgE lived 9 months longer compared with those who had lower or normal IgE levels [22]. This finding may implicate immunologic factors in glioblastoma prognosis [22]. Patients who have glioblastoma and who have higher IgE levels may have better antitumor defenses or less aggressive tumors with weaker anti-immunologic effects; alternatively, IgE itself may have antitumor activity through direct activity on glioma or other nearby cells [22]. Associations between glioma prognosis in relation to atopic allergy, in which IgE is increased, should be studied. As discussed later, there is consistent and compelling evidence of protection against glioma as the result of allergies and immune-related conditions. Further suggesting the importance of immunologic factors in glioblastoma prognosis, a recent report indicates that amplification of interleukin (IL)-6, a cytokine that may promote glioblastoma, is associated significantly with decreased glioblastoma survival [29]. Analyses of atopy, IgE, and cytokines in relation to glioma prognosis may help understand better the complex nature of immunologic response to gliomagenesis, including secreted tumor-specific factors and host immune responses, and such investigations also may have implications for immunologic therapy for glioma. In addition, brain tumors, like all cancers, must evade immune rejection with mechanisms presumably similar to any foreign tissue growth. Future studies also should include the examination of T-cell activities, such as that of T-regulatory cells, which are associated with tissue graft acceptance and brain tumor prognosis [30,31].

*Meningioma*

For benign brain tumors, such as meningioma, there currently are no estimates of American population-based survival probabilities, because these tumors were not registered as part of the SEER program until recently. Population-based data suggest, however, that survival time for patients diagnosed with meningioma in Norway improved between 1963 and 1992 [32] and in Finland between 1953 and 1984 [33]. McCarthy and colleagues [34] estimated that the 5-year survival probability was 69% for meningioma, and 81% among patients ages 21 to 64 years at diagnosis but only 56% among those 65 years of age or older at diagnosis [34]. Patients who had benign meningioma had a 5-year survival probability of 70%, whereas the 5-year survival probability for patients who had malignant meningioma was 55% [34]. Prognostic factors for patients who had meningioma have not been studied thoroughly. Results from a large study of 9000 cases revealed the following prognostic factors for benign meningioma: age, tumor size, and surgical and radiation treatments. In contrast, for malignant meningioma, the prognostic factors included only age and surgical and radiation treatments [34]. Abnormalities of chromosome 14 also may affect meningioma prognosis [35].

## Risk factors

Risk factors for brain tumors are discovered by conducting analytic epidemiologic studies, which usually compare either brain tumor risk in participants with or without certain characteristics (cohort studies) or the histories of participants with or without brain tumors (case–control studies). Results from a cohort study can provide evidence that a modifiable or varying cause (risk factor) preceded the brain tumor, whereas results from a case–control study usually cannot address temporality (the major exception being studies of germline characteristics that clearly precede environmental exposures and brain tumor diagnoses). Epilepsy or seizure disorder (which is associated consistently with glioma risk) is not discussed in this article, because it probably is a result of glioma rather than a cause [36]. Compelling and promising lines of research that have emerged from the brain tumor literature and from descriptive comparisons are discussed.

### Reproductive and menstrual factors

Women have a lower glioma risk (shown in Table 1). Incidence rates from the New York State Cancer Registry suggest that this protection occurs between the approximate ages of menarche and menopause and decreases in postmenopausal age groups [37]; however, as shown in Fig. 5 (which shows the male-to-female ratios of average annual glioma incidence rates according to age group), incidence rates derived from the SEER program suggest increased glioma risk among men within each age group, with the exception of infants; further, the rates among men remain at least 40% greater than those among women for all age groups 30 years and older. Age-adjusted comparisons of postmenopausal women, whose menopause was not induced surgically, with premenopausal women show that postmenopausal women are at greater risk for glioma and acoustic neuroma [38] than are premenopausal women. Results pertaining to parity and glioma risk are mixed, suggesting lower risk among parous women [39,40] or no association [38,41,42]. Two recent studies [41,42] suggest a possible increase in glioma risk as the result of later (14 years or older versus younger than 12 years) age at menarche. Meningioma is approximately twice as common in

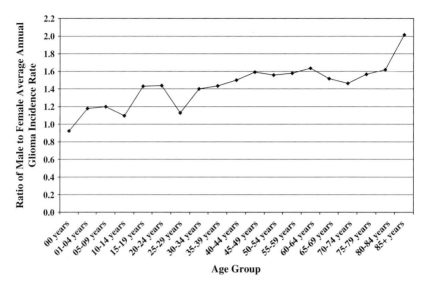

Fig. 5. Ratios of male-to-female average annual glioma incidence rates according to age group. (*Data from* SEER Program. SEER*Stat Database: incidence - SEER 9 Registries Public-Use, Nov 2005 Sub (1973–2003), National Cancer Institute, DCCPS, Surveillance Research Program, Cancer Statistics Branch, released April 2006, based on the November 2005 submission.)

women as in men. Some meningioma tumors express progesterone receptors, and this expression occurs to a greater degree in women [43]. In general, there are consistent results suggesting that, among women of the same age, those who are premenopausal have greater meningioma risk than are those who are postmenopausal. Studies of meningioma risk and age at menarche and parity have produced conflicting results [38,44]. For example, some results concerning parity and age at menarche suggest that estrogen or other reproductive or menstrual hormones may decrease meningioma risk. Further study is required to understand hormone-related factors, especially because some of the findings are opposite of those expected and because menstrual and reproductive factors alone are insufficient to classify lifetime estrogen or other hormonal exposure accurately. Moreover, inconsistent results pertaining to oral contraceptive use and hormone replacement therapy and both glioma [41,42,45] and meningioma [42,45] risks encourage the continued study of the relationships between brain tumor risks and endogenous and exogenous estrogen exposures. Cohort studies of reproductive factors and brain tumor risk among women who have and have not taken estrogen replacement therapy should be conducted.

## Environmental and behavioral risk factors

Because they may be modifiable and because there are strong associations between some modifiable factors (such as tobacco smoking) and cancers of other anatomic sites (such as lung cancer), investigators have examined potential associations between brain tumor risk and environmental and behavioral factors. Only one such factor is associated consistently with brain tumor risk—exposure to therapeutic doses of ionizing radiation.

*Therapeutic doses of ionizing radiation*

Exposure to therapeutic doses of ionizing radiation is the only established potentially modifiable brain tumor risk factor [5,46]. Ionizing radiation used to treat tinea capitis and skin hemangioma in children or infants is associated with relative risks as high as 18 for nerve sheath tumors, 10 for meningioma, and 3 for glioma [5,46]. Children irradiated for treatment of tinea capitis also have a greater risk for pituitary adenoma [47]. There are mixed results concerning exposure to diagnostic and therapeutic readiographs of the head and neck [48,49]; however, radiographs performed 15 to 40 years preceding diagnosis seem to increase meningioma risk [50], as do radiographs performed before age 20 or taken before the year 1945 [51]. A study in a Finnish population showed that second primary brain tumors occur more frequently than expected among patients treated previously for brain tumors with radiation therapy [52]. Survivors of the atomic bombing of Hiroshima have a high incidence of meningioma correlating with the dose of radiation to their brain [53]. These atomic bomb survivors also have higher incidences of glioma, schwannoma, and pituitary tumors, although there is no increased risk for brain tumors among those who were exposed in utero [46]. There are homogenous and strong results suggesting associations between ionizing radiation and brain tumor risk; however, because exposure to high levels of ionizing radiation is rare, these exposures account for only a small percentage of brain tumors.

*Cellular telephone use*

Most early studies of the association between cell phone use and glioma risk generally provide no evidence for this relationship [54]. If the latency period is at least 5 years long, however, then these early studies did not have sufficient numbers of long-term cell phone users to evaluate this relationship adequately. In contrast, several recent studies provide some evidence for an association between long-term cell phone use and glioma that also may be attributed to recall or selection bias [55,56]. The largest population-based case–control study reported to date (1522 glioma cases and 3301 controls) conducted in five Nordic Countries and the United Kingdom [57] found no consistent evidence overall for increased risk for glioma related to use of cell phones nor did they find increased glioma risk in the most highly exposed group. Only one subgroup, that consisting of individuals indicating ipsilateral use (same side of the head as the brain tumor) 10 or more years before the reference date, had an increased risk for glioma, and there was an increasing trend with years since first use on the ipsilateral side. Over the past 2 decades, there have been decreasing levels of nonionizing radiation from cell phones and these levels vary across cell phone types. Further studies are needed to determine whether or not the observed risk represents a biologic effect of nonionizing radiation from cell phones on glioma risk or merely is an artifact. As the number of long-term cell phone users increases, it will be possible to identify increasing numbers of patients who have glioma who are long-term cell phone users and, thus, conduct studies with sufficient statistical power to provide definitive answers to this important public health question.

*Additional environmental and behavioral risk factors with inconclusive, minimal, or no compelling evidence of association with brain tumor risk*

Several environmental and behavioral risk factors may alter brain tumor risk, but there is inconclusive, minimal, or no evidence to establish causality for the following associations: head injury and trauma (for intravascular brain tumors) [58]; head injury and trauma (for nonintravascular brain tumors) [5,58–62]; dietary calcium intake (for glioma) [63,64]; dietary N-nitroso compound intake (for glioma and meningioma) [65–68]; dietary antioxidant intake (for glioma); [64–67]; dietary maternal N-nitroso compound intake (for childhood brain tumors) [5,62]; dietary maternal and early life antioxidant intake (for childhood brain tumors); maternal folate supplementation (for primitive neuroectodermal tumors) [62,69]; tobacco smoking (for glioma and meningioma) [62,66,70]; alcohol consumption (for glioma, meningioma, and childhood brain tumors) [46,71]; and exposure to electromagnetic fields (for childhood and adult brain tumors) [62]. In addition, the literature on occupational risk factors is vast and inconclusive; Wrensch and colleagues [5] summarized this literature; however, there has been no comprehensive review of occupational factors associated with brain tumor risk since 1986. Possible explanations for failure to find consistent and statistically significant findings for the factors listed include the following: small study sample sizes; false-positive results (related to small sample sizes and lack of precise research hypotheses); invalid or imprecise exposure measures (resulting from use of proxy respondents when patients who have brain tumor are unavailable, from errors in exposure history recall, or from lack of validation of verifiable exposures); inherited or developmental variation in metabolic and repair pathways; unaccounted-for protective exposures or conditions (such as allergies, described later); differential diffusion of chemicals across the blood-brain barrier; differentially expressed metabolic and repair pathways in the brain; and disease heterogeneity. It also is possible that failure to find strong and consistent environmental risk factors for brain tumors (except for therapeutic ionizing radiation) may be attributable to the absence of true strong environmental associations. Nonetheless, low brain tumor survival probabilities dictate the continued search for environmental factors that might be altered to prevent disease.

## Genetic factors

Many investigators have turned attention away from environmental and behavioral risk factors and toward genetic risk factors, in part because of the abundance of null or inconclusive findings related to potentially modifiable environmental factors, in part because there is increasing knowledge of the molecular pathology of brain tumors, especially glioma, and in part because of new technologies for examining associations between genotypes and diseases. Although familial aggregation of glioma has been demonstrated, it can be difficult to distinguish shared environmental exposures from inherited characteristics. Grossman and colleagues [72] showed that brain tumors occur in families with no known predisposing hereditary disease and that the pattern of occurrence in many families suggests environmental causes. Results presented by Malmer and coworkers [73], however, suggest that first-degree relatives, and not spouses, have a significantly increased brain tumor risk.

## Rare mutations in penetrant genes and familial aggregation

Brain tumors are believed to develop through the progressive accumulation of genetic or epigenetic alterations that permit cells to evade normal regulatory mechanisms or escape destruction by the immune system. There is strong epidemiologic evidence that genetic factors are associated with brain tumor risk. First, several diseases or syndromes associated with rare mutations in highly penetrant genes (including tuberous sclerosis complex, neurofibromatosis types 1 and 2, nevoid basal-cell carcinoma syndrome, syndromes related to adenomatous polyps, and Li-Fraumeni cancer family syndrome) increase brain tumor risk [5,74]. In a study of 500 patients who had glioma, however, fewer than 1% had a known hereditary syndrome [75]. Although genetic predisposition is considered influential in few brain tumors (5% to 10%), the proportion may be underestimated because some hereditary syndromes are not diagnosed readily and because patients who have brain tumors are not referred routinely to a clinical geneticist. Second, patterns of glioma risk in families, case–control studies, and six Swedish cohorts with overlapping populations are consistent in suggesting potential inheritance. For example, results from one study suggest that approximately 2% of glioma cases may be explained by an autosomal recessive gene [76]; however, a low penetrant dominant gene, and not an autosomal recessive gene, was the more likely explanation for familial clustering in another study [77]. A greater proportion of familial glioma cases overexpress p53 based on immunohistochemistry [78]. The first molecular genetic evidence for familial aggregation of glioma recently was submitted by Paunu and colleagues [79], whose results suggest a novel low-penetrance locus at 15q23-q26.3 among people who have familial glioma in Western Finland. Malmer and colleagues [80] report that glioma and meningioma risks are associated significantly with the CC-CG-CC genotype combination formed by three polymorphims in p53 but only when cases of a family history of cancer are included; however, these results are based on a small number of cases and controls. Familial aggregation of meningioma has been suggested [81,82] but not demonstrated consistently and should be validated through additional studies.

In addition to rare mutations and familial aggregation, Bondy and coworkers [83,84] found that lymphocyte mutagen sensitivity to gamma radiation increases glioma risk; however, these results should be verified because they may be confounded by age, solar exposure, diet, and glioma treatment and because it was not possible to determine whether or not chromatid breaks increased brain tumor risk or whether or not they represented a systemic effect of the brain tumors themselves.

Because only a small proportion of primary brain tumors seems to result from effects of environmental or behavioral factors or from inherited rare mutations in highly penetrant genes, investigators have turned their attention to common polymorphisms in genes that might influence susceptibility to brain tumors in concert with environmental exposures. Genetic alterations that affect detoxification of carcinogens, DNA stability and repair, and cell cycle regulation conceivably could confer genetic susceptibility to brain tumors.

*Glioma and polymorphisms affecting detoxification, DNA stability and repair, and cell cycle regulation*

Cytochrome p450 s (CYP) and GST are involved in the metabolism of many electrophilic compounds, including carcinogens, mutagens, cytotoxic drugs, metabolites and products of reactive oxidation. Studies of CYP and GST have produced mixed results. For example, although one case–control study found that CYP2D6 increased astrocytoma and meningioma risks more than fourfold [85], another found no association [86]. Results from a recent meta-analysis of eight studies, including 1630 glioma cases, 245 meningioma cases, and 7151 controls, suggest that, although the T1 null genotype is associated with nearly double meningioma risk (odds ratio [OR] 1.95; 95% CI, 1.02–3.76), there were no associations between any of the GSTP1 105 and GSTP1 114 single- nucleotide polymorphisms (SNPs) and glioma risk; however, none of the investigators whose work was summarized had conducted haplotype analyses. Wrensch and colleagues [87] found little evidence for a general association of GST polymorphisms with glioma but did show an association of GSTT1 deletion for glioma with p53 mutations. In a large Nordic and British population-based, case–control study (725 glioma cases, 546 meningioma cases, and 1612 controls), Schwartzbaum and colleagues [88] reported no associations between the GSTM3, GSTP1 NQ01, CYP1A1, GSTM1, or GSTT1 polymorphisms and adult brain tumor risk; however, they found a weak association between the G-C (Val-Ala) GSTP1 105/114 haplotype and glioma (OR 0.73; 95% CI, 0.54–0.99).

Because DNA repair is important in maintaining DNA integrity, inherited variation in components of DNA repair pathways has been studied extensively with respect to cancer. Associations with glioma are reported for variants in ERCC1 [89,90], ERCC2 [89,91,92], the nearby gene GLTSCR1 (glioma tumor suppressor candidate of unknown function) [91], PRKDC (also known as XRCC7—a gene involved in nonhomologous end-joining double-strand break repair) [93], and $O^6$methylguanine–DNA methyltransferase (MGMT), a DNA repair enzyme [94,95], but there are too few studies to assess consistency. The AA or AC versus CC genotype in nucleotide 8092 of ERCC1 is shown to increase oligoastrocytoma risk [91], whereas the AA genotype (C to A polymorphism [R156R]) of ERCC2 was more prevalent than the CC or CA genotypes in cases of glioblastoma, astrocytoma, or oligoastrocytoma than in controls [92]. The ERCC2-exon-22 T allele prevalence was 35% in a group of oligodendroglioma cases compared with 18% for controls, and alterations in GLTSCR1 (or a closely linked gene) are associated with oligodendroglioma risk [91]. Wang and colleagues [93] found that the TT genotype of XRCC7 was more common in glioma cases compared with controls. Regarding the MGMT gene, results presented by Wiencke and colleagues [94] suggest that an inherited factor involving the repair of methylation and other alkylation damage may be associated with the development of glioma that have neither TP53 mutations nor TP53 protein overexpression. The combined heterozygote of V1 and a wild allele of the MGMT gene may contribute to the de novo occurrence of glioblastoma [95]. DNA repair is complex, involving more than 130 known genes; therefore, studies focusing on constellations of variants involved in DNA repair pathways and their interactions might help elucidate the roles of variants in gliomagenesis and progression.

Dysregulation of the cell cycle (control of proliferation and apoptosis) is a hallmark feature of most glioma [96], and MDM2 is a key molecule in maintaining the fidelity of this process. In one study [97], the G variant of SNP309 in the MDM2 promoter led to higher expression of MDM2 with concomitant reduced expression of TP53 and was associated significantly with earlier age of tumor development and multiple tumor sites in participants who had Li-Fraumeni syndrome, of which brain tumors are one component. MDM2 seems to regulate TP53 expression negatively [98], and the inverse association between TP53 and MDM2 expression is reported by Wiencke and colleagues [94], among others. The associations between MDM2, TP53, and EGFR remain poorly understood, however, and should be examined in studies with large sample sizes because of the potential need for smaller subgroup analyses.

Inconsistencies in genetic polymorphism studies may result from false-positive associations based on inadequate sample sizes [26] (especially in subgroup analyses) and from confounding by genes with similar functions not accounted for in the analyses. Another possible explanation for inconsistencies is that study populations may consist of different proportions of types of tumors, and genetic risk for certain subtypes could be masked by lack of risk among other subtypes. When these issues are addressed, the potential interaction between genetic polymorphisms with other genetic characteristics and environmental factors can be evaluated properly.

*Glioma, allergy, allergic conditions, infections, and associated immunologic factors*

Persuasive evidence has accumulated over the past decade that immunologic factors related to allergy, allergic conditions, and infections have an impact on glioma and glioblastoma risk. Reduced glioma or glioblastoma risk has been attributed to allergy and allergic conditions [99–105], autoimmune diseases [99,105], reported history of varicella-zoster virus (VZV) infections, and positive IgG to VZV [106–108].

Many studies support that glioma risk is decreased as a result of allergies and immune-related conditions. For example, in a large population-based study (965 glioma cases and 1716 controls) in the United Kingdom, Schoemaker and colleagues [102] report reduced glioma risk as the result of a history of asthma (OR 0.71; 95% CI, 0.54–0.92), hay fever (OR 0.73; 95% CI, 0.59–0.90), eczema (OR 0.74; 95% CI, 0.56–0.97), or other allergies (OR 0.65; 95% CI, 0.47–0.90), and these estimates are similar to those reported in earlier studies. Although the mechanism governing potential protection has not been identified, it may arise from the anti-inflammatory effects of cytokines involved in allergic and autoimmune disease [109]. It also may result from increased tumor immunosurveillance in those who have allergies and autoimmune disease [110] or from suppression of the immune system by the brain tumor [102]. Wiemels and colleagues [103] found that total IgE levels were lower in glioma cases than in controls (OR 0.37; 95% CI, 0.22–0.64); these, along with earlier results [100], support the notion that the relation between allergic disease and glioma risk is complex and varies by allergen and allergic pathology. A problem with the case–control studies used to examine the glioma-allergy association is that because of the low survival probability from glioblastoma, investigators have used many proxy respondents to ascertain information concerning allergic conditions. Confirming the suggestion that proxy reports may not be reliable, Schwartzbaum and colleagues [105] found that proxy respondents reported fewer allergic conditions for index subjects than did self-reporting respondents. In a cohort study where information on allergic conditions was obtained on average 19 years or more before diagnosis of a brain tumor, however, Schwartzbaum and colleagues [105] reported an association between allergies and glioma risk (hazard ratio [HR] 0.45; 95% CI, 0.19–1.07)—excluding low-grade glioma—and between immune-related hospital discharges and glioma risk (HR 0.46; 95% CI, 0.14–1.49).

Moreover, results submitted by Schwartzbaum and colleagues [101] confirmed the inverse association between asthma and glioblastoma; they examined five SNPs in three genes, IL-4 receptor alpha (IL-4RA), IL-13, and ADAM33. The IL-4RA SNP T478C TC, CC and A551G AG, AA were significantly positively associated with glioblastoma (ORs were 1.64 [95% CI, 1.05–2.55] and 1.61 [95% CI, 1.05–2.47]), respectively, whereas the IL-13 SNP C1112T CT, TT was associated inversely with glioblastoma (OR 0.56, 95% CI, 0.33–0.96). It is possible that IL-13 or its shared receptor with IL-4, IL-4RA, plays an independent role in allergic conditions and glioblastoma. Alternatively, some aspect of allergic conditions themselves might reduce glioblastoma or glioma risk. Each of the polymorphism-glioblastoma associations is in the opposite direction of a corresponding polymorphism-asthma association, consistent with previous findings that self-reported asthmatics and people who have allergic conditions are less likely to have glioblastoma than are people who do not report these conditions. This result addresses lingering doubts that associations between allergic conditions and glioblastoma merely are reporting artifacts resulting from recall bias or effects of the tumor on the immune system [101]. These results were confirmed weakly when data from three additional countries—approximately tripling the original number of cases and controls—were added; in addition, Schwartzbaum and colleagues [111] identified an association between the T-G haplotype of IL-4RA and glioblastoma risk. Moreover, their original finding of the association between the IL-13 C1112T SNP and glioblastoma subsequently was confirmed by Wiemels and colleagues [104] in a large case–control study of glioma (456 cases and 541 controls). Furthermore, Wiemels and colleagues [104] report that this same IL-13 SNP was associated inversely with IgE levels in controls ($P = .04$) and observed an association of borderline statistical significance between an IL-4RA haplotype and glioma (OR 1.49; 95% CI, 0.99–2.25). In spite of this molecular evidence of an association between allergic conditions and glioblastoma, further research is needed to evaluate the complete IL-4/IL-13 pathways to determine their potential function in glioblastoma development or progression.

A variety of viruses (papovaviruses, including simian virus 40 [SV40], JC virus, and BK virus; adenoviruses; retroviruses; the herpes viruses; and influenza) and parasitic infections (*Toxoplasma gondii*) also have been investigated in relation to gliomagenesis in experimental animals and limited epidemiologic studies. The potential risk from these agents generally has been addressed inadequately in epidemiologic studies, however [112,113]. With relative consistency, results from two case–control series suggest that prior clinical disease associated with VZV infection and anti-VZV IgG levels may be associated inversely with adult glioma risk [106–108]. It might be the specific nature of the immune system's response to antigens, and not exposure to the antigen per se, that is responsible for this inverse association with glioma [100–103].

With respect to SV40, between 1955 and 1963, an unknown proportion of all inactivated and live polio vaccines distributed was contaminated with SV40 [114]. In Germany, where children were followed over a 20-year period, those inoculated with the polio vaccine contaminated with SV40 had higher occurrences of glioblastoma, medulloblastoma, and some less common brain tumor types than children not given the contaminated vaccine [115]. In the United States, no difference in brain tumor risk was found for glioma or meningioma between the two groups of children [116], but one study reported that the incidence of ependymoma was 37% greater in the children receiving the contaminated vaccine [114]. Results pertaining to infections should be validated in studies in which serologic measurement of viral or bacterial exposure is ascertained before the development of brain tumors and in which there is serologic or symptom-based confirmation of infection.

Results pertaining to HLA–cell surface molecules that modulate immune responses, in part by presenting antigenic peptides to T-lymphocytes, also suggest the importance of immunologic responses in glioma development. Tang and colleagues [117] showed that glioblastoma is associated positively with the HLA genotype B*13 and the HLA haplotype B*07-Cw*07 ($P = .01$ and $P < .001$, respectively) and is associated inversely with the genotype Cw*01 ($P = .05$). If confirmed, these results could explain partially the increased glioblastoma incidence among whites, because B*07 and B*07-Cw*07 are more common among whites. Guerini and colleagues [118] compared a small group of patients who had glioma in Northern Italy with control organ donors from the same region and demonstrated a positive association between HLA DRB1*14 and the presence of symptomatic cerebral glioma (OR 2.48; 95% CI, 1.09–5.45). Facoetti and colleagues [119] found that HLA class I antigens were lost in approximately half of glioblastoma tumors but in only 20% of grade 2 astrocytoma tumors; selective HLA-A2 antigen loss was observed in approximately 80% of glioblastoma lesions and half of the grade 2 astrocytoma tumors; and HLA class I antigen loss was correlated significantly ($P < .025$) with tumor grade. Studies of HLA may contribute to understanding immune escape mechanisms used by glioma, because HLA antigens mediate interactions of tumor cells with the host immune response; further, HLA antigen defects in astrocytoma brain tumors may explain the poor clinical response rates observed in the majority of the T cell-based immunotherapy clinical trials [119].

## Summary

Brain tumors seemed to have increase in incidence over the past 30 years, but the rise probably results mostly from use of new neuroimaging techniques. Treatments have not improved prognosis for the most rapidly fatal brain tumors. Established brain tumor risk factors (exposure to therapeutic ionizing radiation, rare mutations of penetrant genes, and familial history) explain only a small proportion of brain tumors, and only one of these potentially is modifiable. It is likely that genetic and environmental characteristics play a role in familial aggregation of glioma, and these factors have not been identified. Among associations currently being investigated, those of interest include reproductive and menstrual factors for glioma and meningioma, cell phone use for glioma and acoustic neuroma, familial aggregation of meningioma, allergic conditions for glioma, and a variety of inherited polymorphisms potentially associated with glioma. Results from studies based on molecular biomarkers of immunologic factors (eg, antibodies and IgE), although sparse, are promising; future examination of these factors should take place in cohort studies or studies within large health systems with archived specimens to minimize the possibility of tumor growth and treatments affecting the factor of interest; further, to include a sufficient number of participants diagnosed with brain tumors, large studies will be needed. Current research on glioma and polymorphisms associated with allergic conditions and immunologic responses may aid in understanding the complex immunologic modulation of gliomagenesis. Focused a priori hypotheses will be needed for these studies and for studies involving genetic polymorphisms that, in conjunction with environmental carcinogens or behavioral factors, may increase brain tumor risk. In addition to these promising leads, new hypotheses should consider previous findings from well-established risk factors, such as gender, race, and ethnicity. New concepts in brain tumor etiology and clinical management are the goal of such research, with an aim at eradicating this devastating disease.

## References

[1] CBTRUS. Statistical report: Primary Brain Tumors in the United States, 1998–2002. 2005.
[2] SEER. Surveillance, Epidemiology, and End Results (SEER) Program SEER* Stat Database: incidence - SEER 13 Regs Public-Use, Nov 2005 Sub (1992–2003), National Cancer Institute, DCCPS, Surveillance Research Program, Cancer Statistics Branch, released April 2006, based on the November 2005 submission. Available at: www.seer.cancer.gov.
[3] Davis FG, Bruner JM, Surawicz TS. The rationale for standardized registration and reporting of brain and central nervous system tumors in population-based cancer registries. Neuroepidemiology 1997;16(6):308–16.
[4] Helseth A. The incidence of primary central nervous system neoplasms before and after computerized tomography availability. J Neurosurg 1995;83(6):999–1003.
[5] Wrensch M, Minn Y, Chew T, et al. Epidemiology of primary brain tumors: current concepts and review of the literature. Neuro-oncol 2002;4(4):278–99.
[6] Olson S, Law A. Meningiomas and the Polynesian population. ANZ J Surg 2005;75(8): 705–9.
[7] Inskip PD, Linet MS, Heineman EF. Etiology of brain tumors in adults. Epidemiol Rev 1995;17(2):382–414.
[8] Singh GK, Siahpush M. All-cause and cause-specific mortality of immigrants and native born in the United States. Am J Public Health 2001;91(3):392–9.
[9] Lacroix M, Abi-Said D, Fourney DR, et al. A multivariate analysis of 416 patients with glioblastoma multiforme: prognosis, extent of resection, and survival. J Neurosurg 2001; 95(2):190–8.

[10] Lutterbach J, Sauerbrei W, Guttenberger R. Multivariate analysis of prognostic factors in patients with glioblastoma. Strahlenther Onkol 2003;179(1):8–15.

[11] Jeremic B, Milicic B, Grujicic D, et al. Multivariate analysis of clinical prognostic factors in patients with glioblastoma multiforme treated with a combined modality approach. J Cancer Res Clin Oncol 2003;129(8):477–84.

[12] Schwartzbaum J, Lal P, Evanoff W, et al. Presurgical serum albumin levels predict survival time from glioblastoma multiforme. J Neurooncol 1999;43:35–41.

[13] Aldape K, Burger PC, Perry A. Clinicopathologic aspects of 1p/19q loss and the diagnosis of oligodendroglioma. Arch Pathol Lab Med 2007;131(2):242–51.

[14] Ushio Y, Tada K, Shiraishi S, et al. Correlation of molecular genetic analysis of p53, MDM2, p16, PTEN, and EGFR and survival of patients with anaplastic astrocytoma and glioblastoma. Front Biosci 2003;8:e281–8.

[15] Batchelor TT, Betensky RA, Esposito JM, et al. Age-dependent prognostic effects of genetic alterations in glioblastoma. Clin Cancer Res 2004;10(1 Pt 1):228–33.

[16] Stander M, Peraud A, Leroch B, et al. Prognostic impact of TP53 mutation status for adult patients with supratentorial World Health Organization Grade II astrocytoma or oligoastrocytoma: a long-term analysis. Cancer 2004;101(5):1028–35.

[17] Backlund LM, Nilsson BR, Liu L, et al. Mutations in Rb1 pathway-related genes are associated with poor prognosis in anaplastic astrocytomas. Br J Cancer 2005;93(1): 124–30.

[18] Deb P, Sharma MC, Mahapatra AK, et al. Glioblastoma multiforme with long term survival. Neurol India 2005;53(3):329–32.

[19] McLendon RE, Herndon JE 2nd, West B, et al. Survival analysis of presumptive prognostic markers among oligodendrogliomas. Cancer 2005;104(8):1693–9.

[20] Houillier C, Lejeune J, Benouaich-Amiel A, et al. Prognostic impact of molecular markers in a series of 220 primary glioblastomas. Cancer 2006;106(10):2218–23.

[21] Layfield LJ, Willmore C, Tripp S, et al. Epidermal growth factor receptor gene amplification and protein expression in glioblastoma multiforme: prognostic significance and relationship to other prognostic factors. Appl Immunohistochem Mol Morphol 2006; 14(1):91–6.

[22] Wrensch M, Wiencke JK, Wiemels J, et al. Serum IgE, tumor epidermal growth factor receptor expression, and inherited polymorphisms associated with glioma survival. Cancer Res 2006;66(8):4531–41.

[23] Schmidt MC, Antweiler S, Urban N, et al. Impact of genotype and morphology on the prognosis of glioblastoma. J Neuropathol Exp Neurol 2002;61(4):321–8.

[24] Ranuncolo SM, Varela M, Morandi A, et al. Prognostic value of Mdm2, p53 and p16 in patients with astrocytomas. J Neurooncol 2004;68(2):113–21.

[25] Simmons ML, Lamborn KR, Takahashi M, et al. Analysis of complex relationships between age, p53, epidermal growth factor receptor, and survival in glioblastoma patients. Cancer Res 2001;61(3):1122–8.

[26] Wacholder S, Chanock S, Garcia-Closas M, et al. Assessing the probability that a positive report is false: an approach for molecular epidemiology studies. J Natl Cancer Inst 2004; 96(6):434–42.

[27] Ohgaki H, Dessen P, Jourde B, et al. Genetic pathways to glioblastoma: a population-based study. Cancer Res 2004;64(19):6892–9.

[28] Wang L, Wang LE, El-Zein R, et al. Human telomerase genetic variation predicts survival of patients with glioblastoma multiforme [abstract number 2823]. Proc Am Assoc Cancer Res 2005;46.

[29] Tchirkov A, Khalil T, Chautard E, et al. Interleukin-6 gene amplification and shortened survival in glioblastoma patients. Br J Cancer 2007;96(3):474–6.

[30] Fecci PE, Mitchell DA, Whitesides JF, et al. Increased regulatory T-cell fraction amidst a diminished CD4 compartment explains cellular immune defects in patients with malignant glioma. Cancer Res 2006;66(6):3294–302.

[31] Yong Z, Chang L, Mei YX, et al. Role and mechanisms of CD4 + CD25+ regulatory T cells in the induction and maintenance of transplantation tolerance. Transpl Immunol 2007; 17(2):120–9.

[32] Helseth A. Incidence and survival of intracranial meningioma patients in Norway 1963–1992. Neuroepidemiology 1997;16(2):53–9.

[33] Sankila R, Kallio M, Jaaskelainen J, et al. Long-term survival of 1986 patients with intracranial meningioma diagnosed from 1953 to 1984 in Finland. Comparison of the observed and expected survival rates in a population-based series. Cancer 1992;70(6): 1568–76.

[34] McCarthy BJ, Davis FG, Freels S, et al. Factors associated with survival in patients with meningioma. J Neurosurg 1998;88(5):831–9.

[35] Maillo A, Orfao A, Sayagues JM, et al. New classification scheme for the prognostic stratification of meningioma on the basis of chromosome 14 abnormalities, patient age, and tumor histopathology. J Clin Oncol 2003;21(17):3285–95.

[36] Schwartzbaum J, Jonsson F, Ahlbom A, et al. Prior hospitalization for epilepsy, diabetes, and stroke and subsequent glioma and meningioma risk. Cancer Epidemiol Biomarkers Prev 2005;14(3):643–50.

[37] McKinley BP, Michalek AM, Fenstermaker RA, et al. The impact of age and sex on the incidence of glial tumors in New York state from 1976 to 1995. J Neurosurg 2000;93(6): 932–9.

[38] Schlehofer B, Blettner M, Wahrendorf J. Association between brain tumors and menopausal status. J Natl Cancer Inst 1992;84(17):1346–9.

[39] Lambe M, Coogan P, Baron J. Reproductive factors and the risk of brain tumors: a population-based study in Sweden. Int J Cancer 1997;72(3):389–93.

[40] Cantor KP, Lynch CF, Johnson D. Reproductive factors and risk of brain, colon, and other malignancies in Iowa (United States). Cancer Causes Control 1993;4(6):505–11.

[41] Silvera SAN, Miller AB, Rohan TE. Hormonal and reproductive factors and risk of glioma: a prospective cohort study. Int J Cancer 2006;118(5):1321–4.

[42] Hatch EE, Linet MS, Zhang J, et al. Reproductive and hormonal factors and risk of brain tumors in adult females. Int J Cancer 2005;114(5):797–805.

[43] Yu ZY, Wrange O, Haglund B, et al. Estrogen and progestin receptors in intracranial meningiomas. J Steroid Biochem 1982;16(3):451–6.

[44] Jhawar BS, Fuchs CS, Colditz GA, et al. Sex steroid hormone exposures and risk for meningioma. J Neurosurg 2003;99(5):848–53.

[45] Wigertz A, Lonn S, Mathiesen T, et al. Risk of brain tumors associated with exposure to exogenous female sex hormones. Am J Epidemiol 2006;164(7):629–36.

[46] Preston-Martin S. Epidemiology of primary CNS neoplasms. Neurol Clin 1996;14(2): 273–90.

[47] Juven Y, Sadetzki S. A possible association between ionizing radiation and pituitary adenoma: a descriptive study. Cancer 2002;95(2):397–403.

[48] Wrensch M, Miike R, Lee M, et al. Are prior head injuries or diagnostic X-rays associated with glioma in adults? The effects of control selection bias. Neuroepidemiology 2000;19(5): 234–44.

[49] Hardell L, Mild KH, Pahlson A, et al. Ionizing radiation, cellular telephones and the risk for brain tumours. Eur J Cancer Prev 2001;10(6):523–9.

[50] Longstreth WTJ, Phillips LE, Drangsholt M, et al. Dental X-rays and the risk of intracranial meningioma: a population-based case-control study. Cancer 2004;100(5):1026–34.

[51] Preston-Martin S, Yu MC, Henderson BE, et al. Risk factors for meningiomas in men in Los Angeles County. J Natl Cancer Inst 1983;70(5):863–6.

[52] Salminen E, Pukkala E, Teppo L. Second cancers in patients with brain tumours-impact of treatment. Eur J Cancer 1999;35(1):102–5.

[53] Shintani T, Hayakawa N, Hoshi M, et al. High incidence of meningioma among Hiroshima atomic bomb survivors. J Radiat Res (Tokyo) 1999;40(1):49–57.

[54] Ahlbom A, Green A, Kheifets L, et al. Epidemiology of health effects of radiofrequency exposure. Environ Health Perspect 2004;112(17):1741–54.

[55] Hardell L, Carlberg M, Hansson Mild K. Pooled analysis of two case-control studies on use of cellular and cordless telephones and the risk for malignant brain tumours diagnosed in 1997–2003. Int Arch Occup Environ Health 2006;79(8):630–9.

[56] Schuz J, Bohler E, Berg G, et al. Cellular phones, cordless phones, and the risks of glioma and meningioma (Interphone Study Group, Germany). Am J Epidemiol 2006;163(6): 512–20.

[57] Lahkola A, Auvinen A, Raitanen J, et al. Mobile phone use and risk of glioma in 5 North European countries. Int J Cancer 2007;120(8):1769–75.

[58] Inskip PD, Mellemkjaer L, Gridley G, et al. Incidence of intracranial tumors following hospitalization for head injuries (Denmark). Cancer Causes Control 1998;9(1):109–16.

[59] Hu J, Johnson KC, Mao Y, et al. Risk factors for glioma in adults: a case-control study in northeast China. Cancer Detect Prev 1998;22(2):100–8.

[60] Hochberg F, Toniolo P, Cole P. Head trauma and seizures as risk factors of glioblastoma. Neurology 1984;34(11):1511–4.

[61] Preston-Martin S, Pogoda JM, Schlehofer B, et al. An international case-control study of adult glioma and meningioma: the role of head trauma. Int J Epidemiol 1998;27(4): 579–86.

[62] Baldwin RT, Preston-Martin S. Epidemiology of brain tumors in childhood-a review-Toxicol Appl Pharmacol 2004;199(2):118–31.

[63] Tedeschi-Blok N, Schwartzbaum J, Lee M, et al. Dietary calcium consumption and astrocytic glioma: the San Francisco Bay Area Adult Glioma Study, 1991–1995. Nutr Cancer 2001;39(2):196–203.

[64] Hu J, La Vecchia C, Negri E, et al. Diet and brain cancer in adults: a case-control study in northeast China. Int J Cancer 1999;81(1):20–3.

[65] Chen H, Ward MH, Tucker KL, et al. Diet and risk of adult glioma in eastern Nebraska, United States. Cancer Causes Control 2002;13(7):647–55.

[66] Lee M, Wrensch M, Miike R. Dietary and tobacco risk factors for adult onset glioma in the San Francisco Bay Area (California, USA). Cancer Causes Control 1997;8(1): 13–24.

[67] Schwartzbaum JA, Fisher JL, Goodman J, et al. Hypotheses concerning roles of dietary energy, cured meat, and serum tocopherols in adult glioma development. Neuroepidemiology 1999;18(3):156–66.

[68] Preston-Martin S, Henderson BE. N-nitroso compounds and human intracranial tumours. IARC Sci Publ 1984;57:887–94.

[69] Bunin GR, Kuijten RR, Buckley JD, et al. Relation between maternal diet and subsequent primitive neuroectodermal brain tumors in young children. N Engl J Med 1993;329(8): 536–41.

[70] Hu J, Little J, Xu T, et al. Risk factors for meningioma in adults: a case-control study in northeast China. Int J Cancer 1999;83(3):299–304.

[71] Wrensch M, Bondy ML, Wiencke J, et al. Environmental risk factors for primary malignant brain tumors: a review. J Neurooncol 1993;17(1):47–64.

[72] Grossman SA, Osman M, Hruban R, et al. Central nervous system cancers in first-degree relatives and spouses. Cancer Invest 1999;17(5):299–308.

[73] Malmer B, Henriksson R, Gronberg H. Familial brain tumours-genetics or environment? A nationwide cohort study of cancer risk in spouses and first-degree relatives of brain tumour patients. Int J Cancer 2003;106(2):260–3.

[74] Bondy M, Wiencke J, Wrensch M, et al. Genetics of primary brain tumors: a review. J Neurooncol 1994;18(1):69–81.

[75] Wrensch M, Lee M, Miike R, et al. Familial and personal medical history of cancer and nervous system conditions among adults with glioma and controls. Am J Epidemiol 1997;145(7):581–93.

[76] Malmer B, Iselius L, Holmberg E, et al. Genetic epidemiology of glioma. Br J Cancer 2001; 84(3):429–34.

[77] Malmer B, Haraldsson S, Einarsdottir E, et al. Homozygosity mapping of familial glioma in Northern Sweden. Acta Oncol 2005;44(2):114–9.

[78] Malmer B, Brannstrom T, Andersson U, et al. Does a low frequency of P53 and Pgp expression in familial glioma compared to sporadic controls indicate biological differences? Anticancer Res 2002;22(6C):3949–54.

[79] Paunu N, Lahermo P, Onkamo P, et al. A novel low-penetrance locus for familial glioma at 15q23-q26.3. Cancer Res 2002;62(13):3798–802.

[80] Malmer B, Feychting M, Lonn S, et al. p53 Genotypes and risk of glioma and meningioma. Cancer Epidemiol Biomarkers Prev 2005;14(9):2220–3.

[81] Hemminki K, Li X, Collins VP. Parental cancer as a risk factor for brain tumors (Sweden). Cancer Causes Control 2001;12(3):195–9.

[82] Hemminki K, Li X. Familial risks in nervous system tumors. Cancer Epidemiol Biomarkers Prev 2003;12(11 Pt 1):1137–42.

[83] Bondy ML, Kyritsis AP, Gu J, et al. Mutagen sensitivity and risk of gliomas: a case-control analysis. Cancer Res 1996;56(7):1484–6.

[84] Berwick M, Vineis P. Markers of DNA repair and susceptibility to cancer in humans: an epidemiologic review. J Natl Cancer Inst 2000;92(11):874–97.

[85] Elexpuru-Camiruaga J, Buxton N, Kandula V, et al. Susceptibility to astrocytoma and meningioma: influence of allelism at glutathione S-transferase (GSTT1 and GSTM1) and cytochrome P-450 (CYP2D6) loci. Cancer Res 1995;55(19):4237–9.

[86] Kelsey KT, Wrensch M, Zuo ZF, et al. A population-based case-control study of the CYP2D6 and GSTT1 polymorphisms and malignant brain tumors. Pharmacogenetics 1997;7(6):463–8.

[87] Wrensch M, Kelsey KT, Liu M, et al. Glutathione-S-transferase and adult glioma. Cancer Epidemiol Biomarkers Prev 2004;13(3):461–7.

[88] Schwartzbaum JA, Ahlbom A, Lonn S, et al. An international case-control study of glutathione transferase and functionally related polymorphisms and risk of primary adult brain tumors. Cancer Epidemiol Biomarkers Prev 2007;16(3):559–96.

[89] Wrensch M, Kelsey KT, Liu M, et al. ERCC1 and ERCC2 polymorphisms and adult glioma. Neuro Oncol 2005;7(4):495–507.

[90] Chen P, Wiencke J, Aldape K, et al. Association of an ERCC1 polymorphism with adult-onset glioma. Cancer Epidemiol Biomarkers Prev 2000;9(8):843–7.

[91] Yang P, Kollmeyer TM, Buckner K, et al. Polymorphisms in GLTSCR1 and ERCC2 are associated with the development of oligodendrogliomas. Cancer 2005;1(103): 2363–72.

[92] Caggana M, Kilgallen J, Conroy JM, et al. Associations between ERCC2 polymorphisms and gliomas. Cancer Epidemiol Biomarkers Prev 2001;10(4):355–60.

[93] Wang L-E, Bondy ML, Shen H, et al. Polymorphisms of DNA repair genes and risk of glioma. Cancer Res 2004;64(16):5560–3.

[94] Wiencke JK, Aldape K, McMillan A, et al. Molecular features of adult glioma associated with patient race/ethnicity, age, and a polymorphism in O6-methylguanine-DNA-methyltransferase. Cancer Epidemiol Biomarkers Prev 2005;14(7):1774–83.

[95] Inoue R, Isono M, Abe M, et al. A genotype of the polymorphic DNA repair gene MGMT is associated with de novo glioblastoma. Neurol Res 2003;25(8):875–9.

[96] Ichimura K, Ohgaki H, Kleihues P, et al. Molecular pathogenesis of astrocytic tumours. J Neurooncol 2004;70(2):137–60.

[97] Bond GL, Hu W, Bond EE, et al. A single nucleotide polymorphism in the MDM2 promoter attenuates the p53 tumor suppressor pathway and accelerates tumor formation in humans. Cell 2004;119(5):591–602.

[98] Bond GL, Hu W, Levine AJ. MDM2 is a central node in the p53 pathway: 12 years and counting. Curr Cancer Drug Targets 2005;5(1):3–8.

[99] Brenner AV, Linet MS, Fine HA, et al. History of allergies and autoimmune diseases and risk of brain tumors in adults. Int J Cancer 2002;99(2):252–9.

[100] Wiemels JL, Wiencke JK, Sison JD, et al. History of allergies among adults with glioma and controls. Int J Cancer 2002;98(4):609–15.

[101] Schwartzbaum J, Ahlbom A, Malmer B, et al. Polymorphisms associated with asthma are inversely related to glioblastoma multiforme. Cancer Res 2005;65(14):6459–65.

[102] Schoemaker MJ, Swerdlow AJ, Hepworth SJ, et al. History of allergies and risk of glioma in adults. Int J Cancer 2006;119(9):2165–72.

[103] Wiemels JL, Wiencke JK, Patoka J, et al. Reduced immunoglobulin E and allergy among adults with glioma compared with controls. Cancer Res 2004;64(22):8468–73.

[104] Wiemels J, Wiencke J, Kelsey K, et al. Allergy-related polymorphisms influence glioma status and serum IgE levels. Cancer Epidemiol Biomarkers Prev 2007;16(6):1229–35.

[105] Schwartzbaum J, Jonsson F, Ahlbom A, et al. Cohort studies of association between self-reported allergic conditions, immune-related diagnoses and glioma and meningioma risk. Int J Cancer 2003;106(3):423–8.

[106] Wrensch M, Weinberg A, Wiencke J, et al. Does prior infection with varicella-zoster virus influence risk of adult glioma? Am J Epidemiol 1997;145(7):594–7.

[107] Wrensch M, Weinberg A, Wiencke J, et al. Prevalence of antibodies to four herpesviruses among adults with glioma and controls. Am J Epidemiol 2001;154(2):161–5.

[108] Wrensch M, Weinberg A, Wiencke J, et al. History of chickenpox and shingles and prevalence of antibodies to varicella-zoster virus and three other herpesviruses among adults with glioma and controls. Am J Epidemiol 2005;161(10):929–38.

[109] Dinarello CA. Setting the cytokine trap for autoimmunity. Nat Med 2003;9(1):20–2.

[110] Dunn GP, Bruce AT, Ikeda H, et al. Cancer immunoediting: from immunosurveillance to tumor escape. Nat Immun 2002;3(11):991–8.

[111] Schwartzbaum J, Ahlbom A, Lonn S, et al. An international case-control study of interleukin-4Ralpha, interleukin-13 and cyclooxygenase-2 polymorphisms and haplotypes and glioblastoma risk, in press.

[112] Wrensch M, Fisher JL, Schwartzbaum JA, et al. The molecular epidemiology of gliomas in adults. Neurosurg Focus 2005;19(5):1–11.

[113] Schwartzbaum JA, Fisher JL, Aldape KD, et al. Epidemiology and molecular pathology of glioma. Nat Clin Pract Neurol 2006;2(9):494–503, quiz 491 p following 516.

[114] Fisher SG, Weber L, Carbone M. Cancer risk associated with simian virus 40 contaminated polio vaccine. Anticancer Res 1999;19(3B):2173–80.

[115] Geissler E, Staneczek W. SV40 and human brain tumors. Arch Geschwulstforsch 1988; 58(2):129–34.

[116] Strickler HD, Rosenberg PS, Devesa SS, et al. Contamination of poliovirus vaccines with simian virus 40 (1955–1963) and subsequent cancer rates. J Am Med Assoc 1998;279(4): 292–5.

[117] Tang J, Shao W, Dorak MT, et al. Positive and negative associations of human leukocyte antigen variants with the onset and prognosis of adult glioblastoma multiforme. Cancer Epidemiol Biomarkers Prev 2005;14(8):2040–4.

[118] Guerini FR, Agliardi C, Zanzottera M, et al. Human leukocyte antigen distribution analysis in North Italian brain Glioma patients: an association with HLA-DRB1*14. J Neurooncol 2006;77(2):213–7.

[119] Facoetti A, Nano R, Zelini P, et al. Human leukocyte antigen and antigen processing machinery component defects in astrocytic tumors. Clin Cancer Res 2005;11(23):8304–11.

ELSEVIER
SAUNDERS

NEUROLOGIC
CLINICS

Neurol Clin 25 (2007) 891–924

# Molecular Pathogenesis of Adult Brain Tumors and the Role of Stem Cells

Claire M. Sauvageot, PhD[a,b,c],
Santosh Kesari, MD, PhD[a,b,c,d],
Charles D. Stiles, PhD[a,c],*

[a]Department of Cancer Biology, Dana-Farber Cancer Institute,
44 Binney Street, Boston, MA 02115-6084, USA
[b]Department of Neurology, Brigham and Women's Hospital,
75 Francis Street, Boston, MA 02115, USA
[c]Harvard Medical School, 25 Shattuck Street, Boston, MA 02115, USA
[d]Dana-Farber/Brigham and Women's Cancer Center, Center for Neuro-Oncology,
44 Binney Street, Boston, MA 02115, USA

Primary brain tumors are a genetically and phenotypically heterogenous group of neoplasms that vary prognostically as a function of location, pathologic features, and molecular genetics [1]. They are comprised of tumors that originate from within the brain and from structures associated intimately with the brain, including the meninges and ependymal tissues. The prognosis of these tumors ranges from relatively benign (ie, meningiomas) to highly aggressive (ie, glioblastomas [GBMs]) and can affect adults and children with different frequencies. Treatment of these tumor types is dependent on their location, extent of resection, and histologic grade. Benign tumors that are in surgically accessible locations essentially are curable, whereas highly infiltrative tumors generally recur and are treated postoperatively with radiation and chemotherapeutics.

A comprehensive understanding of the molecular and genetic changes that manifest themselves during tumorigenesis is critical for the development of new therapeutic strategies to treat brain tumors. This article reviews the genetic and signaling aberrations that are involved in tumor initiation and progression and concludes with an exploration of the cell-of-origin of these neoplasms. An emphasis is placed on gliomas, meningiomas, and medulloblastomas (MBs), as these represent the bulk of all primary brain tumors in adults.

* Corresponding author. Department of Cancer Biology, Dana-Farber Cancer Institute, 44 Binney Street, Boston, MA 02115-6084.
E-mail address: charles_stiles@dfci.harvard.edu (C.D. Stiles).

0733-8619/07/$ - see front matter © 2007 Elsevier Inc. All rights reserved.
doi:10.1016/j.ncl.2007.07.014

## Gliomas

Gliomas are the most common type of primary brain tumor and are grouped into three major categories—astrocytomas, oligodendrogliomas, and mixed oligoastrocytomas—based on their histologic similarity to normal astrocytes or oligodendrocytes within the nervous system. Gliomas are subgrouped further by the World Health Organization (WHO) into grades based on histologic factors, such as nuclear atypia, mitotic activity, vascular proliferation, and necrosis. Tumor grade is predictive of patient survival.

### Astrocytomas

Astrocytomas account for more than 60% of all primary brain tumors [2] and are classified into four grades. Grade I pilocytic astrocytomas are essentially benign and curable by surgery. Grade II diffuse astrocytomas are characterized by nuclear atypia and have an average survival of 5 years. Grade III anaplastic astrocytomas exhibit high mitotic activity and nuclear atypia and have an average survival of 2 to 5 years, whereas grade IV GBMs are highly infiltrative, proliferative, and necrotic, with an average survival of less than 1 year from diagnosis [3–6]. The poor prognosis of GBMs has not changed in decades, even with advances in neurosurgery, radiation therapy, and chemotherapy. Cumulatively, GBMs are the most common form of gliomas, accounting for more than half of all primary gliomas and representing more than 75% of astrocytomas [4].

### Glioblastoma subtypes

Malignant transformation results from the accumulation of genetic abnormalities, including chromosomal loss, mutations, and gene amplifications and rearrangements. Two subtypes of GBMs are identified that are indistinguishable clinically but that have different genetic profiles. Primary GBMs typically appear in older patients who have no previous history of the disease, whereas secondary GBMs usually manifest themselves in younger patients as low-grade astrocytomas that transform within 5 to 10 years into GBM. Primary and secondary GBMs are characterized by different anomalies within the p53 and retinoblastoma (Rb) cell cycle and apoptosis pathways, as well as changes in the expression of different growth factor receptors and downstream signal generators that normally are involved in developmental processes (Fig. 1).

### Defects in the p53 apoptotic and cell cycle pathway

p53 is a tumor suppressor gene that plays a critical role in apoptosis, cellular responses to DNA damage, cell cycle arrest, and neovascularization (Fig. 2) [7,8]. The importance of p53 in gliomagenesis is illustrated in experiments where reintroduction of wild-type p53 into mutant cells promotes

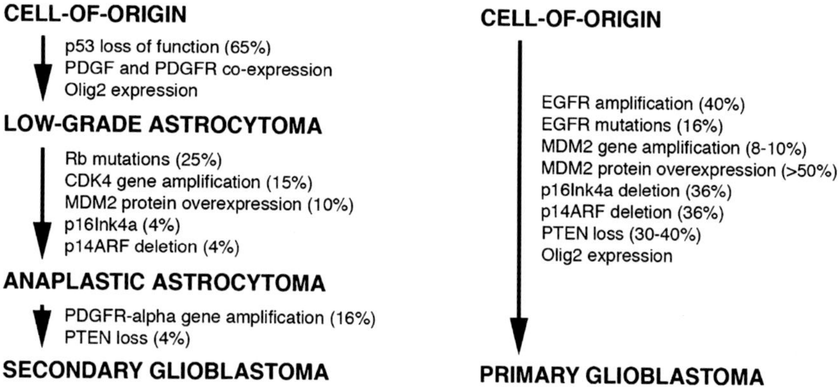

**CELL-OF-ORIGIN**

↓ p53 loss of function (65%)
PDGF and PDGFR co-expression
Olig2 expression

**LOW-GRADE ASTROCYTOMA**

↓ Rb mutations (25%)
CDK4 gene amplification (15%)
MDM2 protein overexpression (10%)
p16Ink4a (4%)
p14ARF deletion (4%)

**ANAPLASTIC ASTROCYTOMA**

↓ PDGFR-alpha gene amplification (16%)
PTEN loss (4%)

**SECONDARY GLIOBLASTOMA**

**CELL-OF-ORIGIN**

↓ EGFR amplification (40%)
EGFR mutations (16%)
MDM2 gene amplification (8-10%)
MDM2 protein overexpression (>50%)
p16Ink4a deletion (36%)
p14ARF deletion (36%)
PTEN loss (30-40%)
Olig2 expression

**PRIMARY GLIOBLASTOMA**

Fig. 1. Molecular and genetic lesions occurring during astrocytoma progression toward primary or secondary GBM.

apoptosis, cell cycle arrest, and suppression of angiogenesis [9,10]. Loss-of-function mutations in the p53 protein are found in more than 65% low-grade astrocytomas, anaplastic astrocytomas, and secondary GBMs [11,12], suggesting that this is an early event in the formation of these tumors. Unlike secondary GBMs, primary GBMs infrequently display mutations in p53 (<10%) [13], although this pathway is deregulated at other levels. Specifically, murine double minute–2 (MDM2) is a protein that is upregulated transcriptionally by p53 and is able to feedback onto p53 to inhibit its activity [14–16]. Approximately 8% to 10% of primary GBMs exhibit *MDM2* gene amplification, and this amplification occurs only in gliomas that do not have p53 mutations [17,18] In addition, more than 50% of primary GBMs show MDM2 protein overexpression compared with only 10% In secondary GBMs [17]. Hence, the MDM2 amplification and overexpression seen in primary GBMs provide an alternate mechanism whereby control of p53 on apoptosis and cell cycle can be bypassed. Finally, more than 35% of primary GBMs have deletions in the p14 alternate reading from (ARF) genetic locus compared with only 4% in secondary GBMs [19]. In a normal cells, ARF functions to inhibit MDM2-induced p53 degradation [20], thereby enhancing apoptosis in a p53-dependent manner, inducing cell cycle arrest and blocking transformation [21–25]. As such, loss of ARF function in GBM results in increased levels of MDM2 and a subsequent decrease in p53 activity. Cumulatively, approximately 75% of GBMs exhibit functional inactivation of the p53 pathway, which results in defects in apoptosis and increased progression through cell cycle [26].

*Defects in the retinoblastoma cell cycle pathway*

Rb is a critical gatekeeper of cell cycle progression by its ability to restrict or allow a cell to progress through the G1 phase of the cell cycle pathway. Hypophosphorylation of Rb maintains the cell in a quiescent state by preventing the transcription of genes important in mitosis. Rb can be

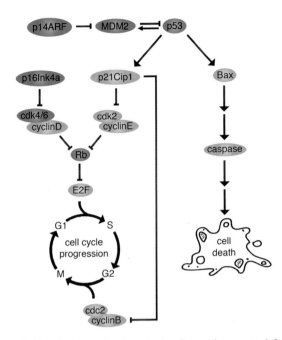

Fig. 2. The p53 and Rb cell cycle and cell death signaling pathways are defective at multiple levels in astrocytomas. Mutations within these pathways result in unimpeded progression through the cell cycle or an inability of the cells to die. Proteins in orange are shown to be mutated, overexpressed, or deleted in astrocytomas. Double arrows indicate multistep stimulation. Bax, BCL2-associated X protein; cdc2, cell division cycle 2.

phosphorylated by cyclin-dependent kinases (CDKs) 4 and 6, which are regulated negatively by CDK inhibitors (CKIs), including $p16^{Ink4a}$ and p21Cip1 [27]. Aberrant entry into the cell cycle pathway can be achieved in tumor cells either by loss of function of Rb or CKIs or by overactivation of CDKs. The transition from low-grade to high-grade astrocytoma is associated with allelic losses on chromosomes 9p and 13q and with amplification of 12q, which are chromosomal loci that house genes associated with the Rb pathway. More specifically, approximately 25% of high-grade gliomas have mutations in Rb [28,29] and 15% exhibit gene amplification of CDK4 [30,31], whereas inactivation of the $p16^{Ink4a}$ CKI occurs in 50% to 70% of these tumors [32,33]. In addition, amplification of CDK6 has been observed in a small subset of tumors [34]. Olig2 is a transcriptional repressor [35,36] that is involved in lineage specification in the nervous system [35–41] and is expressed in astrocytomas regardless of grade [42], suggesting it is an early oncogenic event. A recent article has revealed that Olig2 is required for glioma formation and that it is a direct repressor of the CKI gene, p21Cip1 [43]. As such, an Olig2-mediated decrease of p21Cip1 would result in increased progression through the cell cycle. Many of these mutations generally are mutually exclusive [19,30,34,44,45], resulting in approximately

80% of high-grade gliomas displaying aberrations in their Rb cell cycle pathways. Cumulatively, most of the genetic abnormalities in the Rb pathway manifest themselves in primary and secondary GBM, with the exception of p16$^{Ink4a}$, which is deleted in significantly more primary GBMs than secondary GBMs (36% versus 4%) [19].

*Defects in growth factor signaling*

Growth factor pathways that are involved in normal development of the nervous system and neural stem cells (NSCs) have been shown to be aberrantly regulated in gliomas. In many instances, excessive signaling resulting from the overexpression of either the ligand or the receptor bestows a proliferative and survival advantage to these cells. In other instances, coexpression of cognate ligands and receptors in a single cell result in autocine loops that are involved in transformation and progression. The most common defects in growth factor signaling involve the platelet-derived growth factor (PDGF) and epidermal growth factor (EGF) signaling pathways.

PDGF signaling is involved in the developmental regulation of gliogenesis. The role of PDGF in regulating glial progenitors is illustrated in gain- and loss-of-function mouse models, whereby deletion of the PDGF-A ligand results in reduced numbers of glial progenitors and oligodendrocytes, whereas overexpression of this ligand produces an increase in glial progenitors which subsequently differentiate into oligodendrocytes [46]. Four PDGF ligand genes (A, B, C, and D) are described [47]. The PDGF receptors, consisting of α and β subunits, function by forming noncovalent dimers (α:α, α:β, and β:β), which can be activated by dimers of the ligands—α subunits can associate with either PDGF A, B, or C, whereas the β subunit interacts preferentially with PDGF B and D (reviewed by Li and Eriksson [48]). Coexpression of PDGF ligands with PDGFR-α is common in most glioma cell lines, primary cells, and fresh surgical isolates, whereas PDGFR-β frequently is expressed in glioma and endothelial cells [49–52]. Such coexpression of receptors and ligands within the same cells lead to autocrine loops, which can drive cell proliferation. These autocrine loops are believed to both initiate the transformation process and contribute to the transformed phenotype within these cells [53–55]. In addition to PDGF autocrine loops, PDGF activation in gliomas promotes the upregulation of vascular endothelial growth factor (VEGF), which enhances angiogenesis by promoting pericyte recruitment to neovessels within the tumors [56]. PDGF receptor mRNA expression, which normally is not detectable in the vessels of the normal brain, also is upregulated in proliferating endothelial cells of the tumor vasculature [57], suggesting that the PDGF produced by glioma cells is able to bind neighboring endothelial cells to promote angiogenesis. PDGF ligands and receptors are found in low-grade and high-grade astrocytomas, suggesting that this is an early oncogenic event in secondary GBMs [50]. Overexpression is not associated with gene amplification, although PDGFR-α gene amplification occurs in approximately 16% of high-grade astrocytomas [58]. In addition, PDGFR-α gene amplification is associated with loss of function of p53 [58], placing these two genetic lesions as hallmarks of secondary GBMs.

EGFR is a transmembrane receptor tyrosine kinase that is normally involved in the development of the nervous system by promoting the proliferation of multipotent stem cells [59–62]. Defects in EGFR occur almost exclusively in primary GBMs, where approximately 40% of these tumors feature amplification of the region in chromosome 7 that encodes the EGF receptor (EGFR) gene [63–65]. Overactivity of this receptor results in cellular proliferation, tumor invasiveness, increased angiogenesis and motility, and inhibition of apoptosis [66]. Within tumors exhibiting EGFR amplification, 40% also express a constitutively autophosphorylated variant of the EGFR that lacks the extracellular ligand-binding domain, known as EGFRvIII [63,67–69]. This truncated receptor enhances tumorigenicity by increasing tumor proliferation and invasiveness and decreasing apoptosis [67,70,71]. EGFR amplification is correlated with deletions of the p16$^{Ink4a}$ and p14ARF loci [72,73] and is inversely correlated with p53 inactivation [13].

The effects on proliferation, apoptosis, and angiogenesis following PDGFR and EGFR activation are mediated by the activation of downstream signal transduction pathways, which culminate in the nucleus to affect gene transcription. Common signal transduction pathways activated by these growth factors are the Ras–mitogen-activated protein kinase (MAPK) and the phosphatidylinositol 3 kinase (PI3K)-Akt pathways (Fig. 3). The Ras-MAPK pathway is involved predominately in proliferative responses and cell cycle progression. Although no activating mutations in Ras are documented in astrocytomas [74], elevated Ras activity is common in high-grade astrocytomas [75], presumably because of abnormal activation of upstream receptor tyrosine kinases, such as PDGFR and EGFR. Overactivation of Ras plays a role in tumorigenicity, as inhibition of Ras in glioma cells decrease cellular proliferation in vitro and in vivo [75,76]. The PI3K-Akt pathway is normally involved in inhibition of apoptosis by way of inactivation of the BAD-caspase cell death pathway, as well as cellular proliferation by way of activation of mTOR and S6 kinase. Activating mutations in PI3K are identified in 5% to 7% of GBMs [77,78], which may play a role in the increased proliferation and survival of these tumors. Although no activating mutations of Akt have been identified in astrocytomas, elevated levels of phosphorylated Akt are documented in the majority of GBMs [79], which probably result from a combination of overactivity of receptor tyrosine kinases, PI3K mutations, and loss of phosphatase and tensin homolog deleted on chromosome 10 (PTEN), which normally acts as an inhibitor of this pathway (see discussion later). Activation of the Ras-MAPK and PI3K-Akt pathways may be necessary for astrocytoma progression, as the combined transfer of genes encoding activated Ras and Akt in genetically engineered mice result in GBM formation, whereas the effects of single gene transfer were not sufficient to generate GBMs [79]. Although it is reported that astrocytomas can arise in

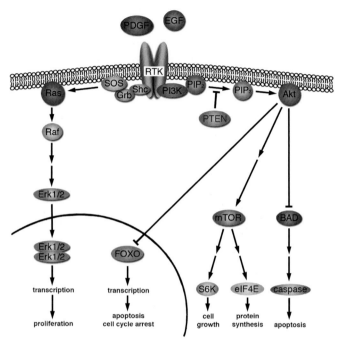

Fig. 3. Activation of receptor tyrosine kinase signaling results in an increase in proliferation and a decrease in apoptosis. Double arrows indicate multistep stimulation. BAD, BCL2-antagonist of cell death; Grb, growth factor receptor-bound protein; ERK, extracellular regulated MAPK; eIF4E, eukaryotic translational initiation factor 4E; FOXO, forkhead box subgroup O; mTOR, target of rapamycin; PIP$_2$, phosphatidylinositol-4,5,-bisphosphate; PIP$_3$, phosphatidylinositol-3,4,5, triophosphate, RTK, receptor tyrosine kinase; Shc, Src homology 2 domain-containing protein; SOS, son of sevenless; S6K, ribosomal protein S6 kinase.

transgenic mice expressing only activated Ras [80], it is highly likely that the PI3K-Akt pathway also may have contributed to this phenotype, as PI3K is a direct Ras effector [81].

PTEN is a tumor suppressor gene [82] that is mutated or deleted in many cancers, including gliomas, prostate, kidney, and breast carcinomas [83]. Structurally, PTEN contains a protein phosphatase domain [82,84], which is important in regulating cell migration and invasion by its activities on focal adhesion kinase [84], and a phosphoinositol phosphatase domain, whose role is to dephosphorylate a lipid second messenger required for activation of the Akt growth and survival pathway [85]. As such, inactivating mutations in PTEN results in increased survival, proliferation, and tumor invasion. Introduction of a wild-type PTEN into glioma cells expressing mutant PTEN causes growth inhibition in vitro and in vivo [86,87], an effect not seen in cells containing endogenous wild-type PTEN. Approximately 30% to 40% of GBMs exhibit mutations within the PTEN tumor suppressor gene [88], which occur almost exclusively in primary GBMs [89]. In addition, in tumors with EGFR amplification, which also occurs in predominately in primary GBMs, simultaneous loss of PTEN is observed [90,91], suggesting that this combination in addition to the loss of p16$^{Ink4a}$ and p14ARF (described previously) are the hallmarks of primary GBMs.

## Oligodendrogliomas

Oligodendrogliomas are diffusely infiltrating tumors whose cells resemble immature oligodendrocytes of the nervous system. They account for more than 4% of all primary brain tumors [92] and represent approximately 20% of all glial tumors [93]. Oligodendrocytomas are classified into two grades—grade II oligodendroglioma, which has a median survival rate of 6 to 10 years [94–96], and grade III anaplastic oligodendroglioma, which has a median survival time of 4 to 5 years [96]. Like astrocytomas, high-grade oligodendrogliomas exhibit more genetic and signaling abnormalities than their low-grade counterparts (Fig. 4).

## Genetic alterations

The main genetic abnormalities associated with oligodendrogliomas are loss of chromosomes 1p and 19q, which occur in approximately 50% to 90% of grade II and grade III tumors [97–101], suggesting that this is an early oncogenic event in the formation of oligodendrogliomas. The 1p and 19q deletions likely result from an unbalanced translocation within these chromosomes [102]. Although extensive mapping of these chromosomes have been undertaken, the tumor-suppressor genes associated with these loci have not yet been identified. In addition, Olig2 is expressed in grade II and grade III tumors [42].

Tumor progression from low-grade to anaplastic oligodendroglioma is associated with similar genetic changes seen during astrocytoma progression, which may represent general oncogenic changes involved in malignant

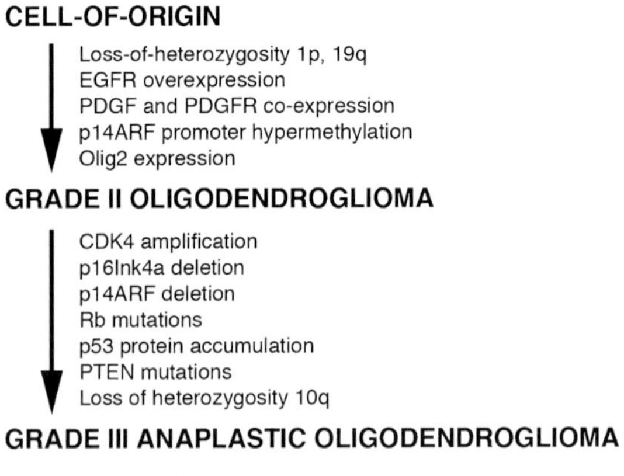

**CELL-OF-ORIGIN**

    Loss-of-heterozygosity 1p, 19q
    EGFR overexpression
    PDGF and PDGFR co-expression
    p14ARF promoter hypermethylation
    Olig2 expression

**GRADE II OLIGODENDROGLIOMA**

    CDK4 amplification
    p16Ink4a deletion
    p14ARF deletion
    Rb mutations
    p53 protein accumulation
    PTEN mutations
    Loss of heterozygosity 10q

**GRADE III ANAPLASTIC OLIGODENDROGLIOMA**

Fig. 4. Molecular and genetic lesions occurring during oligodendroglioma progression.

progression. The Rb cell cycle pathway is altered in 65% of oligodendroglio-mas at the level of CDK4 amplification, mutations in Rb, or homozygous deletions of p16$^{Ink4a}$ [103–105]. Such alterations promote progression through the G1 phase of cell cycle within these cells. Modifications in the p53 apoptosis and cell cycle signaling pathway also occur in high-grade oligodendrogliomas. *p53* gene mutations are seen in approximately 10% to 20% of all oligodendro-cytomas [106–109], with accumulation of the p53 protein occurring in tumors with and without mutations in this genetic locus [109,110]. Although muta-tions in the *p53* gene are not correlated with tumor grade, protein accumula-tion occurs more frequently in anaplastic oligodendrogliomas [109]. p14ARF, whose normal role though the inhibition of MDM2 is to promote p53 activity, shows promoter hypermethylation in 15% to 20% of low-grade and high-grade oligodendrogliomas and deletion in 50% of anaplastic oligodendroglio-mas, compared with only 25% in low-grade tumors [111]. These data suggest that p14ARF promoter methylation is an early event in oligodendroglioma formation, whereas loss of this genetic locus is associated with anaplastic progression. Finally, similar to high-grade astrocytomas, approximately 9% of anaplastic oligodendrogliomas exhibit mutations in PTEN, and more than 20% exhibit loss of the 10q locus which houses PTEN [112,113]. Such mutations, combined with growth factor signal transduction abnormalities (described later), would result in increased proliferation and an inability of cells with these genetic lesions to undergo cell death.

*Defects in growth factor signaling*

Oligodendrogliomas also exhibit abnormalities within the EGFR and PDGFR signal transduction pathways. Unlike astrocytomas, which exhibit EGFR amplification and overexpression only in high-grade tumors, overex-pression of this protein occurs in approximately 50% of low-grade and high-grade oligodendrogliomas [114]. Coexpression of PDGF ligands and the α and β PDGF receptors occurs in almost all oligodendrogliomas [115], suggesting the existence of an autocrine loop within these tumors. Abnormalities within EGFR and PDGFR signaling occur in in low-grade and high-grade oligodendrogliomas, indicating that this is an early onco-genic event in the formation of these tumors. Overexpression of either of these ligands in genetically engineered mouse models has been shown to pro-mote oligodendroglioma tumor formation [116,117]. Tumor formation within these models occurs more rapidly and manifests as higher-grade tu-mors in mice lacking the genes for the Ink4a/ARF loci. This is consistent with the involvement of PDGFR and EGFR in tumor initiation and p16$^{Ink4a}$ and p14ARF in tumor progression.

*Oligoastrocytomas*

As their name implies, oligoastrocytomas are composed of a heteroge-neous population of cells that have characteristics of astrocytomas and oligodendrogliomas. The annual incidence of these tumors ranges from between 9% and 19% of gliomas [118,119]. Oligoastrocytomas are divided into two grades—grade II oligoastrocytomas have a median survival time of 6.3 years compared with 2.8 years observed in anaplastic grade III oligoastrocytomas [120]. As with high-grade astrocytomas and oligodendrogliomas, anaplastic oligoastrocytomas are clinically aggressive and characterized by high mitotic activity, nuclear atypia, and necrosis.

The cellular heterogeneity seen in oligoastrocytomas is reflected in the genetic heterogeneity of these tumors (Fig. 5). Approximately 30% to 50% of oligoastrocytomas exhibit 1p and 19q deletions reminiscent of oligodendrogliomas, whereas a separate 30% of these tumors house genetic anomalies similar to astrocytomas, including mutations in p53 [100,106]. Microdissection of the astrocytoma versus oligodendroglioma components of these tumors have revealed common genetic changes in all components of a given tumor, suggesting that these histologically mixed tumors may arise from a single transforming event [99]. Histologically, those tumors with 1p/19q deletions have a larger fraction of cells with an oligodendroglioma morphology, whereas those with p53 mutations contain more cells resembling astrocytomas. Grade II and grade III oligoastrocytomas express Olig2 protein [42], suggesting this is an early event in tumorigenesis.

Progression from grade II to grade III oligoastrocytomas is characterized by similar transforming events seen in tumor progression of astrocytomas and oligodendrogliomas. These include deletion of the p16$^{Ink4a}$ and p14ARF genetic loci, loss of PTEN, and, in a few cases, amplification of the *EGFR* gene [100].

## Meningiomas

Meningiomas originate from the transformation of meningothelial (arachnoidal) cells and account for approximately 13% to 26% of all primary brain tumors [121]. The large majority of meningiomas are benign and classified as WHO grade I tumors, although 5% to 7% of all

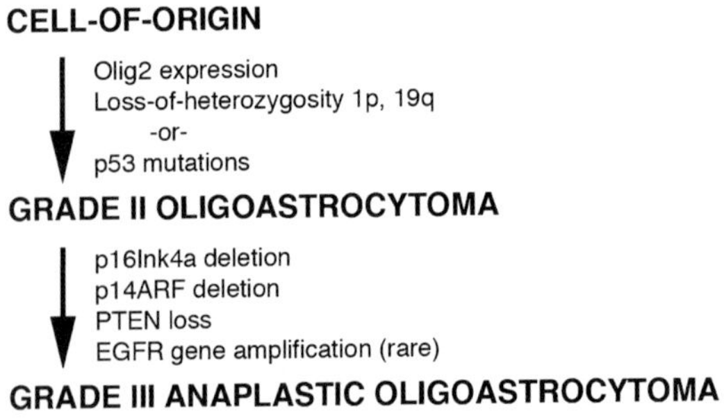

**CELL-OF-ORIGIN**

Olig2 expression
Loss-of-heterozygosity 1p, 19q
-or-
p53 mutations

**GRADE II OLIGOASTROCYTOMA**

p16Ink4a deletion
p14ARF deletion
PTEN loss
EGFR gene amplification (rare)

**GRADE III ANAPLASTIC OLIGOASTROCYTOMA**

Fig. 5. Molecular and genetic lesions occurring during oligoastrocytoma progression.

meningiomas are grade II atypical meningiomas, and 1% to 3% are grade III anaplastic meningiomas [122–126]. Atypical meningiomas are characterized by an increased mitotic index and sheeting architecture, small cell formation, macronucleoli, hypercellularity, or necrosis, whereas anaplastic meningiomas exhibit high mitotic index and frank anaplasia [127]. Increasing tumor grade is associated with shorter survival times [128], with a median survival of 2 years for anaplastic meningioma [125]. Tumor grade also is associated with higher recurrence rates, with grades I, II, and III recurring in 7% to 20%, 29% to 40%, and 50% to 78% of the cases, respectively [124–126,129,130]. Individuals who have neurofibromatosis type 2 (NF-2) or who have been exposed to cranial irradiations have a higher probability of developing meningiomas [127,131].

*Genetic alterations*

The most common cytogenetic change in meningiomas is loss of heterozygosity of chromosome 22, which houses the NF-2 gene (Fig. 6) [132]. Loss of function of NF-2 is an early event in approximately 60% of sporadic meningiomas and occurs in almost all NF-2–associated meningiomas [127,133]. The *NF-2* gene, which is part of the protein 4.1 family, encodes a protein known as merlin or schwannomin, which is involved in linking cell-surface molecules with the actin cytoskeleton [127]. In vitro, merlin is involved in cell growth and motility [134–140], whereas loss of merlin in vivo is associated with increased cell growth and the formation of highly motile and metastatic tumors [141,142]. The role of merlin in meningioma tumor formation

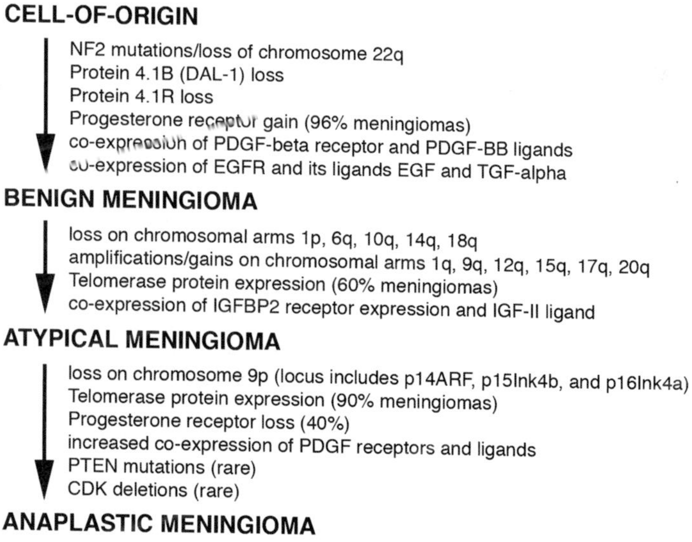

**CELL-OF-ORIGIN**

> NF2 mutations/loss of chromosome 22q
> Protein 4.1B (DAL-1) loss
> Protein 4.1R loss
> Progesterone receptor gain (96% meningiomas)
> co-expression of PDGF-beta receptor and PDGF-BB ligands
> co-expression of EGFR and its ligands EGF and TGF-alpha

**BENIGN MENINGIOMA**

> loss on chromosomal arms 1p, 6q, 10q, 14q, 18q
> amplifications/gains on chromosomal arms 1q, 9q, 12q, 15q, 17q, 20q
> Telomerase protein expression (60% meningiomas)
> co-expression of IGFBP2 receptor expression and IGF-II ligand

**ATYPICAL MENINGIOMA**

> loss on chromosome 9p (locus includes p14ARF, p15Ink4b, and p16Ink4a)
> Telomerase protein expression (90% meningiomas)
> Progesterone receptor loss (40%)
> increased co-expression of PDGF receptors and ligands
> PTEN mutations (rare)
> CDK deletions (rare)

**ANAPLASTIC MENINGIOMA**

Fig. 6. Molecular and genetic lesions occurring during meningioma progression.

is demonstrated by homozygous inactivation of *NF-2* in arachnoidal cells, which results in intracranial meningothelial hyperplasias and meningiomas in approximately 30% of the mice [143]. Another protein 4.1 family member, known either as protein 4.1B or DAL-1, also is implicated in meningioma tumorigenesis, as it is lost in up to 76% in benign and atypical meningiomas and 87% of malignant meningiomas [144,145], and has been shown to have a growth suppressive effect in vitro [144,146]. Loss of protein 4.1R occurs in 40% of meningiomas, whereas 4.1R overexpression in meningioma cell lines results in a reduction in proliferation [147]. These data suggest that the protein 4.1 family of proteins plays a critical role in meningioma formation.

Progression to grade II atypical meningioma is associated with allelic losses of chromosomal arms 1p, 6q, 10q, 14q, and 18q, and gains on 1q, 9q, 12q, 15q, 17q, and 20q [148], although the genes involved in tumor progression at these genetic loci remain to be identified. Approximately two thirds of grade III anaplastic meningiomas have alterations in the tumor suppressor genes $p16^{Ink4a}$, p14ARF, and p15Ink4b [149], with deletions of the first two correlating with shorter survival times [150]. Only rarely have mutations in PTEN and CDK2 been observed in atypical and anaplastic meningiomas [149,151]. Telomerase, an enzyme normally expressed in germ-line and embryonic cells that is involved in stabilizing telomere length, is also associated with tumor progression, with infrequent expression in benign meningiomas (approximately 8%) and higher levels in atypical and anaplastic meningiomas (approximately 60% and approximately 90%, respectively) [152–154]. Progesterone receptors (PRs), which are present in more than 80% of meningiomas [155], also may play a role in the development of these tumors. PR expression in meningiomas is inversely proportional to tumor proliferation and histologic grade, with expression occurring in 96% of benign tumors compared with 40% in malignant meningiomas. PR expression is a favorable prognostic factor for meningiomas, with a loss of PR being a significant predictor of shorter disease-free intervals [156].

*Defects in growth factor signaling*

Growth factor autocrine and paracrine loops also may play a role in meningioma initiation and progression. Coexpression of PDGF ligands and the PDGFR-β receptor occurs in the majority of meningiomas [157], with higher expression correlating with increasing tumor grade [158]. Addition of PDGF-BB to meningioma cells in vitro results in increased proliferation via activation of the MAPK signaling pathway [159], whereas addition of a neutralizing antibody to PDGF-BB blocks this proliferative effect [160]. In addition to PDGF autocrine loops, EGFR and its ligands, EGF and transforming growth factor alpha (TGF-α), are expressed in almost all meningiomas but not in normal meninges [161,162], suggesting a role in meningioma tumorigenesis. Increased TGF-α expression is associated with aggressive meningioma growth and tumor progression [163]. Finally, insulin-like growth factor (IGF)-II and its receptor, IGF binding protein 2 (IGFBP2), are expressed in meningiomas, where a high ligand:receptor ratio is associated with malignant progression [164].

## Medulloblastomas

MBs are an invasive embryonal tumor of the cerebellum that exhibit a tendency to metastasize [165]. Although MB occurs most frequently during childhood, approximately 30% of cases arise in adults [166,167]. MBs are considered WHO grade IV tumors because of their invasive and malignant phenotypes and are grouped into four subtypes based on cell morphology and immunophenotype, consisting of classic, desmoplastic, extensive nodularity and large-cell MBs. Histologic subtype is associated with clinical outcome, with desmoplastic MB having a more favorable outcome than large-cell MB, which is characterized by increased nuclear size and mitotic rates and cytologic anaplasia [168,169]. Adult MBs differ from pediatric MBs in terms of histology, localization, and relapse frequencies. Approximately 50% of adult cases are diagnosed as the more clinically favorable desmoplastic variant compared with only 15% of the childhood cases [170–175]. Unlike pediatric MBs, which are localized predominately in the midline cerebellar vermis and extend into the fourth ventricle, approximately 50% of adult MBs are located laterally within the cerebellar hemispheres [173,176–179], which make them more readily accessible for surgical resection. The event-free survival rates in adults at 5 years of 50% to 60% and at 10 years of 40% to 50% [180] are similar to those observed in children, although late relapses after 5 years remain frequent in adults [171,181].

### Genetic alterations

The most common genetic abnormality in MB consists of an isochromosome of chromosome 17, which arises in approximately 50% of cases [182,183], and which occurs with a higher frequency in classic than in desmoplastic MB [184]. Deletions of the short arm of chromosome 17 also occur in 30% to 45% of cases [185]. Although the tumor suppressor gene, *p53*, is located on 17p and is mutated in many cancer types, only rare mutations in this gene are found in MBs [186–188], suggesting the presence of other as-yet unknown tumor suppressor genes on 17p that may be involved in MB tumorigenesis. Amplification of *MYC*, and to a lesser extent *MYCN*, also is detected in 5% to 10% of MBs [189]. Tumors with lower levels of *MYC* expression have a more favorable clinical outcome [190], consistent with a higher incidence of *MYC* amplification in the more malignant large-cell MB variant [191]. Finally, deletions on chromosomes 1q and 10q are found in approximately 20% to 40% of MBs [192–195], although the genes at these loci implicated in MB have not been unequivocally identified.

*Defects in growth factor signaling*

The main growth factor pathways that are defective in MB are the Sonic hedgehog (Shh), Wingless (Wnt), and ErbB signaling pathways, which are known to be critical for the normal development of the nervous system. The Shh pathway is involved in many aspects of neural development, including neural patterning, axonal guidance, and stem cell maintenance [196]. Signaling within this pathway is initiated by binding of the ligand Shh to its receptor, Patched (PTC), which is a transmembrane receptor that normally suppresses the activity of a protein known as Smoothened (SMO). Activation of SMO releases glioma-associated oncogene homolog-1 (GLI1) from a multiprotein complex that tethers it to microtubules in the cytoplasm, enabling it to enter the nucleus to activate gene transcription (Fig. 7) [197–199]. SMO activation also abolishes cleavage of Gli2 and Gli3, which normally produce truncated transcriptional repressors [197–199]. Hence, within the oncogenic context, PTC can play the role of a tumor suppressor, whereas Shh and SMO are putative oncogenes. Shh signaling was first implicated in cancer after the discovery of germline mutations in the *PTC1* gene in Gorlin's syndrome [200], which leads to a predisposition of several neoplasms, including MB [197,199,201]. Inactivating mutations of *PTC1* have been identified in approximately 8% of sporadic MBs [202–206]. As Shh regulates the proliferation of granule cell precursors in the cerebellum, inactivation of PTC can lead to abnormal proliferation of these progenitor cells and, eventually, tumorigenesis [207]. Activating mutations within Shh and SMO have also been identified in MB, albeit in rare cases [208–210].

The WNT pathway is involved in many aspects of neural development, including patterning, proliferation, orientation, and survival [211]. WNT signaling is mediated by increased β-catenin levels in the cytosol. In the

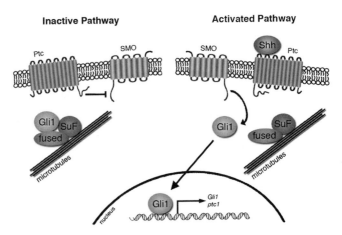

Fig. 7. Shh binding to Ptc removes inhibition of SMO, enabling the release of Gli1 from microtubules and subsequent gene activation. SuF, suppressor of fused.

absence of WNT, β-catenin is sequestered in cadherin-containing cell junctions where it is polyubiquitinated and degraded by a multiprotein complex containing glycogen synthase kinase 3 (GSK-3), adenomatous polyposis coli (APC), and axin. Binding of WNT to the frizzled receptor protein inactivates the GSK-3/APC/axin complex, which decreases polyubiquination of β-catenin, thereby increasing levels of the protein in the cytosol and subsequently in the nucleus, where it can affect gene transcription (Fig. 8). Deregulation of this pathway is involved in many cancers, including MB [212]. Approximately 15% of sporadic MBs exhibit mutations within this pathway, which generally act by blocking the degradation of β-catenin [213–218]. Resulting increases in β-catenin levels enable it to enter the nucleus and activate proliferation genes such as *MYC* and *cyclinD1* [219]. In addition, point mutations in APC have been identified in MBs [215].

ErbB2 is a receptor tyrosine kinase that is involved in cellular proliferation, survival, motility, and differentiation by its ability to activate the Ras-MAPK and PI3K-Akt signaling pathways [220]. Overexpression of ErbB2 or a single point mutation in the transmembrane domain of this receptor can induce tumor formation [220–224]. Although ErbB2 is not expressed in cerebellar granule precursor cells during development [225], 80% of

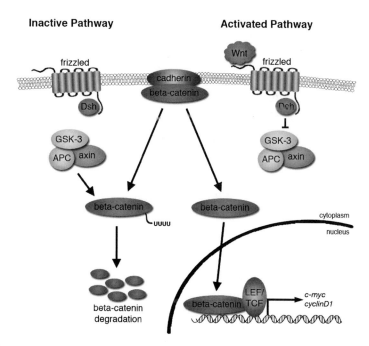

Fig. 8. Wnt activation of the frizzled transmembrane receptor inhibits β-catenin degradation by the GSK-3/APC/axin complex, enabling β-catenin to enter the nucleus and activate the transcription of proliferation-associated genes. Dsh, disheveled; LEF, lymphoid enhancer binding factor; TCF, transcription factor protein; UUUU, ubiquitination.

MBs show expression of ErbB2 [226–228], suggesting it may play a role in tumorigenesis. ErbB2 overexpression in MB is associated with a worse prognosis [226–228]. In addition, the tendency of these tumors to metastisize may be mediated in part by aberrant ErbB2 activation, as ErbB2 overexpression in MB increases cell migration and promotes the upregulation of prometastatic genes [229].

## Cell-of-origin of adult brain tumors

Although the genetic and signaling pathways involved in the progression and malignancy of brain tumors have been relatively well characterized, the cellular origins of these tumors still have not been definitively identified. Tumor recurrence after surgical resection, radiation, and chemotherapeutic treatment occurs in most brain tumors, suggesting that the cells that underlie the malignant growth of these tumors are not targeted efficiently by the current treatment modalities. An understanding of the tumor cell-of-origin may help in the formulation of treatments strategies that are able to target these particular cells, thereby reducing tumor recurrence and increasing survival. There is mounting evidence in the field of cancer biology that the malignant phenotype is propelled by a subset of cells with stem-like qualities [230–232].

### What are stem cells?

Stem cells are defined as cells capable of self-renewal and multipotency. Self-renewal refers to the ability of a cell to generate an identical copy of itself, whereas multipotency refers to the ability of a cell to give rise to all the differentiated cell types within a given tissue. All mature cells within a given tissue arise from a rare population of stem cells that are able to divide asymmetrically to produce mother and daughter cells. The resulting mother cell has equivalent self-renewal and multipotency capabilities as the original stem cell, whereas the daughter cell, frequently referred to as a progenitor cell, has a more limited set of developmental options. Progenitor cells are able to transiently divide before giving rise to the terminally differentiated cells of the tissue.

### Stem cells in the nervous system and in brain tumors

Historically, it has been believed that the cell-of-origin of gliomas must be a mature glial cell, as these were believed to be the only replication competent cells within the adult nervous system capable of acquiring transforming mutations. More recently, neural stem cells (NSCs) have been identified within the adult brain, providing an alternate source of cycling cells capable of transformation. NSCs were identified and isolated by their ability to form neurospheres in serum-free media supplemented with growth factors, such as EGF and FGF2. Removal of these mitogens causes these cells to differentiate into neurons, astrocytes, and oligodendrocytes, revealing their multipotent capabilities. Their ability to self-renew is assessed by clonal expansion of individual cells that can be passaged serially to produce more NSCs capable of differentiating into all mature cell types of the nervous system. NSCs capable of self-renewal and multipotency were identified in germinal areas of the adult nervous system within the subventricular zone and the dentate gyrus of the hippocampus [233–235]. They can be isolated, grown as neurospheres, and driven to differentiate down multiple lineages in vitro [61]. In vivo, these cells proliferate and give rise to all the cell types of the nervous system after implantation into immunodeficient mouse embryos [236,237].

Recent evidence suggests that tumorigenic stem cells also exist within brain tumors. Initial reports showed that NSCs with the ability to grow as neurospheres in vitro and give rise to cells expressing neuronal and glial markers could be isolated from GBM and MB tumors [238–240]. Subsequent experiments revealed that xenotransplantion of neurospheres derived from human brain tumors could form neoplasms that recapitulate the morphology and lineage characteristics of the original tumors, even after serial transplantations. Implantation of as few as 100 of these cells that were shown to express the stem cell marker, CD133, suffices to generate a tumor compared with implantation of $10^5$ CD133-negative cells, which are not able to form a tumor [241], providing evidence that a rare population of tumorigentic stem cells can give rise to the bulk of these heterogeneous tumors. These experiments reveal the existence of tumorigenic stem-like cells within brain tumors but do not exclude the possibility that cycling progenitor cells, or even more differentiated cells, also may play a role in contributing the growth and malignancy of these tumors.

*Mouse models*

Mouse models of gliomas, in which different transforming events are targeted to specific subpopulations of cells within the nervous system, have been created to help clarify the cell-of-origin of gliomas. Although these types of experiments have shown that tumors can arise from progenitor cells and from more differentiated cells, they reveal that progenitor cells are more permissive to oncogenic transformation than differentiated cells such as astrocytes. The most telling of these experiments showed that combined transfer of genes encoding the activated forms of Ras and Akt, which are overactive in astrocytomas, is able to produce gliomas with histologic features of GBM only when targeted to neural progenitors but not differentiated astrocytes [79]. This idea is supported further by data showing that the transforming EGFRvIII gene induces glial tumors more readily when introduced into progenitor cells than in differentiated astrocytes [242], whereas more mature astrocytes are rendered more susceptible to transformation only with additional deletion of the p16$^{Ink4a}$ and p14ARF locus [243]. Furthermore, these Ink4a/ARF$^{-/-}$EGFRvIII astrocytes were able to dediffereniate, reacquire progenitor markers, and even give rise to immature neurons [243]. Finally, reversion of astrocytes to a more undifferentiated state occurs in PDGF-transformed cells that in vivo are able to form mixed gliomas. The tumors formed within this model arise more rapidly and with higher malignancy in an Ink4a/ARF$^{-/-}$ background [116]. These data reveal that malignant transformation occurs more readily in progenitor cells, but that multiple oncogenic pressures can drive more differentiated cells to reacquire progenitor cell phenotypes, which subsequently also can drive tumorigenesis.

*Functional similarities between stem cells and tumor cells*

Several similarities exist between stem cells and tumor cells that further suggest that stem cells, and their daughter progenitor cells, are the cell-of-origin of brain tumors, including extensive proliferation, heterogeneity of progeny, and high motility. NSCs and gliomas are highly proliferative, and the EGFR signaling pathway is involved in this response in both cell types. As described in the previous section, EGF plays a prominent role in promoting the proliferation of gliomas, both as a consequence of EGFR amplification, as well as expression of the constitutively active EGFRvIII variant. Similarly, activation of the EGFR signaling pathway seems necessary for proliferation of NSC within the ventricular zone of the brain, as retroviral overexpression of EGFR in the developing ventricular zone causes NSC proliferation [59], whereas infusion of EGF into the ventricles of the adult brain stimulates the proliferation of transplanted NSCs [60]. In vitro, EGF also is a necessary mitogen for the proliferation of neurosphere cultures.

In addition to their shared proliferative attributes, NSCs and gliomas show a diversity of progeny. As described previously, NSCs are multipotent in vitro and in vivo and can give rise to the heterogeneous population of cells that ultimately make up the mature nervous system. Likewise, gliomas are a heterogeneous population of cells that arise from a very localized transformation event, most likely occurring in a multipotent tumor stem cell, as suggested by the recent identification of CD133$^+$ cancer stem cells that are capable of recapitulating the heterogeneity of the original tumor. Indeed, the clonal origin of a few subtypes of gliomas has been verified after examination of genetic alterations including loss of heterogeneity, immunohistochemical, and mutational analyses, in different areas of a given tumor. In the mixed glioma oligoastrocytoma, for example, identical genetic alterations have been identified in the oligodendroglial and astrocytic components of the tumor [99,244], suggesting multipotency from a common cell of origin. Likewise, in gangliogliomas, clonality is identified in the glial and neuronal components [245] and in gliosarcomas, which exhibit identical mutations in the glial and sarcomatous elements [246]. Although instances exist where clonality cannot be established, which may suggest that independent transformation events in different cells of origin could lead to the heterogeneity exhibited in these tumors, recent evidence reveals that some of the heterogeneity also may arise from progenitors that are recruited to the tumor mass after the original transformation event has occurred [247]. Hence, the heterogeneous progeny of NSCs and gliomas arise from cells with multipotent capabilities.

A cardinal feature of malignant gliomas is their ability to migrate and infiltrate into adjacent regions of the nervous system. Similarly, NSCs and neural progenitors exhibit a migratory capacity in the normal adult brain, consisting of the migration of undifferentiated cells toward the olfactory bulb via the rostral migratory stream [248], and after injury, where progenitor cells are able to migrate from the subventricular zone to the site of injury [249,250]. Once again, this shared phenotype may result from EGF activity. In gliomas, EGFRvIII upregulates effectors of tumor invasion [70], whereas inhibition of EGFR blocks GBM invasion in the brain [251]. Correspondingly in NSCs, constitutive EGFR signaling increases the motility of these cells [252].

*Molecular similarities between stem cells and tumor cells*

In addition to the shared role of EGF in NSCs and glioma cells-of-origin, several proteins that are normally involved in NSC development also are deregulated in gliomas, including PDGF, PTEN, Olig2, and Shh, providing further support for the notion that the origin of gliomas may be NSC and their progenitors. As described previously, coexpression of PDGF ligands and receptors is a common occurrence in brain tumors, resulting in autocrine loops that drive the transformation process. PDGF also plays an important role in regulating glial progenitor proliferation and oligodendrocyte differentiation. During embryogenesis, expression of PDGFR-$\alpha$ in glial progenitors plays a role in the proliferation of glial progenitors, as loss of PDGF results in a reduction of glial progenitors and oligodendrocytes, whereas PDGF overexpression produces more glial progenitors that are able to differentiate into oligodendrocytes [46]. In the adult brain, PDGFR-$\alpha$ expression is restricted to the germinal zone of the brain and, more specifically, is expressed in a subset of subventricular NSCs capable of giving rise to neurospheres and differentiating into neurons and oligodendrocytes. Infusion of PDGF into the lateral ventricles induces the formation of atypical hyperplastic cells that resemble gliomas [253].

The tumor suppressor, PTEN, also is involved in the growth of NSCs and gliomas. It is inactivated in a high percentage of brain tumors, and this inactivation results in increased cell migration, invasion, survival, and proliferation. Correspondingly, PTEN plays a critical role in NSC maintenance and function, as loss of PTEN function in these cells results in increased migration, invasion, and proliferation and a decrease in apoptosis [254,255].

Expression of Olig2 further extends the connection between normal NSCs and gliomas. Olig2 expression is found in all malignant gliomas, is required for glioma formation [42,43], and is expressed in PDGF-induced glioma-like growths [253]. During normal development, Olig2 is expressed in precursor cells within germinal areas of the brain [38,243,256] and is necessary for normal and tumorigenic progenitor cell growth [43].

Finally, the Shh-Gli1 signaling pathway regulates cerebellar granuale precursor cell self-renewal in the cerebellum [207,257,258] and controls the proliferation of precursor cells within the adult germinal zones [259,260]. A variety of primary brain tumors and cell lines, including astrocytomas, oligodendrogliomas, MBs, and GBMs, express Gli1, and inhibition of this pathway inhibits tumor growth [261]. In addition, targeted disruption of the Shh receptor, PTC, results in MBs formation [262]. The parallels between these developmental programs and tumorigenesis lend further evidence that tumor formation results from aberrations of developmental programs normally active in NSCs and their progenitors.

### Localization of stem cell–derived tumors

If NSCs are the cell of origin of brain tumors, then it is expected that these neoplasms be localized preferentially in the germinal areas of the brain. Although this is not the case, much evidence suggests that they arise from these areas and then migrate out to their final locations. In animal models, viral and chemical carcinogens preferentially give rise to tumors in the proliferative subventricular zone of the brain rather than the nonproliferative regions. As these highly invasive tumors grow, their continuity with the subventicular zone becomes increasingly hard to discern [263–266]. This dissociation of transformed cells from germinal areas is consistent with current understanding of stem cell niches (reviewed by Li and Neaves [267]). The germinal areas in which stem cells reside in the mature nervous system are known as niches, and they maintain a homeostatic balance of factors that control the self-renewal and differentiation states of NSCs. Although not yet demonstrated in vertebrate systems, loss of the niche leads to loss of stem cells [268], revealing these cells' dependence on the niche for survival. Tumorigenesis of NSCs may reflect mutations that render the NSC independent of the signals necessary for self-renewal and survival in the niche, thereby enabling it to grow at any location within the brain. The ability of niche-independent NSCs to migrate and grow in aberrant locations of the brain is reminiscent of the highly infiltrative nature of brain tumors.

### Stem cell–targeted therapies

The evidence (summarized previously) strongly suggests that the cells-of-origin of brain tumors are cancer stem cells or transformed progenitor

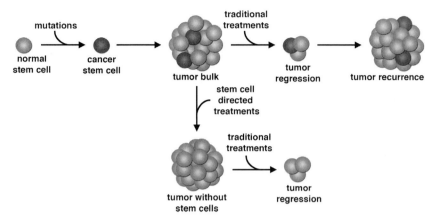

Fig. 9. Stem cell-targeted therapies can diminish tumor recurrence. Mutations that transform normal stem cells into tumor-initiating cells produce tumors composed primarily of cells with limited proliferative capabilities and a minority of stem cell–like cells that can repopulate the whole tumor. Traditional therapies that focus on shrinking the bulk of the tumor may not target the tumor-initiating stem cells, which can result in tumor recurrence. Therapies directed against the cancer stem cells would eliminate the cells capable of repopulating the tumor, resulting in a tumor that cannot grow. The addition of more traditional treatments in conjunction with stem cell–directed therapies cumulatively would result in smaller tumors incapable of recurrence.

cells that arise from these stem cells. Traditional therapies for brain tumors, which frequently result in recurrence, have focused on shrinking the bulk of the tumor (Fig. 9). As cancer stem cells represent only a tiny minority of the tumor bulk, therapies that focus on bulk tumor regression may not eliminate all of these tumor-initiating cells completely, thereby enabling regrowth. Furthermore, the very nature of stem cells may makes them more resistant to current therapies. For example, NSCs express high levels of ATP-binding cassette (ABC) transporters [269,270], which can protect them from chemotherapeutic compounds conventionally administered for brain tumors. Indeed, neurospheres isolated from primary GBMs express higher levels of multidrug resistance-associated proteins than more differentiated cells from the same tumor [271], suggesting they would be more resistant to cytotoxic agents. In addition, CD133+ stem cells isolated from human GBM specimens are more radioresistant than CD133− cells, due to activation of the DNA damage checkpoint response [272]. Hence, therapies targeted specifically against tumorigenic NSCs, such as inhibitors of ABC transporters or of proteins involved in the DNA damage checkpoint response, may be pivotal in preventing recurrence of these tumors. A better understanding of the cell of origin of brain tumors will result in targeted treatment options that may appreciably extend patient survival.

# References

[1] Levin VA, Leibel SA, Gutin PH. Neoplasms of the central nervous system. In: DeVita VT, Hellman S, Rosenberg SA, editors. Cancer: principles and practive of oncology. Philadelphia: Lippincott Williams & Wilkins; 2001.

[2] Cavenee WK, Furnari FB, Nagane M, et al. Diffusely infiltrating astrocytomas. In: Kleihues P, Cavenee WK, editors. Pathology and genetics—tumours of the nervous system. Lyon (France): IARC Press; 2000. p. 10–39.

[3] Burger PC, Vogel FS, Green SB, et al. Glioblastoma multiforme and anaplastic astrocytoma. Pathologic criteria and prognostic implications. Cancer 1985;56(5):1106–11.

[4] CBTRUS. Statistical report: primary brain tumors in the United States, 1998–2002. Chicago: Central Brain Tumor Registry of the United States; Chicago School of Public Health; 2006.

[5] Daumas-Duport C, Scheithauer B, O'Fallon J, et al. Grading of astrocytomas. A simple and reproducible method. Cancer 1988;62(10):2152–65.

[6] Kim TS, Halliday AL, Hedley-Whyte ET, et al. Correlates of survival and the daumas-duport grading system for astrocytomas. J Neurosurg 1991;74(1):27–37.

[7] Bogler O, Huang HJ, Kleihues P, et al. The p53 gene and its role in human brain tumors. Glia 1995;15(3):308–27.

[8] Levine AJ. p53, the cellular gatekeeper for growth and division. Cell 1997;88(3):323–31.

[9] Gomez-Manzano C, Fueyo J, Kyritsis AP, et al. Adenovirus-mediated transfer of the p53 gene produces rapid and generalized death of human glioma cells via apoptosis. Cancer Res 1996;56(4):694–9.

[10] Van Meir EG, Polverini PJ, Chazin VR, et al. Release of an inhibitor of angiogenesis upon induction of wild type p53 expression in glioblastoma cells. Nat Genet 1994;8(2):171–6.

[11] Nozaki M, Tada M, Kobayashi H, et al. Roles of the functional loss of p53 and other genes in astrocytoma tumorigenesis and progression. Neuro Oncol 1999;1(2):124–37.

[12] Watanabe K, Sato K, Biernat W, et al. Incidence and timing of p53 mutations during astrocytoma progression in patients with multiple biopsies. Clin Cancer Res 1997;3(4):523–30.

[13] Watanabe K, Tachibana O, Sata K, et al. Overexpression of the EGF receptor and p53 mutations are mutually exclusive in the evolution of primary and secondary glioblastomas. Brain Pathol 1996;6(3):217–23 [discussion: 223–4].

[14] Haupt Y, Maya R, Kazaz A, et al. Mdm2 promotes the rapid degradation of p53. Nature 1997;387(6630):296–9.

[15] Kubbutat MH, Jones SN, Vousden KH. Regulation of p53 stability by Mdm2. Nature 1997;387(6630):299–303.

[16] Momand J, Zambetti GP, Olson DC, et al. The mdm-2 oncogene product forms a complex with the p53 protein and inhibits p53-mediated transactivation. Cell 1992;69(7):1237–45.

[17] Biernat W, Kleihues P, Yonekawa Y, et al. Amplification and overexpression of MDM2 in primary (de novo) glioblastomas. J Neuropathol Exp Neurol 1997;56(2):180–5.

[18] Reifenberger G, Liu L, Ichimura K, et al. Amplification and overexpression of the MDM2 gene in a subset of human malignant gliomas without p53 mutations. Cancer Res 1993;53(12):2736–9.

[19] Biernat W, Tohma Y, Yonekawa Y, et al. Alterations of cell cycle regulatory genes in primary (de novo) and secondary glioblastomas. Acta Neuropathol (Berl) 1997;94(4):303–9.

[20] Tao W, Levine AJ. P19(ARF) stabilizes p53 by blocking nucleo-cytoplasmic shuttling of Mdm2. Proc Natl Acad Sci U S A 1999;96(12):6937–41.

[21] Kamijo T, Zindy F, Roussel MF, et al. Tumor suppression at the mouse INK4a locus mediated by the alternative reading frame product p19ARF. Cell 1997;91(5):649–59.

[22] Pomerantz J, Schreiber-Agus N, Liegeois NJ, et al. The Ink4a tumor suppressor gene product, p19Arf, interacts with MDM2 and neutralizes MDM2's inhibition of p53. Cell 1998;92(6):713–23.

[23] Quelle DE, Zindy F, Ashmun RA, et al. Alternative reading frames of the INK4a tumor suppressor gene encode two unrelated proteins capable of inducing cell cycle arrest. Cell 1995;83(6):993–1000.

[24] Stott FJ, Bates S, James MC, et al. The alternative product from the human CDKN2A locus, p14(ARF), participates in a regulatory feedback loop with p53 and MDM2. EMBO J 1998;17(17):5001–14.

[25] Zhang Y, Xiong Y, Yarbrough WG. ARF promotes MDM2 degradation and stabilizes p53: ARF-INK4a locus deletion impairs both the Rb and p53 tumor suppression pathways. Cell 1998;92(6):725–34.

[26] Ichimura K, Bolin MB, Goike HM, et al. Deregulation of the p14ARF/MDM2/p53 pathway is a prerequisite for human astrocytic gliomas with G1-S transition control gene abnormalities. Cancer Res 2000;60(2):417–24.

[27] Sherr CJ. Cancer cell cycles. Science 1996;274(5293):1672–7.

[28] Henson JW, Schnitker BL, Correa KM, et al. The retinoblastoma gene is involved in malignant progression of astrocytomas. Ann Neurol 1994;36(5):714–21.

[29] James CD, Carlbom E, Dumanski JP, et al. Clonal genomic alterations in glioma malignancy stages. Cancer Res 1988;48(19):5546–51.

[30] Nishikawa R, Furnari FB, Lin H, et al. Loss of P16INK4 expression is frequent in high grade gliomas. Cancer Res 1995;55(9):1941–5.

[31] Reifenberger G, Reifenberger J, Ichimura K, et al. Amplification of multiple genes from chromosomal region 12q13-14 in human malignant gliomas: preliminary mapping of the amplicons shows preferential involvement of CDK4, SAS, and MDM2. Cancer Res 1994;54(16):4299–303.

[32] James CD, He J, Carlbom E, et al. Chromosome 9 deletion mapping reveals interferon alpha and interferon beta-1 gene deletions in human glial tumors. Cancer Res 1991; 51(6):1684–8.

[33] Olopade OI, Jenkins RB, Ransom DT, et al. Molecular analysis of deletions of the short arm of chromosome 9 in human gliomas. Cancer Res 1992;52(9):2523–9.

[34] Costello JF, Plass C, Arap W, et al. Cyclin-dependent kinase 6 (CDK6) amplification in human gliomas identified using two-dimensional separation of genomic DNA. Cancer Res 1997;57(7):1250–4.

[35] Mizuguchi R, Sugimori M, Takebayashi H, et al. Combinatorial roles of olig2 and neurogenin2 in the coordinated induction of pan-neuronal and subtype-specific properties of motoneurons. Neuron 2001;31(5):757–71.

[36] Novitch BG, Chen AI, Jessell TM. Coordinate regulation of motor neuron subtype identity and pan-neuronal properties by the bHLH repressor Olig2. Neuron 2001;31(5): 773–89.

[37] Furusho M, Ono K, Takebayashi H, et al. Involvement of the Olig2 transcription factor in cholinergic neuron development of the basal forebrain. Dev Biol 2006;293(2):348–57.

[38] Hack MA, Saghatelyan A, de Chevigny A, et al. Neuronal fate determinants of adult olfactory bulb neurogenesis. Nat Neurosci 2005;8(7):865–72.

[39] Lu QR, Sun T, Zhu Z, et al. Common developmental requirement for olig function indicates a motor neuron/oligodendrocyte connection. Cell 2002;109(1):75–86.

[40] Takebayashi H, Nabeshima Y, Yoshida S, et al. The basic helix-loop-helix factor olig2 is essential for the development of motoneuron and oligodendrocyte lineages. Curr Biol 2002;12(13):1157–63.

[41] Zhou Q, Anderson DJ. The bHLH transcription factors OLIG2 and OLIG1 couple neuronal and glial subtype specification. Cell 2002;109(1):61–73.

[42] Ligon KL, Alberta JA, Kho AT, et al. The oligodendroglial lineage marker OLIG2 is universally expressed in diffuse gliomas. J Neuropathol Exp Neurol 2004;63(5):499–509.

[43] Ligon KL, Huillard E, Mehta S, et al. Olig2-regulated lineage-restricted pathway controls replication competence in neural stem cells and malignant glioma. Neuron 2007;53(4): 503–17.

[44] Burns KL, Ueki K, Jhung SL, et al. Molecular genetic correlates of p16, cdk4, and pRb immunohistochemistry in glioblastomas. J Neuropathol Exp Neurol 1998;57(2): 122–30.

[45] Ueki K, Ono Y, Henson JW, et al. CDKN2/p16 or RB alterations occur in the majority of glioblastomas and are inversely correlated. Cancer Res 1996;56(1):150–3.

[46] Calver AR, Hall AC, Yu WP, et al. Oligodendrocyte population dynamics and the role of PDGF in vivo. Neuron 1998;20(5):869–82.

[47] Betsholtz C, Karlsson L, Lindahl P. Developmental roles of platelet-derived growth factors. Bioessays 2001;23(6):494–507.

[48] Li X, Eriksson U. Novel PDGF family members: PDGF-C and PDGF-D. Cytokine Growth Factor Rev 2003;14(2):91–8.

[49] Feldkamp MM, Lau N, Guha A. Signal transduction pathways and their relevance in human astrocytomas. J Neurooncol 1997;35(3):223–48.

[50] Hermanson M, Funa K, Hartman M, et al. Platelet-derived growth factor and its receptors in human glioma tissue: expression of messenger RNA and protein suggests the presence of autocrine and paracrine loops. Cancer Res 1992;52(11):3213–9.

[51] Lokker NA, Sullivan CM, Hollenbach SJ, et al. Platelet-derived growth factor (PDGF) autocrine signaling regulates survival and mitogenic pathways in glioblastoma cells: evidence that the novel PDGF-C and PDGF-D ligands may play a role in the development of brain tumors. Cancer Res 2002;62(13):3729–35.

[52] Maxwell M, Naber SP, Wolfe HJ, et al. Coexpression of platelet-derived growth factor (PDGF) and PDGF-receptor genes by primary human astrocytomas may contribute to their development and maintenance. J Clin Invest 1990;86(1):131–40.

[53] Shamah SM, Stiles CD, Guha A. Dominant-negative mutants of platelet-derived growth factor revert the transformed phenotype of human astrocytoma cells. Mol Cell Biol 1993;13(12):7203–12.

[54] Uhrbom L, Hesselager G, Nister M, et al. Induction of brain tumors in mice using a recombinant platelet-derived growth factor B-chain retrovirus. Cancer Res 1998;58(23): 5275–9.

[55] Westphal M, Ackermann E, Hoppe J, et al. Receptors for platelet derived growth factor in human glioma cell lines and influence of suramin on cell proliferation. J Neurooncol 1991; 11(3):207–13.

[56] Guo P, Hu B, Gu W, et al. Platelet-derived growth factor-B enhances glioma angiogenesis by stimulating vascular endothelial growth factor expression in tumor endothelia and by promoting pericyte recruitment. Am J Pathol 2003;162(4):1083–93.

[57] Jensen RL. Growth factor-mediated angiogenesis in the malignant progression of glial tumors: a review. Surg Neurol 1998;49(2):189–95 [discussion: 196].

[58] Hermanson M, Funa K, Koopmann J, et al. Association of loss of heterozygosity on chromosome 17p with high platelet-derived growth factor alpha receptor expression in human malignant gliomas. Cancer Res 1996;56(1):164–71.

[59] Burrows RC, Wancio D, Levitt P, et al. Response diversity and the timing of progenitor cell maturation are regulated by developmental changes in EGFR expression in the cortex. Neuron 1997;19(2):251–67.

[60] Fricker-Gates RA, Winkler C, Kirik D, et al. EGF infusion stimulates the proliferation and migration of embryonic progenitor cells transplanted in the adult rat striatum. Exp Neurol 2000;165(2):237–47.

[61] Reynolds BA, Weiss S. Generation of neurons and astrocytes from isolated cells of the adult mammalian central nervous system. Science 1992;255(5052):1707–10.

[62] Zhu G, Mehler MF, Mabie PC, et al. Developmental changes in progenitor cell responsiveness to cytokines. J Neurosci Res 1999;56(2):131–45.

[63] Ekstrand AJ, James CD, Cavenee WK, et al. Genes for epidermal growth factor receptor, transforming growth factor alpha, and epidermal growth factor and their expression in human gliomas in vivo. Cancer Res 1991;51(8):2164–72.

[64] Libermann TA, Nusbaum HR, Razon N, et al. Amplification, enhanced expression and possible rearrangement of EGF receptor gene in primary human brain tumours of glial origin. Nature 1985;313(5998):144–7.

[65] Libermann TA, Nusbaum HR, Razon N, et al. Amplification and overexpression of the EGF receptor gene in primary human glioblastomas. J Cell Sci Suppl 1985;3:161–72.

[66] Shinojima N, Tada K, Shiraishi S, et al. Prognostic value of epidermal growth factor receptor in patients with glioblastoma multiforme. Cancer Res 2003;63(20):6962–70.

[67] Nishikawa R, Ji XD, Harmon RC, et al. A mutant epidermal growth factor receptor common in human glioma confers enhanced tumorigenicity. Proc Natl Acad Sci U S A 1994; 91(16):7727–31.

[68] Steck PA, Lee P, Hung MC, et al. Expression of an altered epidermal growth factor receptor by human glioblastoma cells. Cancer Res 1988;48(19):5433–9.

[69] Wong AJ, Ruppert JM, Bigner SH, et al. Structural alterations of the epidermal growth factor receptor gene in human gliomas. Proc Natl Acad Sci U S A 1992;89(7):2965–9.

[70] Lal A, Glazer CA, Martinson HM, et al. Mutant epidermal growth factor receptor up-regulates molecular effectors of tumor invasion. Cancer Res 2002;62(12):3335–9.

[71] Nagane M, Coufal F, Lin H, et al. A common mutant epidermal growth factor receptor confers enhanced tumorigenicity on human glioblastoma cells by increasing proliferation and reducing apoptosis. Cancer Res 1996;56(21):5079–86.

[72] Hayashi Y, Ueki K, Waha A, et al. Association of EGFR gene amplification and CDKN2 (p16/MTS1) gene deletion in glioblastoma multiforme. Brain Pathol 1997;7(3):871–5.

[73] Hegi ME, zur Hausen A, Ruedi D, et al. Hemizygous or homozygous deletion of the chromosomal region containing the p16INK4a gene is associated with amplification of the EGF receptor gene in glioblastomas. Int J Cancer 1997;73(1):57–63.

[74] Bos JL. ras oncogenes in human cancer: a review. Cancer Res 1989;49(17):4682–9.

[75] Guha A, Feldkamp MM, Lau N, et al. Proliferation of human malignant astrocytomas is dependent on Ras activation. Oncogene 1997;15(23):2755–65.

[76] Kurimoto M, Hirashima Y, Hamada H, et al. In vitro and in vivo growth inhibition of human malignant astrocytoma cells by the farnesyltransferase inhibitor B1620. J Neurooncol 2003;61(2):103–12.

[77] Hartmann C, Bartels G, Gehlhaar C, et al. PIK3CA mutations in glioblastoma multiforme. Acta Neuropathol (Berl) 2005;109(6):639–42.

[78] Knobbe CB, Trampe-Kieslich A, Reifenberger G. Genetic alteration and expression of the phosphoinositol-3-kinase/Akt pathway genes PIK3CA and PIKE in human glioblastomas. Neuropathol Appl Neurobiol 2005;31(5):486–90.

[79] Holland EC, Celestino J, Dai C, et al. Combined activation of Ras and Akt in neural progenitors induces glioblastoma formation in mice. Nat Genet 2000;25(1):55–7.

[80] Ding H, Roncari L, Shannon P, et al. Astrocyte-specific expression of activated p21-ras results in malignant astrocytoma formation in a transgenic mouse model of human gliomas. Cancer Res 2001;61(9):3826–36.

[81] Rodriguez-Viciana P, Warne PH, Dhand R, et al. Phosphatidylinositol-3-OH kinase as a direct target of Ras. Nature 1994;370(6490):527–32.

[82] Myers MP, Stolarov JP, Eng C, et al. P-TEN, the tumor suppressor from human chromosome 10q23, is a dual-specificity phosphatase. Proc Natl Acad Sci U S A 1997;94(17): 9052–7.

[83] Steck PA, Pershouse MA, Jasser SA, et al. Identification of a candidate tumour suppressor gene, MMAC1, at chromosome 10q23.3 that is mutated in multiple advanced cancers. Nat Genet 1997;15(4):356–62.

[84] Tamura M, Gu J, Matsumoto K, et al. Inhibition of cell migration, spreading, and focal adhesions by tumor suppressor PTEN. Science 1998;280(5369):1614–7.

[85] Maehama T, Dixon JE. The tumor suppressor, PTEN/MMAC1, dephosphorylates the lipid second messenger, phosphatidylinositol 3,4,5-trisphosphate. J Biol Chem 1998; 273(22):13375–8.

[86] Cheney IW, Johnson DE, Vaillancourt MT, et al. Suppression of tumorigenicity of glioblastoma cells by adenovirus-mediated MMAC1/PTEN gene transfer. Cancer Res 1998; 58(11):2331–4.

[87] Furnari FB, Lin H, Huang HS, et al. Growth suppression of glioma cells by PTEN requires a functional phosphatase catalytic domain. Proc Natl Acad Sci U S A 1997;94(23): 12479–84.

[88] Wang SI, Puc J, Li J, et al. Somatic mutations of PTEN in glioblastoma multiforme. Cancer Res 1997;57(19):4183–6.

[89] Tohma Y, Gratas C, Biernat W, et al. PTEN (MMAC1) mutations are frequent in primary glioblastomas (de novo) but not in secondary glioblastomas. J Neuropathol Exp Neurol 1998;57(7):684–9.

[90] Lang FF, Miller DC, Koslow M, et al. Pathways leading to glioblastoma multiforme: a molecular analysis of genetic alterations in 65 astrocytic tumors. J Neurosurg 1994;81(3): 427–36.

[91] von Deimling A, Louis DN, von Ammon K, et al. Association of epidermal growth factor receptor gene amplification with loss of chromosome 10 in human glioblastoma multiforme. J Neurosurg 1992;77(2):295–301.

[92] Mork SJ, Lindegaard KF, Halvorsen TB, et al. Oligodendroglioma: incidence and biological behavior in a defined population. J Neurosurg 1985;63(6):881–9.

[93] DeAngelis LM. Brain tumors. N Engl J Med 2001;344(2):114–23.

[94] Dehghani F, Schachenmayr W, Laun A, et al. Prognostic implication of histopathological, immunohistochemical and clinical features of oligodendrogliomas: a study of 89 cases. Acta Neuropathol (Berl) 1998;95(5):493–504.

[95] Heegaard S, Sommer HM, Broholm H, et al. Proliferating cell nuclear antigen and Ki-67 immunohistochemistry of oligodendrogliomas with special reference to prognosis. Cancer 1995;76(10):1809–13.

[96] Shaw EG, Scheithauer BW, O'Fallon JR, et al. Oligodendrogliomas: the mayo clinic experience. J Neurosurg 1992;76(3):428–34.

[97] Bello MJ, Leone PE, Vaquero J, et al. Allelic loss at 1p and 19q frequently occurs in association and may represent early oncogenic events in oligodendroglial tumors. Int J Cancer 1995;64(3):207–10.

[98] Bello MJ, Vaquero J, de Campos JM, et al. Molecular analysis of chromosome 1 abnormalities in human gliomas reveals frequent loss of 1p in oligodendroglial tumors. Int J Cancer 1994;57(2):172–5.

[99] Kraus JA, Koopmann J, Kaskel P, et al. Shared allelic losses on chromosomes 1p and 19q suggest a common origin of oligodendroglioma and oligoastrocytoma. J Neuropathol Exp Neurol 1995;54(1):91–5.

[100] Reifenberger J, Reifenberger G, Liu L, et al. Molecular genetic analysis of oligodendroglial tumors shows preferential allelic deletions on 19q and 1p. Am J Pathol 1994;145(5): 1175–90.

[101] von Deimling A, Louis DN, von Ammon K, et al. Evidence for a tumor suppressor gene on chromosome 19q associated with human astrocytomas, oligodendrogliomas, and mixed gliomas. Cancer Res 1992;52(15):4277–9.

[102] Jenkins RB, Blair H, Ballman KV, et al. A t(1;19)(q10;p10) mediates the combined deletions of 1p and 19q and predicts a better prognosis of patients with oligodendroglioma. Cancer Res 2006;66(20):9852–61.

[103] Bigner SH, Rasheed BK, Wiltshire R, et al. Morphologic and molecular genetic aspects of oligodendroglial neoplasms. Neuro Oncol 1999;1(1):52–60.

[104] Cairncross JG, Ueki K, Zlatescu MC, et al. Specific genetic predictors of chemotherapeutic response and survival in patients with anaplastic oligodendrogliomas. J Natl Cancer Inst 1998;90(19):1473–9.

[105] Watanabe T, Yokoo H, Yokoo M, et al. Concurrent inactivation of RB1 and TP53 pathways in anaplastic oligodendrogliomas. J Neuropathol Exp Neurol 2001;60(12):1181–9.

[106] Maintz D, Fiedler K, Koopmann J, et al. Molecular genetic evidence for subtypes of oligoastrocytomas. J Neuropathol Exp Neurol 1997;56(10):1098–104.

[107] Ohgaki H, Eibl RH, Wiestler OD, et al. p53 mutations in nonastrocytic human brain tumors. Cancer Res 1991;51(22):6202–5.

[108] Reifenberger J, Ring GU, Gies U, et al. Analysis of p53 mutation and epidermal growth factor receptor amplification in recurrent gliomas with malignant progression. J Neuropathol Exp Neurol 1996;55(7):822–31.

[109] Hagel C, Laking G, Laas R, et al. Demonstration of p53 protein and TP53 gene mutations in oligodendrogliomas. Eur J Cancer 1996;32A(13):2242–86.

[110] Kros JM, Godschalk JJ, Krishnadath KK, et al. Expression of p53 in oligodendrogliomas. J Pathol 1993;171(4):285–90.

[111] Watanabe T, Nakamura M, Yonekawa Y, et al. Promoter hypermethylation and homozygous deletion of the p14ARF and p16INK4a genes in oligodendrogliomas. Acta Neuropathol (Berl) 2001;101(3):185–9.

[112] Duerr EM, Rollbrocker B, Hayashi Y, et al. PTEN mutations in gliomas and glioneuronal tumors. Oncogene 1998;16(17):2259–64.

[113] Sasaki H, Zlatescu MC, Betensky RA, et al. PTEN is a target of chromosome 10q loss in anaplastic oligodendrogliomas and PTEN alterations are associated with poor prognosis. Am J Pathol 2001;159(1):359–67.

[114] Reifenberger J, Reifenberger G, Ichimura K, et al. Epidermal growth factor receptor expression in oligodendroglial tumors. Am J Pathol 1996;149(1):29–35.

[115] Di Rocco F, Carroll RS, Zhang J, et al. Platelet-derived growth factor and its receptor expression in human oligodendrogliomas. Neurosurgery 1998;42(2):341–6.

[116] Dai C, Celestino JC, Okada Y, et al. PDGF autocrine stimulation dedifferentiates cultured astrocytes and induces oligodendrogliomas and oligoastrocytomas from neural progenitors and astrocytes in vivo. Genes Dev 2001;15(15):1913–25.

[117] Weiss WA, Burns MJ, Hackett C, et al. Genetic determinants of malignancy in a mouse model for oligodendroglioma. Cancer Res 2003;63(7):1589–95.

[118] Helseth A, Mork SJ. Neoplasms of the central nervous system in Norway. III. Epidemiological characteristics of intracranial gliomas according to histology. APMIS 1989;97(6): 547–55.

[119] Jaskolsky D, Zawirski M, Papierz W, et al. Mixed gliomas. Their clinical course and results of surgery. Zentralbl Neurochir 1987;48(2):120–3.

[120] Shaw EG, Scheithauer BW, O'Fallon JR, et al. Mixed oligoastrocytomas: a survival and prognostic factor analysis. Neurosurgery 1994;34(4):577–82 [discussion: 582].

[121] Louis DN, Scheithauer BW, Budka H, et al. Meningiomas. In: Kleihues P, Cavenee WK, editors. Pathology and genetics–tumours of the nervous system. Lyon (France): IARC Press; 2000. p. 176–84.

[122] Jaaskelainen J, Haltia M, Servo A. Atypical and anaplastic meningiomas: radiology, surgery, radiotherapy, and outcome. Surg Neurol 1986;25(3):233–42.

[123] Mahmood A, Caccamo DV, Tomecek FJ, et al. Atypical and malignant meningiomas: a clinicopathological review. Neurosurgery 1993;33(6):955–63.

[124] Maier H, Ofner D, Hittmair A, et al. Classic, atypical, and anaplastic meningioma: three histopathological subtypes of clinical relevance. J Neurosurg 1992;77(4):616–23.

[125] Perry A, Scheithauer BW, Stafford SL, et al. "Malignancy" in meningiomas: a clinicopathologic study of 116 patients, with grading implications. Cancer 1999;85(9):2046–56.

[126] Perry A, Stafford SL, Scheithauer BW, et al. Meningioma grading: an analysis of histologic parameters. Am J Surg Pathol 1997;21(12):1455–65.

[127] Perry A, Gutmann DH, Reifenberger G. Molecular pathogenesis of meningiomas. J Neurooncol 2004;70(2):183–202.

[128] Kallio M, Sankila R, Hakulinen T, et al. Factors affecting operative and excess long-term mortality in 935 patients with intracranial meningioma. Neurosurgery 1992; 31(1):2–12.

[129] Jaaskelainen J, Haltia M, Laasonen E, et al. The growth rate of intracranial meningiomas and its relation to histology. An analysis of 43 patients. Surg Neurol 1985;24(2): 165–72.

[130] Kolles H, Niedermayer I, Schmitt C, et al. Triple approach for diagnosis and grading of meningiomas: histology, morphometry of Ki-67/Feulgen stainings, and cytogenetics. Acta Neurochir (Wien) 1995;137(3–4):174–81.

[131] Kleinschmidt-DeMasters BK, Lillehei KO. Radiation-induced meningioma with a 63-year latency period. Case report. J Neurosurg 1995;82(3):487–8.

[132] Zang KD. Cytological and cytogenetical studies on human meningioma. Cancer Genet Cytogenet 1982;6(3):249–74.

[133] Lamszus K. Meningioma pathology, genetics, and biology. J Neuropathol Exp Neurol 2004;63(4):275–86.

[134] Gutmann DH, Hirbe AC, Haipek CA. Functional analysis of neurofibromatosis 2 (NF2) missense mutations. Hum Mol Genet 2001;10(14):1519–29.

[135] Gutmann DH, Sherman L, Seftor L, et al. Increased expression of the NF2 tumor suppressor gene product, merlin, impairs cell motility, adhesionand spreading. Hum Mol Genet 1999;8(2):267–75.

[136] Ikeda K, Saeki Y, Gonzalez-Agosti C, et al. Inhibition of NF2-negative and NF2-positive primary human meningioma cell proliferation by overexpression of merlin due to vector-mediated gene transfer. J Neurosurg 1999;91(1):85–92.

[137] Lallemand D, Curto M, Saotome I, et al. NF2 deficiency promotes tumorigenesis and metastasis by destabilizing adherens junctions. Genes Dev 2003;17(9):1090–100.

[138] Morrison H, Sherman LS, Legg J, et al. The NF2 tumor suppressor gene product, merlin, mediates contact inhibition of growth through interactions with CD44. Genes Dev 2001; 15(8):968–80.

[139] Shaw RJ, Paez JG, Curto M, et al. The Nf2 tumor suppressor, merlin, functions in rac-dependent signaling. Dev Cell 2001;1(1):63–72.

[140] Sherman L, Xu HM, Geist RT, et al. Interdomain binding mediates tumor growth suppression by the NF2 gene product. Oncogene 1997;15(20):2505–9.

[141] Giovannini M, Robanus-Maandag E, van der Valk M, et al. Conditional biallelic Nf2 mutation in the mouse promotes manifestations of human neurofibromatosis type 2. Genes Dev 2000;14(13):1617–30.

[142] McClatchey AI, Saotome I, Mercer K, et al. Mice heterozygous for a mutation at the Nf2 tumor suppressor locus develop a range of highly metastatic tumors. Genes Dev 1998;12(8): 1121–33.

[143] Kalamarides M, Niwa-Kawakita M, Leblois H, et al. Nf2 gene inactivation in arachnoidal cells is rate-limiting for meningioma development in the mouse. Genes Dev 2002;16(9): 1060–5.

[144] Gutmann DH, Donahoe J, Perry A, et al. Loss of DAL-1, a protein 4.1-related tumor suppressor, is an important early event in the pathogenesis of meningiomas. Hum Mol Genet 2000;9(10):1495–500.

[145] Perry A, Cai DX, Scheithauer BW, et al. Merlin, DAL-1, and progesterone receptor expression in clinicopathologic subsets of meningioma: a correlative immunohistochemical study of 175 cases. J Neuropathol Exp Neurol 2000;59(10):872–9.

[146] Gutmann DH, Hirbe AC, Huang ZY, et al. The protein 4.1 tumor suppressor, DAL-1, impairs cell motility, but regulates proliferation in a cell-type-specific fashion. Neurobiol Dis 2001;8(2):266–78.

[147] Robb VA, Li W, Gascard P, et al. Identification of a third protein 4.1 tumor suppressor, protein 4.1R, in meningioma pathogenesis. Neurobiol Dis 2003;13(3):191–202.

[148] Weber RG, Bostrom J, Wolter M, et al. Analysis of genomic alterations in benign, atypical, and anaplastic meningiomas: toward a genetic model of meningioma progression. Proc Natl Acad Sci U S A 1997;94(26):14719–24.

[149] Bostrom J, Meyer-Puttlitz B, Wolter M, et al. Alterations of the tumor suppressor genes CDKN2A (p16(INK4a)), p14(ARF), CDKN2B (p15(INK4b)), and CDKN2C (p18(INK4c)) in atypical and anaplastic meningiomas. Am J Pathol 2001;159(2):661–9.

[150] Perry A, Banerjee R, Lohse CM, et al. A role for chromosome 9p21 deletions in the malignant progression of meningiomas and the prognosis of anaplastic meningiomas. Brain Pathol 2002;12(2):183–90.

[151] Peters N, Wellenreuther R, Rollbrocker B, et al. Analysis of the PTEN gene in human meningiomas. Neuropathol Appl Neurobiol 1998;24(1):3–8.

[152] Falchetti ML, Larocca LM, Pallini R. Telomerase in brain tumors. Childs Nerv Syst 2002; 18(3–4):112–7.

[153] Langford LA, Piatyszek MA, Xu R, et al. Telomerase activity in ordinary meningiomas predicts poor outcome. Hum Pathol 1997;28(4):416–20.

[154] Simon M, Park TW, Leuenroth S, et al. Telomerase activity and expression of the telomerase catalytic subunit, hTERT, in meningioma progression. J Neurosurg 2000;92(5): 832–40.

[155] Blaauw G, Blankenstein MA, Lamberts SW. Sex steroid receptors in human meningiomas. Acta Neurochir (Wien) 1986;79(1):42–7.

[156] Hsu DW, Efird JT, Hedley-Whyte ET. Progesterone and estrogen receptors in meningiomas: prognostic considerations. J Neurosurg 1997;86(1):113–20.

[157] Maxwell M, Galanopoulos T, Hedley-Whyte ET, et al. Human meningiomas co-express platelet-derived growth factor (PDGF) and PDGF-receptor genes and their protein products. Int J Cancer 1990;46(1):16–21.

[158] Yang SY, Xu GM. Expression of PDGF and its receptor as well as their relationship to proliferating activity and apoptosis of meningiomas in human meningiomas. J Clin Neurosci 2001;8(Suppl 1):49–53.

[159] Johnson MD, Woodard A, Kim P, et al. Evidence for mitogen-associated protein kinase activation and transduction of mitogenic signals by platelet-derived growth factor in human meningioma cells. J Neurosurg 2001;94(2):293–300.

[160] Todo T, Adams EF, Fahlbusch R, et al. Autocrine growth stimulation of human meningioma cells by platelet-derived growth factor. J Neurosurg 1996;84(5):852–8 [discussion: 858–9].

[161] Carroll RS, Black PM, Zhang J, et al. Expression and activation of epidermal growth factor receptors in meningiomas. J Neurosurg 1997;87(2):315–23.

[162] Torp SH, Helseth E, Dalen A, et al. Expression of epidermal growth factor receptor in human meningiomas and meningeal tissue. APMIS 1992;100(9):797–802.

[163] Hsu DW, Efird JT, Hedley-Whyte ET. MIB-1 (Ki-67) index and transforming growth factor-alpha (TGF alpha) immunoreactivity are significant prognostic predictors for meningiomas. Neuropathol Appl Neurobiol 1998;24(6):441–52.

[164] Nordqvist AC, Peyrard M, Pettersson H, et al. A high ratio of insulin-like growth factor II/insulin-like growth factor binding protein 2 messenger RNA as a marker for anaplasia in meningiomas. Cancer Res 1997;57(13):2611–4.

[165] Giangaspero F, Bigner SH, Kleihues P, et al. Medulloblastoma. In: Kleihues P, Cavenee WK, editors. Pathology and genetics—tumours of the nervous system. Lyon (France): IARC Press; 2000. p. 129–37.

[166] Arseni C, Ciurea AV. Statistical survey of 276 cases of medulloblastoma (1935–1978). Acta Neurochir (Wien) 1981;57(3–4):159–62.

[167] Roberts RO, Lynch CF, Jones MP, et al. Medulloblastoma: a population-based study of 532 cases. J Neuropathol Exp Neurol 1991;50(2):134–44.

[168] Eberhart CG, Kepner JL, Goldthwaite PT, et al. Histopathologic grading of medulloblastomas: a pediatric oncology group study. Cancer 2002;94(2):552–60.

[169] Perry A. Medulloblastomas with favorable versus unfavorable histology: how many small blue cell tumor types are there in the brain? Adv Anat Pathol 2002;9(6):345–50.

[170] Bloom HJ. Medulloblastoma: prognosis and prospects. Int J Radiat Oncol Biol Phys 1977; 2(9–10):1031–3.

[171] Carrie C, Lasset C, Alapetite C, et al. Multivariate analysis of prognostic factors in adult patients with medulloblastoma. Retrospective study of 156 patients. Cancer 1994;74(8): 2352–60.

[172] Chatty EM, Earle KM. Medulloblastoma. A report of 201 cases with emphasis on the relationship of histologic variants to survival. Cancer 1971;28(4):977–83.

[173] Haie C, Schlienger M, Constans JP, et al. Results of radiation treatment of medulloblastoma in adults. Int J Radiat Oncol Biol Phys 1985;11(12):2051–6.

[174] Kretschmar CS, Tarbell NJ, Kupsky W, et al. Pre-irradiation chemotherapy for infants and children with medulloblastoma: a preliminary report. J Neurosurg 1989;71(6): 820–5.

[175] Park TS, Hoffman HJ, Hendrick EB, et al. Medulloblastoma: clinical presentation and management. Experience at the hospital for sick children, toronto, 1950-1980. J Neurosurg 1983;58(4):543–52.

[176] Aragones MP, Magallon R, Piqueras C, et al. Medulloblastoma in adulthood: prognostic factors influencing survival and recurrence. Acta Neurochir (Wien) 1994;127(1–2):65–8.

[177] Bloom HJ, Bessell EM. Medulloblastoma in adults: a review of 47 patients treated between 1952 and 1981. Int J Radiat Oncol Biol Phys 1990;18(4):763–72.

[178] Carrie C, Lasset C, Blay JY, et al. Medulloblastoma in adults: survival and prognostic factors. Radiother Oncol 1993;29(3):301–7.

[179] Prados MD, Warnick RE, Wara WM, et al. Medulloblastoma in adults. Int J Radiat Oncol Biol Phys 1995;32(4):1145–52.

[180] Brandes AA, Palmisano V, Monfardini S. Medulloblastoma in adults: clinical characteristics and treatment. Cancer Treat Rev 1999;25(1):3–12.

[181] Frost PJ, Laperriere NJ, Wong CS, et al. Medulloblastoma in adults. Int J Radiat Oncol Biol Phys 1995;32(4):951–7.

[182] Bigner SH, Mark J, Friedman HS, et al. Structural chromosomal abnormalities in human medulloblastoma. Cancer Genet Cytogenet 1988;30(1):91–101.

[183] Griffin CA, Hawkins AL, Packer RJ, et al. Chromosome abnormalities in pediatric brain tumors. Cancer Res 1988;48(1):175–80.

[184] Nicholson JC, Ross FM, Kohler JA, et al. Comparative genomic hybridization and histological variation in primitive neuroectodermal tumours. Br J Cancer 1999;80(9):1322–31.

[185] Cogen PH, McDonald JD. Tumor suppressor genes and medulloblastoma. J Neurooncol 1996;29(1):103–12.

[186] Adesina AM, Nalbantoglu J, Cavenee WK. p53 gene mutation and mdm2 gene amplification are uncommon in medulloblastoma. Cancer Res 1994;54(21):5649–51.

[187] Alderson L, Fetell MR, Sisti M, et al. Sentinel lesions of primary CNS lymphoma. J Neurol Neurosurg Psychiatry 1996;60(1):102–5.

[188] Ohgaki H, Eibl RH, Schwab M, et al. Mutations of the p53 tumor suppressor gene in neoplasms of the human nervous system. Mol Carcinog 1993;8(2):74–80.

[189] Brandes AA, Paris MK. Review of the prognostic factors in medulloblastoma of children and adults. Crit Rev Oncol Hematol 2004;50(2):121–8.

[190] Grotzer MA, Hogarty MD, Janss AJ, et al. MYC messenger RNA expression predicts survival outcome in childhood primitive neuroectodermal tumor/medulloblastoma. Clin Cancer Res 2001;7(8):2425–33.

[191] Brown HG, Kepner JL, Perlman EJ, et al. "Large cell/anaplastic" medulloblastomas: a pediatric oncology group study. J Neuropathol Exp Neurol 2000;59(10):857–65.

[192] Blaeker H, Rasheed BK, McLendon RE, et al. Microsatellite analysis of childhood brain tumors. Genes Chromosomes Cancer 1996;15(1):54–63.

[193] Kraus JA, Koch A, Albrecht S, et al. Loss of heterozygosity at locus F13B on chromosome 1q in human medulloblastoma. Int J Cancer 1996;67(1):11–5.

[194] Reardon DA, Michalkiewicz E, Boyett JM, et al. Extensive genomic abnormalities in childhood medulloblastoma by comparative genomic hybridization. Cancer Res 1997;57(18): 4042–7.

[195] Scheurlen WG, Schwabe GC, Joos S, et al. Molecular analysis of childhood primitive neuroectodermal tumors defines markers associated with poor outcome. J Clin Oncol 1998; 16(7):2478–85.

[196] Fuccillo M, Joyner AL, Fishell G. Morphogen to mitogen: the multiple roles of hedgehog signalling in vertebrate neural development. Nat Rev Neurosci 2006;7(10):772–83.

[197] McMahon AP, Ingham PW, Tabin CJ. Developmental roles and clinical significance of hedgehog signaling. Curr Top Dev Biol 2003;53:1–114.

[198] Ruiz i Altaba A, Palma V, Dahmane N. Hedgehog-gli signalling and the growth of the brain. Nat Rev Neurosci 2002;3(1):24–33.

[199] Ruiz i Altaba A, Sanchez P, Dahmane N. Gli and hedgehog in cancer: tumours, embryos and stem cells. Nat Rev Cancer 2002;2(5):361–72.

[200] Hahn H, Wicking C, Zaphiropoulous PG, et al. Mutations of the human homolog of drosophila patched in the nevoid basal cell carcinoma syndrome. Cell 1996;85(6):841–51.

[201] Taipale J, Beachy PA. The hedgehog and wnt signalling pathways in cancer. Nature 2001; 411(6835):349–54.

[202] Pietsch T, Waha A, Koch A, et al. Medulloblastomas of the desmoplastic variant carry mutations of the human homologue of drosophila patched. Cancer Res 1997;57(11):2085–8.

[203] Raffel C, Jenkins RB, Frederick L, et al. Sporadic medulloblastomas contain PTCH mutations. Cancer Res 1997;57(5):842–5.

[204] Vorechovsky I, Tingby O, Hartman M, et al. Somatic mutations in the human homologue of drosophila patched in primitive neuroectodermal tumours. Oncogene 1997;15(3):361–6.

[205] Wolter M, Reifenberger J, Sommer C, et al. Mutations in the human homologue of the drosophila segment polarity gene patched (PTCH) in sporadic basal cell carcinomas of the skin and primitive neuroectodermal tumors of the central nervous system. Cancer Res 1997; 57(13):2581–5.

[206] Zurawel RH, Allen C, Chiappa S, et al. Analysis of PTCH/SMO/SHH pathway genes in medulloblastoma. Genes Chromosomes Cancer 2000;27(1):44–51.

[207] Wechsler-Reya RJ, Scott MP. Control of neuronal precursor proliferation in the cerebellum by sonic hedgehog. Neuron 1999;22(1):103–14.

[208] Lam CW, Xie J, To KF, et al. A frequent activated smoothened mutation in sporadic basal cell carcinomas. Oncogene 1999;18(3):833–6.

[209] Oro AE, Higgins KM, Hu Z, et al. Basal cell carcinomas in mice overexpressing sonic hedgehog. Science 1997;276(5313):817–21.

[210] Reifenberger J, Wolter M, Weber RG, et al. Missense mutations in SMOH in sporadic basal cell carcinomas of the skin and primitive neuroectodermal tumors of the central nervous system. Cancer Res 1998;58(9):1798–803.

[211] Li F, Chong ZZ, Maiese K. Winding through the WNT pathway during cellular development and demise. Histol Histopathol 2006;21(1):103–24.

[212] Polakis P. Wnt signaling and cancer. Genes Dev 2000;14(15):1837–51.

[213] Baeza N, Masuoka J, Kleihues P, et al. AXIN1 mutations but not deletions in cerebellar medulloblastomas. Oncogene 2003;22(4):632–6.

[214] Eberhart CG, Tihan T, Burger PC. Nuclear localization and mutation of beta-catenin in medulloblastomas. J Neuropathol Exp Neurol 2000;59(4):333–7.

[215] Huang H, Mahler-Araujo BM, Sankila A, et al. APC mutations in sporadic medulloblastomas. Am J Pathol 2000;156(2):433–7.

[216] Koch A, Waha A, Tonn JC, et al. Somatic mutations of WNT/wingless signaling pathway components in primitive neuroectodermal tumors. Int J Cancer 2001;93(3):445–9.

[217] Yokota N, Nishizawa S, Ohta S, et al. Role of wnt pathway in medulloblastoma oncogenesis. Int J Cancer 2002;101(2):198–201.

[218] Zurawel RH, Chiappa SA, Allen C, et al. Sporadic medulloblastomas contain oncogenic beta-catenin mutations. Cancer Res 1998;58(5):896–9.

[219] Henderson BR, Fagotto F. The ins and outs of APC and beta-catenin nuclear transport. EMBO Rep 2002;3(9):834–9.

[220] Yarden Y, Sliwkowski MX. Untangling the ErbB signalling network. Nat Rev Mol Cell Biol 2001;2(2):127–37.

[221] Muller WJ, Sinn E, Pattengale PK, et al. Single-step induction of mammary adenocarcinoma in transgenic mice bearing the activated c-neu oncogene. Cell 1988;54(1):105–15.

[222] Padhy LC, Shih C, Cowing D, et al. Identification of a phosphoprotein specifically induced by the transforming DNA of rat neuroblastomas. Cell 1982;28(4):865–71.

[223] Segatto O, King CR, Pierce JH, et al. Different structural alterations upregulate in vitro tyrosine kinase activity and transforming potency of the erbB-2 gene. Mol Cell Biol 1988; 8(12):5570–4.

[224] Weiner DB, Liu J, Cohen JA, et al. A point mutation in the neu oncogene mimics ligand induction of receptor aggregation. Nature 1989;339(6221):230–1.

[225] Gilbertson RJ, Clifford SC, MacMeekin W, et al. Expression of the ErbB-neuregulin signaling network during human cerebellar development: implications for the biology of medulloblastoma. Cancer Res 1998;58(17):3932–41.

[226] Gajjar A, Hernan R, Kocak M, et al. Clinical, histopathologic, and molecular markers of prognosis: toward a new disease risk stratification system for medulloblastoma. J Clin Oncol 2004;22(6):984–93.

[227] Gilbertson R, Wickramasinghe C, Hernan R, et al. Clinical and molecular stratification of disease risk in medulloblastoma. Br J Cancer 2001;85(5):705–12.

[228] Gilbertson RJ, Perry RH, Kelly PJ, et al. Prognostic significance of HER2 and HER4 coexpression in childhood medulloblastoma. Cancer Res 1997;57(15):3272–80.

[229] Hernan R, Fasheh R, Calabrese C, et al. ERBB2 up-regulates S100A4 and several other prometastatic genes in medulloblastoma. Cancer Res 2003;63(1):140–8.

[230] Al-Hajj M, Wicha MS, Benito-Hernandez A, et al. Prospective identification of tumorigenic breast cancer cells. Proc Natl Acad Sci U S A 2003;100(7):3983–8.

[231] Bonnet D, Dick JE. Human acute myeloid leukemia is organized as a hierarchy that originates from a primitive hematopoietic cell. Nat Med 1997;3(7):730–7.

[232] Collins AT, Berry PA, Hyde C, et al. Prospective identification of tumorigenic prostate cancer stem cells. Cancer Res 2005;65(23):10946–51.

[233] Eriksson PS, Perfilieva E, Bjork-Eriksson T, et al. Neurogenesis in the adult human hippocampus. Nat Med 1998;4(11):1313–7.

[234] Johansson CB, Svensson M, Wallstedt L, et al. Neural stem cells in the adult human brain. Exp Cell Res 1999;253(2):733–6.

[235] Sanai N, Tramontin AD, Quinones-Hinojosa A, et al. Unique astrocyte ribbon in adult human brain contains neural stem cells but lacks chain migration. Nature 2004; 427(6976):740–4.

[236] Tamaki S, Eckert K, He D, et al. Engraftment of sorted/expanded human central nervous system stem cells from fetal brain. J Neurosci Res 2002;69(6):976–86.

[237] Uchida N, Buck DW, He D, et al. Direct isolation of human central nervous system stem cells. Proc Natl Acad Sci U S A 2000;97(26):14720–5.

[238] Hemmati HD, Nakano I, Lazareff JA, et al. Cancerous stem cells can arise from pediatric brain tumors. Proc Natl Acad Sci U S A 2003;100(25):15178–83.

[239] Ignatova TN, Kukekov VG, Laywell ED, et al. Human cortical glial tumors contain neural stem-like cells expressing astroglial and neuronal markers in vitro. Glia 2002;39(3): 193–206.

[240] Singh SK, Clarke ID, Terasaki M, et al. Identification of a cancer stem cell in human brain tumors. Cancer Res 2003;63(18):5821–8.

[241] Singh SK, Hawkins C, Clarke ID, et al. Identification of human brain tumour initiating cells. Nature 2004;432(7015):396–401.

[242] Holland EC, Hively WP, DePinho RA, et al. A constitutively active epidermal growth factor receptor cooperates with disruption of G1 cell-cycle arrest pathways to induce glioma-like lesions in mice. Genes Dev 1998;12(23):3675–85.

[243] Bachoo RM, Maher EA, Ligon KL, et al. Epidermal growth factor receptor and Ink4a/Arf: convergent mechanisms governing terminal differentiation and transformation along the neural stem cell to astrocyte axis. Cancer Cell 2002;1(3):269–77.

[244] Dong ZQ, Pang JC, Tong CY, et al. Clonality of oligoastrocytomas. Hum Pathol 2002; 33(5):528–35.

[245] Zhu JJ, Leon SP, Folkerth RD, et al. Evidence for clonal origin of neoplastic neuronal and glial cells in gangliogliomas. Am J Pathol 1997;151(2):565–71.

[246] Biernat W, Aguzzi A, Sure U, et al. Identical mutations of the p53 tumor suppressor gene in the gliomatous and the sarcomatous components of gliosarcomas suggest a common origin from glial cells. J Neuropathol Exp Neurol 1995;54(5):651–6.

[247] Assanah M, Lochhead R, Ogden A, et al. Glial progenitors in adult white matter are driven to form malignant gliomas by platelet-derived growth factor-expressing retroviruses. J Neurosci 2006;26(25):6781–90.

[248] Lois C, Alvarez-Buylla A. Long-distance neuronal migration in the adult mammalian brain. Science 1994;264(5162):1145–8.

[249] Goings GE, Sahni V, Szele FG. Migration patterns of subventricular zone cells in adult mice change after cerebral cortex injury. Brain Res 2004;996(2):213–26.

[250] Hayashi T, Iwai M, Ikeda T, et al. Neural precursor cells division and migration in neonatal rat brain after ischemic/hypoxic injury. Brain Res 2005;1038(1):41–9.

[251] Penar PL, Khoshyomn S, Bhushan A, et al. Inhibition of epidermal growth factor receptor-associated tyrosine kinase blocks glioblastoma invasion of the brain. Neurosurgery 1997; 40(1):141–51.

[252] Boockvar JA, Kapitonov D, Kapoor G, et al. Constitutive EGFR signaling confers a motile phenotype to neural stem cells. Mol Cell Neurosci 2003;24(4):1116–30.

[253] Jackson EL, Garcia-Verdugo JM, Gil-Perotin S, et al. PDGFR alpha-positive B cells are neural stem cells in the adult SVZ that form glioma-like growths in response to increased PDGF signaling. Neuron 2006;51(2):187–99.

[254] Groszer M, Erickson R, Scripture-Adams DD, et al. Negative regulation of neural stem/progenitor cell proliferation by the Pten tumor suppressor gene in vivo. Science 2001; 294(5549):2186–9.

[255] Li L, Liu F, Salmonsen RA, et al. PTEN in neural precursor cells: regulation of migration, apoptosis, and proliferation. Mol Cell Neurosci 2002;20(1):21–9.

[256] Menn B, Garcia-Verdugo JM, Yaschine C, et al. Origin of oligodendrocytes in the subventricular zone of the adult brain. J Neurosci 2006;26(30):7907–18.

[257] Dahmane N, Ruiz i Altaba A. Sonic hedgehog regulates the growth and patterning of the cerebellum. Development 1999;126(14):3089–100.

[258] Wallace VA. Purkinje-cell-derived sonic hedgehog regulates granule neuron precursor cell proliferation in the developing mouse cerebellum. Curr Biol 1999;9(8):445–8.

[259] Machold R, Hayashi S, Rutlin M, et al. Sonic hedgehog is required for progenitor cell maintenance in telencephalic stem cell niches. Neuron 2003;39(6):937–50.

[260] Palma V, Lim DA, Dahmane N, et al. Sonic hedgehog controls stem cell behavior in the postnatal and adult brain. Development 2005;132(2):335–44.

[261] Dahmane N, Sanchez P, Gitton Y, et al. The sonic hedgehog-gli pathway regulates dorsal brain growth and tumorigenesis. Development 2001;128(24):5201–12.

[262] Goodrich LV, Milenkovic L, Higgins KM, et al. Altered neural cell fates and medulloblastoma in mouse patched mutants. Science 1997;277(5329):1109–13.

[263] Hopewell JW. The subependymal plate and the genesis of gliomas. J Pathol 1975;117(2): 101–3.

[264] Lantos PL, Cox DJ. The origin of experimental brain tumours: a sequential study. Experientia 1976;32(11):1467–8.

[265] Vick NA, Lin MJ, Bigner DD. The role of the subependymal plate in glial tumorigenesis. Acta Neuropathol (Berl) 1977;40(1):63–71.

[266] Zhu Y, Guignard F, Zhao D, et al. Early inactivation of p53 tumor suppressor gene cooperating with NF1 loss induces malignant astrocytoma. Cancer Cell 2005;8(2):119–30.

[267] Li L, Neaves WB. Normal stem cells and cancer stem cells: the niche matters. Cancer Res 2006;66(9):4553–7.

[268] Xie T, Spradling AC. A niche maintaining germ line stem cells in the drosophila ovary. Science 2000;290(5490):328–30.

[269] Islam MO, Kanemura Y, Tajria J, et al. Functional expression of ABCG2 transporter in human neural stem/progenitor cells. Neurosci Res 2005;52(1):75–82.

[270] Islam MO, Kanemura Y, Tajria J, et al. Characterization of ABC transporter ABCB1 expressed in human neural stem/progenitor cells. FEBS Lett 2005;579(17):3473–80.

[271] Salmaggi A, Boiardi A, Gelati M, et al. Glioblastoma-derived tumorospheres identify a population of tumor stem-like cells with angiogenic potential and enhanced multidrug resistance phenotype. Glia 2006;54(8):850–60.

[272] Bao S, Wu Q, McLendon RE, et al. Glioma stem cells promote radioresistance by preferential activation of the DNA damage response. Nature 2006;444(7120):756–60.

ELSEVIER
SAUNDERS

NEUROLOGIC
CLINICS

Neurol Clin 25 (2007) 925–946

# Genetic Causes of Brain Tumors: Neurofibromatosis, Tuberous Sclerosis, von Hippel-Lindau, and Other Syndromes

Christopher J. Farrell, MD[a],
Scott R. Plotkin, MD, PhD[b,c],*

[a]Department of Neurosurgery, White 502, Massachusetts General Hospital and Harvard Medical School, 55 Fruit Street, Boston, MA 02114, USA
[b]Department of Neurology, Massachusetts General Hospital and Harvard Medical School, 55 Fruit Street, Boston, MA, USA
[c]Pappas Center for Neuro-Oncology, Yawkey 9E, 55 Fruit Street, Boston, MA 02114, USA

Several familial syndromes are associated with an increased incidence of nervous system tumors. Recognition of these syndromes is critical to provide optimal clinical care and genetic counseling to affected patients and their families. Identification of the genetic defects responsible for these relatively uncommon disorders has led to the improved understanding of critical molecular pathways involved in tumorigenesis and has contributed to the emergence of molecularly targeted therapeutics against cancer.

The hereditary syndromes and diseases included in this review are limited to those associated with brain tumors: neurofibromatosis 1 (NF1), neurofibromatosis 2 (NF2), tuberous sclerosis complex (TSC), von Hippel-Lindau disease (VHL), and the less frequently encountered Cowden disease and Li-Fraumeni, Turcot's, and Gorlin's syndromes. Most of these disorders are inherited in an autosomal dominant fashion, and the genes involved function primarily as tumor suppressors. Consistent with Knudson's [1] "two-hit hypothesis," germline mutations in these genes result in increased susceptibility to tumor formation following development of a secondary somatic mutation and loss of heterozygosity.

———————
* Corresponding author. Pappas Center for Neuro-Oncology, Yawkey 9E, 55 Fruit Street, Boston, MA 02114.
  E-mail address: splotkin@partners.org (S.R. Plotkin).

**Neurofibromatosis 1**

*Clinical features*

NF1, also called von Recklinghausen's disease or peripheral neurofibromatosis, is the most common neurogenetic disorder, with a birth incidence of 1 in 3000 to 1 in 4000 [2,3]. NF1 is an autosomal dominant disorder with full penetrance and extreme phenotypic variability within and between families. About half of all patients have new mutations and clinically unaffected parents.

Tumors of the nervous system associated with NF1 include neurofibromas and gliomas. Neurofibromas are benign tumors derived from the nerve sheath and contain multiple cell types including Schwann cells, perineural fibroblasts, and mast cells embedded in large qualities of extracellular matrix and collagen. Neurofibromas grow within the nerve bundle and do not usually have a surrounding capsule. By puberty, more than 80% of NF1 patients develop neurofibromas [4] that can be cutaneous, subcutaneous, or deep in location. Spinal neurofibromas are common but seldom require intervention. Intracranial neurofibromas are exceedingly rare; in contrast, neurofibromas of the head and neck are common.

T2-weighted changes on cranial MRI (unidentified bright objects, or UBOs) are found in more than half of children who have NF1, especially in the brainstem, cerebellum, and basal ganglia, and have no known clinical significance. Pilocytic astrocytomas, though less uniformly seen in NF1 patients than neurofibromas, are also closely associated with NF1. Pilocytic astrocytomas are classified as World Health Organization grade 1 tumors. They have low cellularity and exhibit a biphasic pattern that includes compact areas with bipolar piloid cells and Rosenthal fibers in addition to loose-textured microcystic areas. Although they may appear in any part of the brain, pilocytic astrocytomas show a preference for the optic nerve, chiasm, and tract and the adjacent hypothalamus (ie, optic pathway gliomas) (Fig. 1). Optic-pathway gliomas are identified in about 15% of patients who have NF1; in most cases, such disease is limited to nonprogressive enlargement of the structure. Symptomatic optic gliomas occur in only 4% of patients [4] and manifest as proptosis, visual loss, or precocious puberty. Children younger than 7 years are at greatest risk, although older children and adults may rarely present with symptomatic tumors [5].

Nonoptic gliomas also occur at increased frequency in NF1. The prevalence in patients younger than 50 years is 100 times greater than expected according to Surveillance, Epidemiology, and End Results estimates for this age group [6]. The most common sites include the brainstem (49%), cerebral hemispheres (21%), and basal ganglia (14%); histologies include low-grade and high-grade tumors [7].

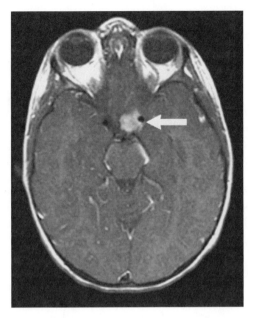

Fig. 1. Axial postcontrast MRI of a patient who has NF1. Note the enhancement within the optic chiasm (*arrow*) consistent with optic glioma.

## Molecular genetics and pathogenesis

The *NF1* locus maps to chromosome 17q11.2, covering 335 kilobases (kb) of genomic DNA divided into at least 60 exons with an open reading frame of 8454 base pairs. Neurofibromin, the most common gene product, is a 2818–amino acid protein found to have a GTPase–activating protein domain that functions to silence the RAS in its activated form. Loss-of-function mutations of the *NF1* gene are associated with increased RAS activity and with the occurrence of benign and malignant tumors, suggesting a tumor suppressor function for the gene [8,9]. The demonstration of *NF1* mutations or "second hits" in NF1-related tumors has been complicated by the heterogeneous pathologic composition of neurofibromas. The presence of Schwann cells, fibroblasts, vascular structures, and mast cells suggests that *NF1* is lost in a single cell type that then recruits other wild-type elements into the tumor. Supporting this hypothesis, loss of *NF1* in Schwann cells alone is sufficient to generate tumors in mice [10] and can be demonstrated in Schwann cells but not fibroblasts from human tumors [11].

Recently, the mammalian target of rapamycin (mTOR) pathway was shown to be aberrantly activated in *NF1*-deficient primary cells and in human tumors [12,13]. This activation is mediated by the phosphorylation and inactivation of the TSC2-encoded protein tuberin. Tumor cell lines derived from NF1 patients are highly sensitive to rapamycin, and increased levels of mTOR pathway activation is reported in human NF1-associated pilocytic astrocytomas.

*Diagnostic criteria and therapy*

The diagnostic criteria developed by the National Institutes of Health (NIH) Consensus Conference in 1987 and updated in 1997 require the presence of at least two of the following clinical features to confirm a diagnosis of NF1: six or more café-au-lait macules, two or more neurofibromas or one plexiform neurofibroma, freckling in the axillary or inguinal regions, optic pathway glioma, two or more Lisch nodules, a distinctive bony lesion such as sphenoid dysplasia or thinning of the long bone cortex, and a first-degree relative who has NF1 [14]. At age 2 years, 50% of individuals who have NF1 will fulfill diagnostic criteria, and this number increases to 97% by age 8 years. Essentially, all patients who have classic NF1 meet diagnostic criteria by the time they reach age 20 years [4]. Mutational analysis of the *NF1* gene has improved drastically in recent years and can identify 95% of causative mutations in patients who have classic NF1 [15]. It can be used to offer preimplantation genetic diagnosis or prenatal testing in families affected by NF1 but should not be used to confirm a diagnosis in patients who meet clinical criteria.

Screening for symptomatic optic glioma includes annual ophthalmologic examination between ages 2 and 7 years and review of growth and sexual development to identify precocious puberty (ie, hypothalamic involvement). Ophthalmologic assessment should include measures of visual acuity and color vision; visual evoked potentials are not recommended [5]. Routine laboratory investigations are not needed for patients who have NF1, and imaging studies of the brain and spine can be reserved for those who have unexplained or progressive symptoms.

Current therapy for NF1 remains primarily surgical; however, recent research has pointed to potential future medical options. Patients who have symptomatic optic gliomas should be followed closely, with therapy reserved for lesions that are progressive. Current treatment options for progressive tumors include chemotherapy such as carboplatin/vincristine or temozolomide. Surgery should be considered for patients who have painful proptosis and blindness or who have hydrocephalus from chiasmal lesions. Similarly, radiation therapy is reserved for patients who progress through chemotherapy, given the risk of developing moyamoya disease [16], endocrinologic dysfunction, and cognitive problems. In addition, radiation has been associated with increased risk of malignant transformation of the optic pathway glioma [17].

Asymptomatic, homogenously enhancing lesions outside the optic pathway can be followed serially by MRI without intervention. Tumor growth or new symptoms should prompt a consideration of surgical sampling to establish tumor grade. In general, high-grade tumors are treated in a fashion similar to sporadic tumors. Radiation therapy should be deferred in low-grade tumors, if possible, for reasons outlined above. The recent finding that the mTOR pathway may be involved in the development of tumors in NF1 has raised interest in investigating a possible therapeutic role for mTOR inhibitors such as rapamycin (sirolimus), which is currently approved by the Food and Drug Administration for use as an immunosuppressant.

## Neurofibromatosis 2

### Clinical features

NF2, also called central neurofibromatosis, is significantly less common than NF1, with a birth incidence of 1 in 25,000 to 1 in 40,000 [18]. NF2 is transmitted in autosomal dominant fashion with full penetrance. Like NF1, about half of all patients have new mutations and clinically unaffected parents. NF2 is characterized by the predisposition to develop multiple tumors including schwannomas, meningiomas, and spinal cord gliomas. The average age of onset of symptoms is between 17 and 21 years and typically precedes a formal diagnosis of NF2 by 5 to 8 years. Features of eighth nerve dysfunction (deafness, tinnitus, or imbalance) are the most common presenting symptoms in adults but occur in only a minority of pediatric patients. In younger patients, presenting signs include cranial nerve dysfunction, peripheral nerve dysfunction, myelopathy, seizures, skin tumors, café-au-lait macules, and juvenile cataracts.

Vestibular schwannomas are the hallmark of NF2 and invariably develop in patients who have the disorder. Schwannomas of nonvestibular cranial nerves and spinal nerves are common (Fig. 2). NF2-related schwannomas are histologically benign, but malignant peripheral nerve sheath tumors may occur in patients who have received prior radiation therapy. About 50% of all patients who have NF2 develop intracranial meningiomas (Fig. 3). Optic sheath meningiomas occur in 4% to 8% of patients who have NF2 and are a disproportionate cause of decreased visual acuity. Meningiomas associated with NF2 are almost universally benign histologically. Spinal ependymomas and astrocytomas in patients who have NF2 present as intramedullary spinal cord lesions and occur in up to 53% of patients. Two-thirds of patients who have ependymomas have multiple tumors. The cervicomedullary junction or cervical spine is most commonly involved (63%–82%), followed by the thoracic spine (36%–44%). The brain and lumbar spine, common sites for sporadic tumors, are rarely involved. Radiographic evidence of tumor progression occurs in less than 10% of patients, and progressive neurologic dysfunction requiring surgical intervention occurs in 12% to 20% of patients.

### Molecular genetics and pathogenesis

The *NF2* gene was mapped to chromosome 22 in 1987 [19,20] and then identified by two independent groups in 1993 [21,22]. The *NF2* gene is

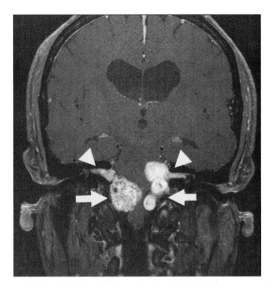

Fig. 2. Coronal postcontrast MRI of a patient who has NF2. Note the bilateral vestibular schwannomas (*arrowheads*) extending through the internal auditory canals and the schwannomas of the lower cranial nerves (*arrows*).

composed of 17 exons spanning 110 kb. There are three alternative messenger RNA species (7 kb, 4.4 kb, and 2.6 kb) due to the variable length of the 3′ untranslated region. The predominant *NF2* gene product is a 595–amino acid protein and a member of the 4.1 family of cytoskeletal proteins termed

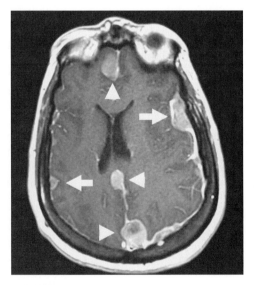

Fig. 3. Axial postcontrast MRI of an NF2 patient who has multiple meningiomas located along the falx (*arrowheads*) and convexities bilaterally (*arrows*).

"merlin" (*m*oezin, *e*zrin, *r*adixin-like protein) to emphasize its relationship to various cytoskeletal proteins. The protein links membrane-associated proteins to the actin cytoskeleton, thereby acting as an interface with the extracellular environment [23].

The NF2 protein functions as a true tumor suppressor: loss of both copies of the gene results in tumor growth. Inactivation of the NF2 gene can be detected in the vast majority of sporadic schwannomas [24] and in about 50% to 60% of sporadic meningiomas. Despite significant progress in understanding the role of the *NF2* gene product, the molecular mechanism by which loss of the NF2 protein leads to tumorigenesis has not been fully elucidated. Recent data suggest that the protein has an important role in the regulation of receptor tyrosine kinases and in maintenance of contact-dependent inhibition of proliferation [23].

## Diagnostic criteria and management

Clinical criteria for the diagnosis of NF2 were first formulated at the NIH Consensus Conference on NF1 and NF2 in 1987 and revised in 1991. Under NIH criteria, a diagnosis of NF2 is based on (1) the presence of bilateral vestibular schwannomas or (2) a family history of NF2 plus a unilateral vestibular schwannoma or any two other tumors typically associated with NF2 [14,25]. Thus, only patients who have bilateral vestibular schwannomas or a family history can qualify for a diagnosis under NIH criteria. Patients who lack these criteria but have multiple features associated with NF2 represent a diagnostic dilemma. For this reason, revised criteria were proposed by the Manchester group in 1992 and by the National Neurofibromatosis Foundation in 1997. The relative merits of these criteria continue to be debated by researchers.

Comprehensive mutational analysis of the *NF2* gene identifies a causative mutation in about 70% of affected individuals. The presence of large deletions, mutations in promoter or intronic regions, and somatic mosaicism contributes to the difficulty in identifying a mutation in all patients. As with NF1, genetic testing can be used for family planning but should not be used to confirm a clinical diagnosis.

Initial evaluation of patients who have or are at risk for NF2 should include testing to confirm a diagnosis and to identify potential problems. A medical history should include questions about auditory and vestibular function, focal neurologic symptoms, skin tumors, seizures, headache, and visual symptoms. A family history should explore unexplained neurologic and audiologic symptoms in all first-degree relatives. MRI of the brain should include gadolinium and include axial and coronal thin cuts through the brainstem to identify vestibular schwannomas. MRI of the cervical spine should be performed, given the predilection of ependymomas for this site. Some clinicians recommend imaging of the thoracic and lumbar spine, whereas others reserve these examinations for patients who have neurologic symptoms referable to these locations. Ophthalmologic examination serves to identify characteristic lesions such as lens opacities, retinal hamartomas, or epiretinal membranes. A complete neurologic examination serves as a baseline for future comparison and may assist in the selection of sites within the nervous system that require further imaging studies. Audiology (including pure-tone threshold and word recognition) and brainstem evoked responses document eighth cranial nerve dysfunction related to vestibular schwannomas and set a baseline for future comparisons.

After initial diagnosis, patients should be seen relatively frequently (every 3–6 months) until the growth rate and biologic behavior of the tumors are determined. Consultation with an experienced surgeon after initial diagnosis is often helpful for presymptomatic patients (ie, those who have adequate hearing) to discuss the feasibility of hearing-sparing surgery. Most patients who do not have acute problems can be followed on an annual basis. Evaluation at these visits should include complete neurologic examination; MRI of the brain, with thin cuts through the brainstem; MRI of symptomatic lesions outside the brain, if present; audiology; and brainstem evoked responses. Ophthalmologic evaluation should be performed in selected patients who have visual impairment or facial weakness. Yearly audiology serves to document changes in pure-tone threshold and word recognition. This information can be helpful in planning early surgical intervention for vestibular schwannomas and in counseling patients about possible deafness. Changes in brainstem auditory evoked responses may precede hearing loss. The frequency with which routine spinal imaging is obtained varies among clinics but is clearly indicated in patients who have new or progressive symptoms referable to the spinal cord.

The approach to management of NF2-associated tumors differs from that of sporadic tumors. The surgical removal of every lesion is not possible or advisable, and the primary goal is to preserve function and maximize quality of life. Surgery is the mainstay for treatment of NF2-related tumors. Surgery is clearly indicated for patients who have significant brainstem or spinal cord compression or who have obstructive hydrocephalus. In patients who have little or no neurologic dysfunction related to their tumors, watchful waiting may allow patients to retain neurologic function for many years [26].

Indications for surgical resection of other tumors are less well defined. In general, schwannomas of other cranial nerves are slow growing and produce few symptoms. Surgical resection in these patients should be reserved for those who have unacceptable neurologic symptoms or rapid tumor growth. Patients who have meningiomas typically have more than one tumor, and resection of all lesions is often not advisable. The benefit of surgery must be carefully weighed against potential complications. As a general rule, indications for resection include rapid tumor growth and worsening neurologic symptoms. Intervention for spinal cord tumors is necessary in a minority of patients [27]. Surgery is more often required in patients who have extramedullary tumors (59%) versus intramedullary tumors (12%) [28].

Radiation is often used as adjuvant therapy for treatment of sporadic brain tumors. Treatment outcomes for patients who have NF2-related vestibular schwannomas are worse than for patients who have sporadic tumors [29]. More recently, fractionated stereotactic radiotherapy has been advocated to minimize the risk of hearing loss. The actuarial 5-year local control rate using this technique is 93%, and the hearing-preservation rate is 64% [30]. The role of adjuvant radiation in other tumors such as meningiomas and ependymomas is not established, but most of these tumors demonstrate benign histology and can be controlled surgically. No case series have been published on treatment of NF2-related meningiomas.

Most clinicians prefer surgical extirpation of tumors when possible and reserve radiation treatment for tumors that are not surgically accessible. This practice is based on the experience that radiation therapy makes subsequent resection of vestibular schwannomas and function of auditory brainstem implants more difficult [31]. In addition, there are reports of malignant transformation of NF2-associated schwannomas after radiation treatment and indirect evidence of increased numbers of malignancy in NF2 patients who have received radiation [32,33]. At the present time, there is no effective chemotherapy for treatment of NF2-related tumors.

## Tuberous sclerosis complex

### Clinical features

TSC is one of the more common hereditary disorders affecting the central nervous system (CNS), with an incidence of approximately 1 in 6,000 live births [34]. Epilepsy and cognitive disability are the most common and debilitating neurologic manifestations of the syndrome [35–37], but disease expression can vary broadly. Other characteristic manifestations of TSC include dermatologic abnormalities such as facial angiofibroma (adenoma sebaceum), hypomelanotic macules (ash-leaf spots), ungual fibromas, and shagreen patches [38]. Visceral findings typically consist of renal angiomyolipoma, pulmonary lymphangiomatosis, and cardiac rhabdomyomas [39–41].

Within the CNS, prominent lesions include cortical tubers, subependymal nodules, and subependymal giant cell astrocytomas (SEGAs). Cortical tubers are benign hamartomas thought to result from disordered cellular differentiation and migration. They are detectable in approximately 95% of TSC patients and are histologically composed of dysplastic neurons and glial cells along with the presence of giant cells. These large eosinophilic cells are considered the hallmark pathologic feature of TSC and have been shown to be of mixed glioneuronal lineage [42]. Subependymal nodules also represent hamartomatous growths and can be located throughout the lateral ventricles. The radiographic appearance of cortical tubers and subependymal nodules varies with patient age and progressive calcification but typically appear as multiple nonenhancing lesions on MRI. Although these lesions do not undergo malignant transformation, about 5% to 15% of TSC patients may develop SEGAs that are believed to develop from accelerated growth of subependymal nodules [43]. These benign tumors usually progress during adolescence and have a predilection for the region of the foramen of Monro (Fig. 4). Due to the potential for obstructive hydrocephalus, surveillance imaging is important for the early detection and treatment of these lesions before the onset of clinical deterioration.

*Molecular genetics and pathogenesis*

Extensive linkage analysis of families that have TSC revealed that the syndrome was heterogeneous and localizable to gene abnormalities on two distinct chromosomes. Subsequently, the *TSC1* and *TSC2* genes were identified on chromosomes 9q34 and 16p13, respectively. A wide variety of germline mutations for *TSC1* and *TSC2* has been observed, and nearly 70% of reported cases of TSC are sporadic. Of interest, *TSC2* mutations are present at rates higher than expected in these sporadic cases and associated with a more severe clinical phenotype [44].

The genetic variability of TSC is explained by analysis of the functional activity of the gene products of *TSC1* (hamartin) and *TSC2* (tuberin). Within the cytoplasm, hamartin and tuberin associate to form a heterodimer that acts as a critical regulator of cell cycle progression by way of inhibition

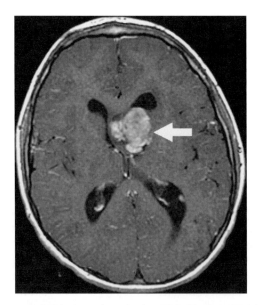

Fig. 4. Axial postcontrast MRI of a patient who has TSC. The large SEGA (*arrow*) is located near the foramen of Monro and causes obstructive hydrocephalus.

of the mTOR pathway [45]. Under normal circumstances, the hamartin/ tuberin suppressor complex is disrupted in response to growth factors and nutrients, which enables increased activation of mTOR and subsequent promotion of cellular growth through mRNA translation and ribosome biosynthesis. In TSC, mutations of *TSC1* and *TSC2* result in failure to inactivate mTOR and unregulated cell growth. SEGAs demonstrate biallelic inactivation of *TSC1* or *TSC2*, supporting the concept that loss of function of the tuberin/hamartin complex underlies tumorigenesis [46]. In contrast, cortical tubers do not consistently harbor two mutations. An alternative mechanism such as haploinsufficiency at the *TSC1* or *TSC2* locus may lead to tuber formation [47]. In addition, *TSC1* and *TSC2* have been implicated in rapamycin-independent pathways that may be important in tumor formation and phenotypic variance.

## Diagnostic criteria and management

Diagnostic criteria for the TSC were revised in 1998 [48]. Clinical diagnosis is supported by the presence of two major features or one major feature plus two additional minor features. Genetic testing is available, but due to the complexity of the disorder, mutational analysis may be associated with an increased false-negative rate and is usually only performed in situations in which the clinical diagnosis is unclear.

Practical management of patients who have TSC involves treatment of seizure disorder and vigilant surveillance for the development of disabling tumors including renal angiomyolipomas and SEGAs. Seizures are primarily treated with anticonvulsants and ketogenic diets, although infantile spasms may prove medically refractory [49]. Surgical treatment of epilepsy can often be complicated by the presence of multiple lesions in eloquent cortical areas and the difficulty of accurate localization of epileptogenic foci. Successful surgical treatment has been described for some patients, however, and the use of more invasive monitoring techniques may allow for better localization [50]. It remains to be seen whether early and more aggressive treatment of seizures will result in improved cognitive outcomes.

Surveillance with brain MRI is recommended every 1 to 3 years to monitor for SEGAs [51]. Indications for surgical resection of SEGAs include obstructive hydrocephalus, increased intracranial pressure, tumor progression, and the presence of focal neurologic deficits referable to the tumor. The mainstay of treatment for symptomatic SEGAs is surgical resection, and gross total resection is considered curative for these benign tumors. Due to their intraventricular location, however, surgical morbidity is common and gross total resection may not be possible. A recent study of SEGAs treated surgically demonstrated significant postoperative neurologic deficits in 2 of 11 patients and gross total resection in only 6 patients [43]. New chemotherapeutic agents based on the role of *TSC1* and *TSC2* in the mTOR pathway may soon provide an alternative to operative intervention. In a recent small clinical study, 4 patients who had SEGAs were treated with rapamycin; all lesions exhibited regression on serial imaging [52].

## Von Hippel-Lindau disease

### Clinical features

VHL is an autosomal dominant hereditary syndrome predisposing to the development of a variety of benign and malignant tumors, including hemangioblastomas of the brain and spinal cord. The incidence of VHL is estimated to be 1 in 31,000 to 1 in 39,000 live births [53]. Characteristic lesions outside of the CNS include retinal hemangioblastomas, clear cell renal carcinoma, pancreatic neuroendocrine tumors, and pheochromocytomas, in addition to benign cysts in multiple organs. Hemangioblastomas are highly vascular, histologically benign tumors composed of endothelial and stromal elements that have a predilection for the posterior fossa (cerebellum and brainstem) and spinal cord. They may occur sporadically or as part of VHL, with recent studies indicating that 20% to 38% of cerebellar hemangioblastomas are VHL associated [54,55]. Radiographic imaging typically reveals a cystic lesion with a strongly enhancing mural nodule (Fig. 5). Vascular flow voids may be seen, confirming the vascularity of these tumors.

No pathologic differences exist between sporadic and VHL-associated hemangioblastomas; both are believed to result from identical mutations within the *VHL* gene. Patients who have VHL, however, typically develop neurologic symptoms at an earlier age and are more likely to harbor multiple cerebellar lesions [55,56]. Symptoms are usually related to dysfunction of the cerebellar hemispheres, including ataxia and dysmetria, but more acute symptoms may be associated with development of obstructive hydrocephalus. Spinal cord hemangioblastomas are less frequently encountered than cerebellar lesions, but their presence is more correlative with the presence of VHL. The identification of a spinal hemangioblastoma should prompt a high degree of suspicion for VHL [55].

Between 11% and 16% of patients who have VHL also develop tumors of the endolymphatic sac or duct within the temporal bone [56]. Although these tumors are histologically benign, they may be locally invasive and result in significant neurologic disability including deafness and dysequilibrium. Hearing loss is usually irreversible and may be chronic (from enlarging tumors) or acute (from intralabyrinthine hemorrhage, hydrops formation, or both) [57]. Additional common presenting features of endolymphatic sac tumors include tinnitus, aural fullness, vertigo, and facial nerve paresis [57].

### Molecular genetics and pathogenesis

In 1993, the responsible gene (*VHL*) was mapped to the short arm of chromosome 3 [58]. The encoded protein of the *VHL* gene (pVHL)

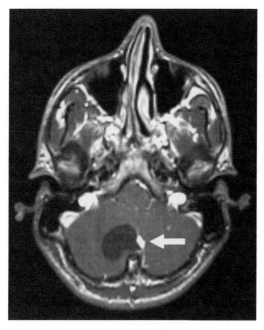

Fig. 5. Axial postcontrast MRI of a patient who has VHL. There is a typical-appearing hemangioblastoma within the cerebellar hemisphere consisting of a cystic lesion with a small, intensely enhancing mural nodule (*arrow*).

functions as a tumor suppressor, and further characterization has revealed a role in angiogenesis through regulation of hypoxia-inducible genes. Inactivation of pVHL results in overexpression of hypoxia-inducible factor, leading to increased levels of downstream targets including vascular endothelial growth factor (VEGF), platelet-derived growth factor, and erythropoietin. Other mechanisms by which pVHL disruption leads to tumor formation are less clear but include interactions with the extracellular matrix and cytoskeleton and control of the cell cycle [59].

*Diagnostic criteria and management*

Recognition of VHL in patients presenting with CNS hemangioblastomas is imperative to ensure appropriate monitoring for other associated malignancies including renal cell carcinoma. Clinical criteria for the diagnosis of VHL include the presence of multiple hemangioblastomas or a single hemangioblastoma plus a characteristic visceral lesion. If a family history of VHL is present, only one hemangioblastoma or visceral lesion is needed to make the diagnosis. Although the diagnosis of VHL can be made clinically, definitive molecular testing is now available through approved diagnostic laboratories and may provide additional genotype-phenotype information. For example, missense *VHL* mutations (type 2) are typically not associated with pheochromocytoma development, as opposed to deletions or other mutations that result in a truncated pVHL (type 1) [60,61]. In addition, genetic testing can be used for family planning.

Treatment of cerebellar and spinal hemangioblastomas is primarily by surgical resection. Despite their benign histology, a recurrence rate of 17% for cerebellar lesions has been reported, likely related to the difficulty in completely resecting these lesions within the posterior fossa [55]. This report also demonstrated that long-term surveillance is important in VHL patients, because 67% developed new CNS lesions during the follow-up period [55].

Regular otologic examinations and high-resolution imaging through the temporal bone are recommended to allow for early detection of endolymphatic sac tumors. Because these tumors frequently present with acute and irreversible hearing loss, early detection allows for surgical removal of these tumors with hearing preservation [57].

Improved understanding of the function of the *VHL* gene product has enabled clinical translation and the development of targeted therapeutics. Antiangiogenesis inhibitors including antibodies directed against VEGF and small-molecule inhibitors of VEGF receptors are currently being employed in a number of clinical trials for clear cell renal carcinoma and have led to improvement in survival in phase III trials [62]. Further studies will be needed to address whether these agents are similarly effective against hemangioblastomas, although initial experiences in a very small number of patients have shown promise [63].

## Cowden disease

### Clinical features

Cowden disease is an autosomal dominant disorder characterized by the presence of hamartomas in multiple organ systems including the CNS and by an increased predisposition to cancers of the breast, thyroid, and endometrium. Although the incidence of the disorder has been estimated at 1 in 200,000 [64], this likely represents an underestimate, given the disorder's variable expression and often subtle cutaneous signs. The hallmark cutaneous features of Cowden disease include trichilemmomas. Within the CNS, the pathognomonic feature is the presence of Lhermitte-Duclos disease (LDD; National Comprehensive Cancer Network Guidelines 2006), although other associations include macrocephaly, heterotopias, seizures, vascular abnormalities, and mental retardation.

LDD is a space-occupying lesion of the cerebellar cortex that most commonly presents as headaches, nausea, vomiting, and ataxia. Secondary obstructive hydrocephalus may result from impingement on the fourth ventricle. Histopathologically, LDD is characterized by the replacement and expansion of the internal granular layer with hypertrophic neurons and by the loss of Purkinje cells and increased myelination within the molecular layer [65]. The hamartomatous nature of LDD is suggested by the absence of mitoses, atypia, or proliferation within pathologic specimens from affected patients.

Although the definitive diagnosis of LDD is made histopathologically, the unique features of LDD allow for an accurate diagnosis to be made by radiographic imaging. MRI reveals a well-circumscribed, nonenhancing area of cerebellar folia enlargement. T2-hyperintensity is normally present, and the involved cerebellar cortex has a striated, laminated appearance often described as "tiger striped" [66].

*Molecular genetics and pathogenesis*

In 1996, the genetic basis for Cowden disease was identified as germline mutations in the *PTEN* gene on chromosome 10 [64]. The product of the *PTEN* gene is a phosphatase that inhibits signal transduction within the phosphatidylinositol 3-kinase (PI3K)/AKT pathway that controls many important processes including cellular growth, migration, differentiation, and apoptosis. Mutations in *PTEN* also lead to increased activation of the downstream target mTOR, and increased activation of AKT and mTOR have been demonstrated in immunohistochemical analyses from most adult-onset LDD patients. Conversely, samples from childhood LDD reveal normal levels of PTEN activity, and germline *PTEN* mutations are not observed; childhood LDD is not considered a manifestation of Cowden disease [65,67].

*Diagnostic criteria and management*

The most recent guidelines for the diagnosis of Cowden disease consider adult-onset LDD as pathognomonic for the disorder. Pediatric LDD, in contrast, is likely an isolated syndrome unrelated to Cowden disease. The association between LDD and Cowden disease represents a significant advancement because Cowden disease has frequently been under-recognized in patients treated for LDD, and diagnosis of Cowden disease is imperative because of the high risk of systemic cancers in affected patients. Lifetime risks for the development of breast cancer and thyroid cancer have been estimated to be 25% to 50% and 10%, respectively, emphasizing the importance of appropriate screening measures [68].

Although LDD represents a benign lesion, it frequently demonstrates progressive growth, and surgical resection is considered the only effective means of treatment. Recurrences are common and most likely due to difficulty in identifying distinct borders between normal and affected cortex during surgical resection [65]. Symptoms from LDD result from hypertrophy of individual cells rather than cellular proliferation, and concordantly, radiation therapy has not been effective in achieving regression of these lesions. Demonstration of increased mTOR activity within LDD samples suggests that mTOR inhibitors may be effective.

## Li-Fraumeni syndrome

### Clinical features

Li-Fraumeni syndrome (LFS) is a hereditary disorder that predisposes to a wide variety of early-onset tumors including breast cancer, sarcomas, leukemia, adrenocortical carcinoma, and brain tumors. Sarcomas and premenopausal breast cancer are the most frequent cancers associated with LFS, although approximately 13% of LFS kindreds with *TP53* mutations develop nervous system tumors [69]. Astrocytic tumors are the most commonly reported brain tumors, although medulloblastomas and supratentorial primitive neuroectodermal tumors may also occur. In addition, tumors of the peripheral nervous system including neuroblastoma have also been observed in LFS families. The mean age of onset for brain tumors in LFS with *TP53* mutations is 16 years [69].

### Molecular genetics and pathogenesis

Germline mutations in the *TP53* have been identified as the underlying genetic defect in approximately 70% of LFS individuals [70]. The diverse tumor suppressor functions of *TP53*'s gene product, p53, have been extensively characterized due its aberrant expression in a large number of sporadic human cancers, and critical roles for p53 have been determined in cell cycle arrest, DNA repair, and apoptosis. Germline mutations in the checkpoint kinase gene, *CHEK2*, have been identified in a small percentage of *TP53*-negative families [71,72]. The CHEK2 protein causes cell cycle arrest in response to DNA damage; however, several subsequent analyses of LFS families have not confirmed an underlying role for *CHEK2* [73].

### Diagnostic criteria and management

Diagnosis of LFS includes the following criteria: a proband with a sarcoma before age 45 years, a first-degree relative who has any cancer diagnosed before age 45 years, and another first- or second-degree relative who has a sarcoma at any age or any other cancer diagnosed before age 45 years. A less stringent definition of the syndrome is referred to as the Li-Fraumeni–like variant, and germline mutations in TP53 have been identified in 22% to 40% of these families [74].

Treatment of brain tumors associated with LFS is similar to that for sporadic tumors, although LFS patients should be monitored for the development of secondary malignancies following administration of DNA-damaging agents such as ionizing radiation or most chemotherapeutics [75].

## Turcot's syndrome

### Clinical features

Turcot's syndrome refers to the rare association of brain tumors and colorectal polyposis. Two forms of hereditary colorectal cancer have been established: familial adenomatous polyposis (FAP) and hereditary nonpolyposis colorectal cancer (HNPCC). FAP is characterized by the development of hundreds to thousands of polyps in the colon and rectum during adolescence. Although these polyps are benign, eventual progression to malignancy typically occurs by age 35 to 40 years. The absolute risk of an individual who has FAP developing a brain tumor is low, but the relative risk is significantly elevated compared with the general population [76,77]. Pooled data on families that have FAP indicate that medulloblastomas are most common (60%), followed by astrocytomas (14%) and ependymoma (10%). In contrast, patients who have HNPCC usually develop fewer adenomatous polyps, but these polyps are typically larger and more likely to represent adenocarcinomas. Affected patients have an increased incidence of extracolonic malignancies, including primary glial tumors such as glioblastoma.

### Molecular genetics and pathogenesis

The complex molecular basis for Turcot's syndrome was first reported in 1995 [76]. Tumors in patients who have FAP result from mutations in the *APC* gene on chromosome 5, whereas HNPCC-related tumors result from mutations in a series of DNA-mismatch repair (MMR) genes. The primary mechanism by which mutations in the APC protein is believed to result in tumorigenesis is through disruption of the WNT signaling pathway, a pathway that is also commonly disrupted in sporadic colorectal cancers and medulloblastomas. Most affected HNPCC families have mutations in the *hMSH2* and *hMLH1* genes, but additional mutations have also been described in other MMR genes, including *hPMS1*, *hPMS2*, and *hMSH6* [76]. Germline mutations in all of these MMR genes result in the characteristic finding of microsatellite instability, a consequence of failure to repair mismatched nucleotides during DNA replication and subsequent misalignment of DNA strands [76]. Such mutations have been identified as a cause of sporadic high-grade gliomas in young individuals [78].

### Diagnostic criteria and management

Turcot's syndrome is typically diagnosed clinically in the patient who has a primary CNS tumor and evidence of colorectal polyposis. Genetic confirmation studies are available to differentiate mutations in MMR genes (Turcot's syndrome type 1) from *APC* mutations (Turcot's syndrome type 2), a distinction that is most relevant in affected patients who have attenuated forms of FAP and fewer adenomatous polyps.

Although Turcot's syndrome represents a rare disorder, patients who have FAP or HNPCC and develop neurologic symptoms must be thoroughly investigated. Treatment of brain tumors in this population is similar to that for sporadic tumors; however, treatment with DNA-damaging agents such as ionizing radiation should be used with caution due to the increased risk of secondary malignancies.

## Gorlin's syndrome

### Clinical features

Gorlin's syndrome, also called nevoid basal cell carcinoma syndrome, is an autosomal dominant disorder with an estimated prevalence of 1 in 57,000 to 1 in 164,000 [79,80]. The frequency of new mutations in the absence of a family history is about 50%. The syndrome includes multiple basal cell carcinomas, jaw cysts, partial absence of the stratum corneum on the hands and feet (palmar/plantar pits), dural calcifications, rib abnormalities, and brain tumors. The lifetime risk for developing medulloblastomas in Gorlin's syndrome is about 3% to 5%, and Gorlin's syndrome is identified in 1% to 2% of patients who have medulloblastomas [81]. In addition, these tumors tend to occur at an earlier age than their sporadic counterparts, and medulloblastomas may often represent the initial tumor manifestation of Gorlin's syndrome [81]. Dural calcifications and meningiomas are found in up to 70% and 5%, respectively, of patients who have Gorlin's syndrome [82].

### Molecular genetics and pathogenesis

Gorlin's syndrome is linked to germline mutation of the human homolog of the *Drosophila melanogaster Patched* gene (*PTCH*) on chromosome 9q [83]. The protein product of *PTCH* is a transmembrane receptor for the secreted ligand sonic hedgehog (SHH), which is essential for cerebellar development. In the absence of SHH, PTCH exists as an inactive form in association with the transmembrane receptor smoothened (SMO). Binding of SHH to PTCH releases the inhibition of SMO and allows it to transduce freely within the SHH signaling pathway. The majority of *PTCH* mutations result in a truncated protein product with resultant unregulated activation of this pathway [84].

### Diagnostic criteria and management

Most patients who have Gorlin's syndrome are diagnosed on the basis of compatible clinical findings. Exon scanning of the *PTCH* gene of 106 unrelated pedigrees submitted to a DNA diagnostics laboratory identified mutations in 47 kindreds (44%). Pedigrees with only a single feature of Gorlin's syndrome, including patients who have multiple basal cell carcinomas, did not have mutations in *PTCH*. Management of patients who have Gorlin's syndrome–associated medulloblastomas is similar to that for sporadic tumors; however, careful consideration should be given to radiation planning due to the predisposition for radiation-induced tumors. Future treatment of sporadic medulloblastomas and those associated with Gorlin's syndrome may include the use of small molecule inhibitors of the SHH pathway. Although the use of these molecules has not yet been reported in clinical trials, these inhibitors have appeared extremely effective in preclinical murine models [85].

## References

[1] Knudson AG Jr. Mutation and cancer: statistical study of retinoblastoma. Proc Natl Acad Sci U S A 1971;68(4):820–3.

[2] Friedman JM. Epidemiology of neurofibromatosis type 1. Am J Med Genet 1999;89(1):1–6.

[3] Lammert M, Friedman JM, Kluwe L, et al. Prevalence of neurofibromatosis 1 in German children at elementary school enrollment. Arch Dermatol 2005;141(1):71–4.

[4] DeBella K, Szudek J, Friedman JM. Use of the National Institutes of Health criteria for diagnosis of neurofibromatosis 1 in children. Pediatrics 2000;105(3 Pt 1):608–14.

[5] Listernick R, Ferner RE, Liu GT, et al. Optic pathway gliomas in neurofibromatosis-1: controversies and recommendations. Ann Neurol 2007;61(3):189–98.

[6] Gutmann DH, Rasmussen SA, Wolkenstein P, et al. Gliomas presenting after age 10 in individuals with neurofibromatosis type 1 (NF1). Neurology 2002;59(5):759–61.

[7] Guillamo JS, Creange A, Kalifa C, et al. Prognostic factors of CNS tumours in Neurofibromatosis 1 (NF1): a retrospective study of 104 patients. Brain 2003;126(Pt 1):152–60.

[8] Serra E, Puig S, Otero D, et al. Confirmation of a double-hit model for the NF1 gene in benign neurofibromas. Am J Hum Genet 1997;61(3):512–9.

[9] Gutmann DH, Donahoe J, Brown T, et al. Loss of neurofibromatosis 1 (NF1) gene expression in NF1-associated pilocytic astrocytomas. Neuropathol Appl Neurobiol 2000;26(4):361–7.

[10] Zhu Y, Ghosh P, Charnay P, et al. Neurofibromas in NF1: Schwann cell origin and role of tumor environment. Science 2002;296(5569):920–2.

[11] Serra E, Rosenbaum T, Winner U, et al. Schwann cells harbor the somatic NF1 mutation in neurofibromas: evidence of two different Schwann cell subpopulations. Hum Mol Genet 2000;9(20):3055–64.

[12] Johannessen CM, Reczek EE, James MF, et al. The NF1 tumor suppressor critically regulates TSC2 and mTOR. Proc Natl Acad Sci U S A 2005;102(24):8573–8.

[13] Dasgupta B, Yi Y, Chen DY, et al. Proteomic analysis reveals hyperactivation of the mammalian target of rapamycin pathway in neurofibromatosis 1-associated human and mouse brain tumors. Cancer Res 2005;65(7):2755–60.

[14] NIH Consensus Conference. Neurofibromatosis. Conference statement. National Institutes of Health Consensus Development Conference. Arch Neurol 1988;45(5):575–8.

[15] Messiaen LM, Callens T, Mortier G, et al. Exhaustive mutation analysis of the NF1 gene allows identification of 95% of mutations and reveals a high frequency of unusual splicing defects. Hum Mutat 2000;15(6):541–55.

[16] Ullrich NJ, Robertson R, Kinnamon DD, et al. Moyamoya following cranial irradiation for primary brain tumors in children. Neurology 2007;68(12):932–8.

[17] Sharif S, Ferner R, Birch JM, et al. Second primary tumors in neurofibromatosis 1 patients treated for optic glioma: substantial risks after radiotherapy. J Clin Oncol 2006;24(16): 2570–5.

[18] Evans DG, Moran A, King A, et al. Incidence of vestibular schwannoma and neurofibromatosis 2 in the North West of England over a 10-year period: higher incidence than previously thought. Otol Neurotol 2005;26(1):93–7.

[19] Rouleau GA, Wertelecki W, Haines JL, et al. Genetic linkage of bilateral acoustic neurofi-
     bromatosis to a DNA marker on chromosome 22. Nature 1987;329(6136):246–8.
[20] Wertelecki W, Rouleau GA, Superneau DW, et al. Neurofibromatosis 2: clinical and DNA
     linkage studies of a large kindred. N Engl J Med 1988;319(5):278–83.
[21] Trofatter JA, MacCollin MM, Rutter JL, et al. A novel moesin-, ezrin-, radixin-like gene is
     a candidate for the neurofibromatosis 2 tumor suppressor. Cell 1993;72(5):791–800.
[22] Rouleau GA, Merel P, Lutchman M, et al. Alteration in a new gene encoding a putative
     membrane-organizing protein causes neuro-fibromatosis type 2. Nature 1993;363(6429):
     515–21.
[23] McClatchey AI, Giovannini M. Membrane organization and tumorigenesis–the NF2 tumor
     suppressor, Merlin. Genes Dev 2005;19(19):2265–77.
[24] Jacoby LB, MacCollin M, Barone R, et al. Frequency and distribution of NF2 mutations in
     schwannomas. Genes Chromosomes Cancer 1996;17(1):45–55.
[25] Mulvihill JJ, Parry DM, Sherman JL, et al. NIH conference. Neurofibromatosis 1 (Reckling-
     hausen disease) and neurofibromatosis 2 (bilateral acoustic neurofibromatosis). An update.
     Ann Intern Med 1990;113(1):39–52.
[26] Liu R, Fagan P. Facial nerve schwannoma: surgical excision versus conservative manage-
     ment. Ann Otol Rhinol Laryngol 2001;110(11):1025–9.
[27] Mautner VF, Tatagiba M, Lindenau M, et al. Spinal tumors in patients with neurofibroma-
     tosis type 2: MR imaging study of frequency, multiplicity, and variety. AJR Am J Roent-
     genol 1995;165(4):951–5.
[28] Patronas NJ, Courcoutsakis N, Bromley CM, et al. Intramedullary and spinal canal tumors
     in patients with neurofibromatosis 2: MR imaging findings and correlation with genotype.
     Radiology 2001;218(2):434–42.
[29] Fuss M, Debus J, Lohr F, et al. Conventionally fractionated stereotactic radiotherapy
     (FSRT) for acoustic neuromas. Int J Radiat Oncol Biol Phys 2000;48(5):1381–7.
[30] Combs SE, Volk S, Schulz-Ertner D, et al. Management of acoustic neuromas with fraction-
     ated stereotactic radiotherapy (FSRT): long-term results in 106 patients treated in a single
     institution. Int J Radiat Oncol Biol Phys 2005;63(1):75–81.
[31] Slattery WH III, Brackmann DE. Results of surgery following stereotactic irradiation for
     acoustic neuromas. Am J Otol 1995;16(3):315–9.
[32] Baser ME, Evans DG, Jackler RK, et al. Neurofibromatosis 2, radiosurgery and malignant
     nervous system tumours. Br J Cancer 2000;82(4):998.
[33] Thomsen J, Mirz F, Wetke R, et al. Intracranial sarcoma in a patient with neurofibromatosis
     type 2 treated with gamma knife radiosurgery for vestibular schwannoma. Am J Otol 2000;
     21(3):364–70.
[34] Osborne JP, Fryer A, Webb D. Epidemiology of tuberous sclerosis. Ann N Y Acad Sci 1991;
     615:125–7.
[35] Goh S, Kwiatkowski DJ, Dorer DJ, et al. Infantile spasms and intellectual outcomes in
     children with tuberous sclerosis complex. Neurology 2005;65(2):235–8.
[36] Jozwiak S, Goodman M, Lamm SH. Poor mental development in patients with tuberous
     sclerosis complex: clinical risk factors. Arch Neurol 1998;55(3):379–84.
[37] Hunt A. Tuberous sclerosis: a survey of 97 cases. III: family aspects. Dev Med Child Neurol
     1983;25(3):353–7.
[38] Jozwiak S, Schwartz RA, Janniger CK, et al. Skin lesions in children with tuberous sclerosis
     complex: their prevalence, natural course, and diagnostic significance. Int J Dermatol 1998;
     37(12):911–7.
[39] Jozwiak S, Kawalec W, Dluzewska J, et al. Cardiac tumours in tuberous sclerosis: their
     incidence and course. Eur J Pediatr 1994;153(3):155–7.
[40] Castro M, Shepherd CW, Gomez MR, et al. Pulmonary tuberous sclerosis. Chest 1995;
     107(1):189–95.
[41] Webb DW, Kabala J, Osborne JP. A population study of renal disease in patients with
     tuberous sclerosis. Br J Urol 1994;74(2):151–4.

[42] Mizuguchi M, Takashima S. Neuropathology of tuberous sclerosis. Brain Dev 2001;23(7): 508–15.

[43] Goh S, Butler W, Thiele EA. Subependymal giant cell tumors in tuberous sclerosis complex. Neurology 2004;63(8):1457–61.

[44] Dabora SL, Jozwiak S, Franz DN, et al. Mutational analysis in a cohort of 224 tuberous sclerosis patients indicates increased severity of TSC2, compared with TSC1, disease in multiple organs. Am J Hum Genet 2001;68(1):64–80.

[45] Tee AR, Fingar DC, Manning BD, et al. Tuberous sclerosis complex-1 and -2 gene products function together to inhibit mammalian target of rapamycin (mTOR)-mediated downstream signaling. Proc Natl Acad Sci U S A 2002;99(21):13571–6.

[46] Chan JA, Zhang H, Roberts PS, et al. Pathogenesis of tuberous sclerosis subependymal giant cell astrocytomas: biallelic inactivation of TSC1 or TSC2 leads to mTOR activation. J Neuropathol Exp Neurol 2004;63(12):1236–42.

[47] Jansen FE, Notenboom RGE, Nellist M, et al. Differential localization of hamartin and tuberin and increased S6 phosphorylation in a tuber. Neurology 2004;63(7):1293–5.

[48] Roach ES, Gomez MR, Northrup H. Tuberous sclerosis complex consensus conference: revised clinical diagnostic criteria. J Child Neurol 1998;13(12):624–8.

[49] Kossoff EH, Thiele EA, Pfeifer HH, et al. Tuberous sclerosis complex and the ketogenic diet. Epilepsia 2005;46(10):1684–6.

[50] Weiner HL, Ferraris N, LaJoie J, et al. Epilepsy surgery for children with tuberous sclerosis complex. J Child Neurol 2004;19(9):687–9.

[51] Hyman MH, Whittemore VH. National Institutes of Health consensus conference: tuberous sclerosis complex. Arch Neurol 2000;57(5):662–5.

[52] Franz DN, Leonard J, Tudor C, et al. Rapamycin causes regression of astrocytomas in tuberous sclerosis complex. Ann Neurol 2006;59(3):490–8.

[53] Maher ER, Iselius L, Yates JR, et al. Von Hippel-Lindau disease: a genetic study. J Med Genet 1991;28(7):443–7.

[54] Neumann HP, Eggert HR, Weigel K, et al. Hemangioblastomas of the central nervous system. A 10-year study with special reference to von Hippel-Lindau syndrome. J Neurosurg 1989;70(1):24–30.

[55] Conway JE, Chou D, Clatterbuck RE, et al. Hemangioblastomas of the central nervous system in von Hippel-Lindau syndrome and sporadic disease. Neurosurgery 2001;48(1). 55–62.

[56] Slater A, Moore NR, Huson SM. The natural history of cerebellar hemangioblastomas in von Hippel-Lindau disease. AJNR Am J Neuroradiol 2003;24(8):1570–4.

[57] Lonser RR, Kim HJ, Butman JA, et al. Tumors of the endolymphatic sac in von Hippel-Lindau disease. N Engl J Med 2004;350(24):2481–6.

[58] Latif F, Tory K, Gnarra J, et al. Identification of the von Hippel-Lindau disease tumor suppressor gene. Science 1993;260(5112):1317–20.

[59] Kim WY, Kaelin WG. Role of VHL gene mutation in human cancer. J Clin Oncol 2004; 22(24):4991–5004.

[60] Maher ER, Webster AR, Richards FM, et al. Phenotypic expression in von Hippel-Lindau disease: correlations with germline VHL gene mutations. J Med Genet 1996; 33(4):328–32.

[61] Stolle C, Glenn G, Zbar B, et al. Improved detection of germline mutations in the von Hippel-Lindau disease tumor suppressor gene. Hum Mutat 1998;12(6):417–23.

[62] Motzer RJ, Hutson TE, Tomczak P, et al. Sunitinib versus interferon alfa in metastatic renal-cell carcinoma. N Engl J Med 2007;356(2):115–24.

[63] Madhusudan S, Deplanque G, Braybrooke JP, et al. Antiangiogenic therapy for von Hippel-Lindau disease. JAMA 2004;291(8):943–4.

[64] Nelen MR, Kremer H, Konings IB, et al. Novel PTEN mutations in patients with Cowden disease: absence of clear genotype-phenotype correlations. Eur J Hum Genet 1999;7(3): 267–73.

[65] Abel TW, Baker SJ, Fraser MM, et al. Lhermitte-Duclos disease: a report of 31 cases with immunohistochemical analysis of the PTEN/AKT/mTOR pathway. J Neuropathol Exp Neurol 2005;64(4):341–9.

[66] Kulkantrakorn K, Awwad EE, Levy B, et al. MRI in Lhermitte-Duclos disease. Neurology 1997;48(3):725–31.

[67] Zhou XP, Marsh DJ, Morrison CD, et al. Germline inactivation of PTEN and dysregulation of the phosphoinositol-3-kinase/Akt pathway cause human Lhermitte-Duclos disease in adults. Am J Hum Genet 2003;73(5):1191–8.

[68] Eng C. Will the real Cowden syndrome please stand up: revised diagnostic criteria. J Med Genet 2000;37(11):828–30.

[69] Olivier M, Goldgar DE, Sodha N, et al. Li-Fraumeni and related syndromes: correlation between tumor type, family structure, and TP53 genotype. Cancer Res 2003;63(20):6643–50.

[70] Varley JM, McGown G, Thorncroft M, et al. Germ-line mutations of TP53 in Li-Fraumeni families: an extended study of 39 families. Cancer Res 1997;57(15):3245–52.

[71] Bell DW, Varley JM, Szydlo TE, et al. Heterozygous germ line hCHK2 mutations in Li-Fraumeni syndrome. Science 1999;286(5449):2528–31.

[72] Vahteristo P, Tamminen A, Karvinen P, et al. p53, CHK2, and CHK1 genes in Finnish families with Li-Fraumeni syndrome: further evidence of CHK2 in inherited cancer predisposition. Cancer Res 2001;61(15):5718–22.

[73] Sodha N, Houlston RS, Bullock S, et al. Increasing evidence that germline mutations in CHEK2 do not cause Li-Fraumeni syndrome. Hum Mutat 2002;20(6):460–2.

[74] Varley JM. Germline TP53 mutations and Li-Fraumeni syndrome. Hum Mutat 2003;21(3): 313–20.

[75] Evans DGR, Birch JM, Ramsden RT, et al. Malignant transformation and new primary tumours after therapeutic radiation for benign disease: substantial risks in certain tumour prone syndromes. J Med Genet 2006;43(4):289–94.

[76] Hamilton SR, Liu B, Parsons RE, et al. The molecular basis of Turcot's syndrome. N Engl J Med 1995;332(13):839–47.

[77] Attard TM, Giglio P, Koppula S, et al. Brain tumors in individuals with familial adenomatous polyposis: a cancer registry experience and pooled case report analysis. Cancer 2007; 109(4):761–6.

[78] Leung SY, Chan TL, Chung LP, et al. Microsatellite instability and mutation of DNA mismatch repair genes in gliomas. Am J Pathol 1998;153(4):1181–8.

[79] Farndon PA, Del Mastro RG, Evans DG, et al. Location of gene for Gorlin syndrome. Lancet 1992;339(8793):581–2.

[80] Shanley S, Ratcliffe J, Hockey A, et al. Nevoid basal cell carcinoma syndrome: review of 118 affected individuals. Am J Med Genet 1994;50(3):282–90.

[81] Evans DG, Farndon PA, Burnell LD, et al. The incidence of Gorlin syndrome in 173 consecutive cases of medulloblastoma. Br J Cancer 1991;64(5):959–61.

[82] Kimonis VE, Goldstein AM, Pastakia B, et al. Clinical manifestations in 105 persons with nevoid basal cell carcinoma syndrome. Am J Med Genet 1997;69(3):299–308.

[83] Hahn H, Wicking C, Zaphiropoulous PG, et al. Mutations of the human homolog of Drosophila patched in the nevoid basal cell carcinoma syndrome. Cell 1996;85(6):841–51.

[84] Wicking C, Shanley S, Smyth I, et al. Most germ-line mutations in the nevoid basal cell carcinoma syndrome lead to a premature termination of the PATCHED protein, and no genotype-phenotype correlations are evident. Am J Hum Genet 1997;60(1):21–6.

[85] Romer JT, Kimura H, Magdaleno S, et al. Suppression of the Shh pathway using a small molecule inhibitor eliminates medulloblastoma in Ptc1(+/-)p53(-/-) mice. Cancer Cell 2004;6(3):229–40.

NEUROLOGIC
CLINICS

Neurol Clin 25 (2007) 947–973

# Advanced MRI of Adult Brain Tumors

Geoffrey S. Young, MD[a,b,*]

[a]*Department of Radiology, Brigham and Women's Hospital,
75 Francis Street, Boston, MA 02115, USA*
[b]*Harvard Medical School, Boston, MA 02115, USA*

Over the last decade, advanced magnetic resonance (MR) techniques that produce image contrast reflecting attributes of tissue physiology and microstructure have begun to be widely applied in clinical brain tumor imaging at major academic centers. These techniques are all adapted from, and must be interpreted in the context of, conventional MRI techniques based on the fundamental physical properties of tissue protons—proton density, T1, T2, T2*, and delayed permeability—that produce image contrasts reflecting gross anatomy on a scale of 500 μm or greater.

This article introduces the preliminary clinical experience that guides the neurooncologic application of the most established of these techniques. Because the article is directed primarily at clinical neurologists and neurooncologists rather than neuroradiologists, the physical or physiologic principles underlying these techniques are not discussed in any detail, but the references for each section should provide an entry point to the more technical literature for the interested reader. Also, although the rapidly expanding literature describes dozens of advanced techniques currently under investigation, this discussion is limited to the most widely available, practical, and robust techniques: diffusion-weighted imaging (DWI), perfusion-weighted imaging MRI (PMR), dynamic contrast-enhanced T1 permeability imaging (T1P), diffusion-tensor imaging (DTI), and MR spectroscopy (MRS). It may help to note that PMR is also variously known as "perfusion-weighted imaging," "MR perfusion," "perfusion MR," and "dynamic susceptibility contrast imaging." T1P is also known as "dynamic contrast-enhanced imaging," among other terms. MRS is also known as "chemical shift imaging." The techniques themselves, the available hardware and software, and the clinical literature and practice are evolving so rapidly that this

---

* Department of Radiology, Brigham and Women's Hospital, 75 Francis St., Boston, MA 02115.
*E-mail address:* gsyoung@partners.org

0733-8619/07/$ - see front matter © 2007 Elsevier Inc. All rights reserved.
doi:10.1016/j.ncl.2007.07.010 *neurologic.theclinics.com*

introduction will inevitably be out of date in important aspects even as this article goes to press.

Although qualitative interpretation of basic brain tumor MRI (including T2-weighted images and gadolinium [Gd]-enhanced T1-weighted images), remains the backbone of brain tumor imaging, in a significant number of cases, these techniques fail to allow confident and correct differential diagnosis, grading, and monitoring of brain tumor [1]. Thus, the immediate goals of tumor imaging include (1) initial differential diagnosis, to aid in the distinction of newly diagnosed brain tumors from non-neoplastic conditions such as tumefactive demyelination and ischemia and to aid in the differentiation of glioma from extra-axial neoplasm and metastasis; (2) preoperative therapeutic planning, to provide an estimate of tumor grade and to guide biopsy, resection, and local ablative therapy; and (3) therapeutic follow-up, to monitor disease progression and therapeutic response, including the differentiation of recurrent tumor from delayed radiation necrosis. These goals are related to but distinct from the scientific goals of advanced imaging that include a better understanding of the pathophysiology of brain tumor and improved prediction of therapeutic response.

## Brain tumor cellularity: diffusion-weighted imaging

DWI contrast reflects the brownian motion of tissue water. Because the mean path length of water diffusion within each tissue voxel, characterized by the "apparent diffusion coefficient" (ADC), is determined by tissue barriers to diffusion on a scale of roughly 10 μm, the ADC in brain tissue is principally determined by tissue cellularity, as measured by the intracellular volume fraction and extracellular volume fractions [2,3].

### Diffusion-weighted imaging differential diagnosis

DWI has a sensitivity and specificity of over 90% for distinguishing epidermoid (low ADC) from arachnoid cyst (high ADC) and distinguishing abscess (low ADC) from necrotic tumor (high ADC). The viscous keratin and cholesterol in epidermoid and the viscous and cellular pus in abscess produce a very low ADC that distinguishes these lesions from increased diffusivity in necrotic tumor and from normal or slightly low diffusivity in demyelinating plaque [4–7].

A low ADC in an intra-axial neoplasm should raise suspicion of lymphoma or metastasis, depending on the conventional MRI appearance, because the higher cellularity of these tumors generally produces an ADC that is significantly lower than that of glioma [8,9]. In an extra-axial lesion, meningioma and dural metastasis should be considered; however, although most gliomas have a much higher ADC (related to their lower cellularity), a number of case reports and several larger series have demonstrated a low ADC in a small number of glioblastomas (GBM). The resulting significant overlap among ADC values in the three tumor types reinforces the need to integrate DWI with other advanced and conventional neuroimaging data for accurate clinical interpretation (Fig. 1) [8,10–12].

*Diffusion-weighted imaging in preoperative grading and surgical planning*

An inverse correlation between minimum ADC (ADC$_{min}$) and tumor cellularity has been verified by histology in a wide variety of tumors, including high- and low-grade glioma, lymphoma, medulloblastoma, meningioma, and metastases [8,13–17]. Within meningioma, a lower ADC has been demonstrated in atypical and malignant versus typical subtypes, but it is unfortunate that the overlap of the two groups precludes the use of the ADC for differentiation in individual patients [16]. In glioma, however, a number of groups have found that ADC$_{min}$ values below a cutoff in the range of 1.7 to 2.5 can be used to distinguish high-grade glioma from low-grade glioma [18,19]. Again, overlap between tumor grades mandates that ADC$_{min}$ information be combined with other advanced and conventional MRI data to reliably distinguish high-grade from low-grade glioma [9,18,20,21].

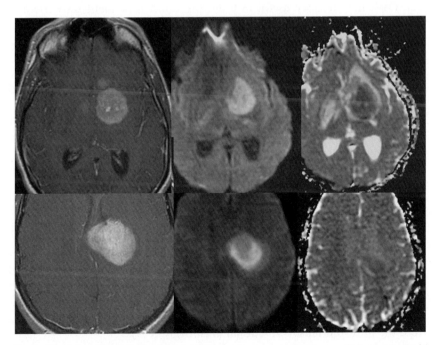

Fig. 1. T1 with contrast (*left*), DWI (*middle*), and apparent diffusion coefficient map (*right*) demonstrate markedly reduced diffusivity within a homogeneously enhancing periventricular lesion that extends across the corpus callosum (*top row*). Although this is strongly suggestive of primary central nervous system lymphoma, highly cellular GBM do occur (*bottom row*), so correlation with perfusion imaging is strongly indicated to assist in differential diagnosis.

Furthermore, $ADC_{min}$ and tumor cellularity prove to be variable among tumors of a given grade, especially in high-grade glioma [22]. Although the presence of necrosis, hemorrhage, and calcification may contribute to the spread of the tumor ADC observed in each tumor grade, it seems likely that in large part, the heterogeneity of $ADC_{min}$ within tumor grade reflects heterogeneity of cellularity among tumors of the same grade. This heterogeneity of cellularity within tumors of the same grade limits the utility of DWI as a surrogate for histopathology but raises the possibility that $ADC_{min}$ could help to substratify tumors within grade, as suggested by a recent report stating that ADC estimates of cellularity accurately predict radiation responsiveness in glioma and metastasis [23].

*Diffusion-weighted imaging monitoring of therapeutic response*

On immediate postoperative MRI, ischemia at the margin of surgical resection or elsewhere [24] and pyogenic infection can produce a focally reduced ADC that is important to detect and can generally be distinguished from tumor based on the signal intensity on DWI, the morphology of the area, correlation with other pulse sequences, and correlation with history [25]. DWI may be very useful in following tumor treatment response and subsequent recurrence in individual patients because cytotoxic radiation and chemotherapy reduce tumor cellularity and thus increase the ADC within a given area of tumor [14,15,26–28]. The relative insensitivity of a glioma ADC to steroid therapy contrasts with a pronounced effect of steroids on enhancement, edema, and permeability and a debatable effect on blood volumes [29], suggesting that despite technical issues related to serial longitudinal registration of echoplanar data, DWI will remain valuable for tumor follow-up. A novel way of presenting longitudinal DWI follow-up data, called "functional diffusion mapping," has recently received considerable attention, but it remains to be seen whether this method adds value compared with more straightforward methods of data presentation (Fig. 2) [30,31].

## Tissue microstructural derangement: diffusion-tensor imaging

DTI is similar to DWI but involves the collection of additional data necessary to define the tensor (vector) describing the preferential direction and magnitude of water diffusion [32,33]. The degree to which water diffusion in tissue is facilitated in one direction and hindered in another—referred to as "diffusion anisotropy"—is often characterized by a scalar value derived from the diffusion tensor: fractional anisotropy (FA).

*Diffusion-tensor imaging in preoperative guidance*

Because the myelin sheaths of white matter are one of the principal barriers to extracellular water diffusion in the brain, DTI allows a very sensitive

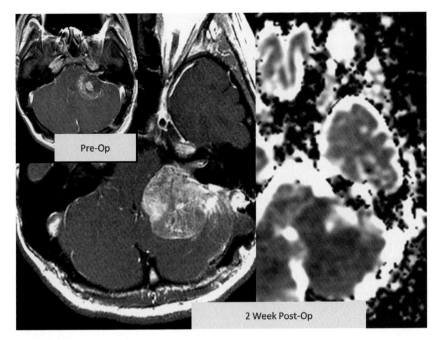

Fig. 2. Gd-enhanced T1-weighted images (*above left*) before and 2 weeks after surgical resection demonstrate surprisingly rapid increase in size of the enhancing mass. The very low diffusivity seen in the mass on the ADC map (*far right*) confirmed high cellularity of the lesion, consistent with rapid recurrence of medulloblastoma.

depiction of the orientation and integrity of white matter tracts. Various algorithms have been developed to trace white matter tracts by connecting the principal direction or directions of preferred diffusivity in each voxel to those of adjoining voxels. Especially when integrated with functional MRI, these tractography techniques have been used successfully to identify the location of eloquent white matter tracts displaced by tumor and to predict the degree of postoperative functional impairment based on intraoperative injury to these tracts [34–38].

*Diffusion-tensor imaging in differential diagnosis*

Although glioma cells infiltrate widely throughout the brain, anatomic MRI or positron emission tomography is not able to accurately characterize the extent of tumor infiltration beyond the area of abnormal T2 and cannot distinguish abnormal T2 related to infiltrative tumor from vasogenic edema. Because glioma infiltration disrupts the organization of the white matter tracts, FA and other anisotropy measures derived from DTI promise to allow definition of the degree of this tumor infiltration.

Some but not all recent studies have suggested that DTI can aid in the distinction of vasogenic edema surrounding metastases and meningioma from nonenhancing tumor infiltration in glioma. The mixed success of the published reports suggests that the angular resolution, b-value, and signal-to-noise ratio achieved by a given DTI protocol will be critical determinants of the concentration of tumor that can be detected within white matter [39,40].

*Diffusion-tensor imaging in glioma grading*

Initial experience with DTI tractography revealed a continuous increase in organization of the white matter in proportion to the distance from the enhancing glioma core [34], but efforts to use DTI to define the margins of glioma white matter invasion have yielded mixed results [22,41–45]. Because white matter adjacent to glioma generally contains different proportions of vasogenic edema and tumor infiltration at different distances from the center of the tumor, it is difficult to define an unbiased region of interest for valid grouped data analysis. This difficulty is compounded by the challenge of obtaining a pathologic "gold standard," because extensive biopsy of grossly intact white matter around tumors is ethically unacceptable.

*Diffusion-tensor imaging in tumor follow-up*

Preliminary reports using FA in combination with ADC for differentiation of tumor recurrence from radiation necrosis have also been published, but the contribution of anisotropy measures remains to be fully defined [46]. Based on promising initial results in differentiating infiltrative tumor from vasogenic edema and in characterizing the extent of glioma white matter infiltration by FA, early reports of the development of a "fiber coherence index" and a number of other measures promise to allow more sensitive assessment of white matter microstructural disorganization than FA, by employing more sophisticated analyses of the directional information available from high-diffusion direction DTI (Fig. 3) [39,42,47–49].

## Metabolite imaging in brain tumor: spectroscopy

MRS techniques essentially allow nuclear MR (NMR) spectroscopy to be performed in vivo, albeit at much lower field strength and sensitivity than in synthetic chemistry laboratory NMR scanners. As in NMR, proton MRS assays the number of each chemically distinct proton ($^1H_0$) species present in each voxel by detecting slight differences in the NMR frequency ("chemical shift") of each proton nucleus that result from shielding by the surrounding covalent bond electron cloud. The differences in proton resonance frequency are displayed on the x-axis of each spectrum (graph) in units of parts per million of the resonance frequency of a standard reference compound, rather than in hertz, to produce spectra that are

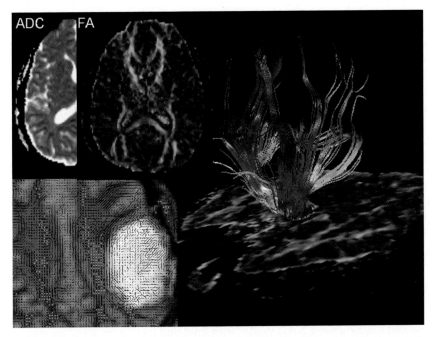

Fig. 3. FA color map and ADC maps (*upper left, as labeled*) from one subject demonstrate the dramatically increased sensitivity to the structure of myelinated white matter tracks obtained with DTI. Principal eigenvectors from diffusion-tensor tractography overlayed on anatomic MRI (*lower left*) from a different subject demonstrates displacement of white matter tracts by glioma Tractogram from a third subject (*right*) illustrates the standard technique for displaying DTI data for surgical planning. (FA and tractogram images courtesy of Kelvin Wong, PhD, using Philips Pride Software at Jockey Club MRI Center, University of Hong Kong.)

comparable across field strengths. Because clinical MRS is not directly quantifiable, the y-axis of the graph represents arbitrary units of signal intensity scaled relative to the highest peak [50,51]. Simultaneous interrogation of two-dimensional (2D) or three-dimensional (3D) arrays of small voxels is referred to as 2D or 3D MR spectroscopic imaging (2D-MRSI or 3D-MRSI, respectively). 2D- or 3D-MRSI data can be used to produce impressive color "metabolite maps" that depict the spatial distribution of the different peak heights, areas, or peak ratios that can be derived from these spectra but are of limited use for clinical diagnosis because the primary data can only be assessed from the spectral graphs.

Although numerous peaks are observed, the principal peaks seen in brain tumor MRS at 1.5 T include branch chain amino acids (0.9–1.0 ppm), lipid (0.9–1.5 ppm), lactate (1.3 ppm), alanine (1.5 ppm), *n*-acetyl aspartate (NAA; 2.0 ppm), choline (3.2 ppm), creatine (3.0 ppm and 3.9 ppm), and myoinositol (3.6 ppm). Note that creatine produces two resonant peaks because it contains two chemically nonequivalent species of protons, and that the lipid and amino acid peaks are broad because each contains a large number of different molecules with numerous nonequivalent protons. For this reason, amino acids, lactate, and lipid peaks overlap. When distinction between these is critical, a combination of short and intermediate or intermediate and long echo time spectra can be used to distinguish these species based on phase cycling of their peaks with respect to NAA, creatine, and choline. NAA is a marker of neuronal number and function, creatine a marker of energy metabolism and stores, and choline a marker of membrane synthesis and degradation ("membrane turnover"). All processes that injure neurons decrease NAA; all processes that injure glia or stimulate glial division increase choline; all processes that disrupt aerobic glycolysis result in lactate formation; and all processes that produce necrosis release lipid and decrease creatine [52–54]. Because the normal concentrations of these metabolites vary by anatomic location and because the relative signal detected from a given concentration of each metabolite varies with echo time chosen for a spectroscopy sequence, reference to spectra of normal-appearing voxels is critical for clinical interpretation of MRS [55–59].

*Magnetic resonance spectroscopy in differential diagnosis*

Although the typical pattern of glioma spectra is well defined—high choline and low or absent NAA peaks, with lipid and lactate peaks often seen in GBM—studies of MRS for prediction of tumor histology have not shown sufficient specificity to make this a clinically useful adjunct in most cases. MRS of extra-axial tumors that do not arise from glial precursors, such as meningioma, generally reveal very high choline and no NAA because the tumors contain no neurons. Although the presence of a very high alanine peak in a subset of meningioma can be useful to suggest the diagnosis, a recent well-controlled study suggests that the presence of low levels of alanine detected in up to 80% of meningioma is not useful because it is detected in similar frequency in metastases and schwannoma [60]. This pattern may aid in the differentiation of large meningioma from peripheral-enhancing intra-axial neoplasms, particularly when MRS is used in combination with perfusion imaging (as described later), but has proved unreliable in the differentiation of metastases from GBM because both may show high choline, absent or very low NAA, and high lactate and lipid peaks.

Extensive investigation has failed to demonstrate that MRS adds value in differential diagnosis of tumor types or of tumor from non-neoplastic processes such as demyelination, ischemia, and gliosis [61–64]. The lack of specificity of the principal MRS markers explains this limitation. A large choline peak suggesting increased membrane turnover may be seen in neoplasia with rapid membrane formation and seen in demyelination or ischemia with rapid membrane breakdown. All three processes may injure neuronal function or integrity, reducing the NAA peak; ischemia and neoplasia may result in anaerobic metabolism and necrosis, producing lactate and lipid peaks. One notable exception to this rule is the distinction of abscess from rim-enhancing tumor by demonstrating amino acids within the contents of the cyst, a finding that is essentially diagnostic of the presence of activated polymorphonuclear leukocytes, and thus of bacterial or, less likely, parasitic infection (Fig. 4) [5,65].

*Magnetic resonance spectroscopy in preoperative glioma grading and operative guidance*

Although MRS has not proved to be a reliable aid to tumor differential diagnosis, qualitative or quantitative detection of high choline/NAA peak height ratios has been shown in a number of studies to be predictive of the presence of high-grade tumor [19,66]. Similarly, the presence of lipid/lactate in untreated glioma suggests the presence of necrotic grade IV tumor [19,67]. Although there is considerable overlap between high-and low-grade tumor spectra, meticulously acquired spectra revealing choline/NAA ratios above 1.5 or analogous thresholds developed for choline/NAA ratios have been shown to improve the accuracy of anatomic MRI prediction of tumor grade [68–70]. Although more technically robust and cost-effective perfusion and permeability techniques have significantly reduced the use of MRS for

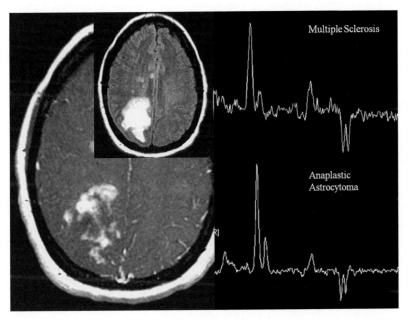

Fig. 4. Two spectra (echo time, 144 milliseconds) from patients who have heterogeneously enhancing white matter lesions. The indistinguishable spectra demonstrate elevated choline, low NAA, and moderate lactate. One spectrum represents tumefactive multiple sclerosis (MS); the other anaplastic astrocytoma. In anaplastic astrocytoma, choline elevation represents new membrane production, whereas in MS, it represents membrane injury. The patient whose images are shown in the top right spectrum turned out to have MS, but the comparison starkly illustrates the limitations of MR spectroscopy for differential diagnosis of new lesions.

tumor grade estimation, lesions suggestive of oligodendroglioma remain a notable exception because (as discussed later) high blood volume is seen even in low-grade oligodendroglioma, limiting the usefulness of perfusion for grading [71–74]. Also, some investigators have suggested that MRS may be especially useful compared with perfusion in patients in whom tumor recurrence is mixed with radiation necrosis, but this hypothesis is very difficult to prove because of the lack of appropriate gold standards [75].

The use of MRS to target biopsies to areas with high choline/NAA ratios has been reported to increase the accuracy of tumor biopsy by targeting areas of metabolically active tumor within areas of heterogeneous glioma, thus reducing the false-negative rate [76,77]. Similar methods have been used to guide stereotactic radiosurgery [78–80]. The true utility of MRS for these applications is difficult to assess with certainty because precise correlation of tissue pathology with anatomic location on MRI is difficult and the efficacy of surgical, radiosurgical, and focal ablative therapy is poor.

A recent report showed that glioma may decrease whole-brain NAA 30% more than can be explained by the visible tumor burden, suggesting that decreased whole-brain NAA may reflect the global burden of infiltrative tumor [81]. Because infiltration is a feature of glioma that cannot be detected reliably with current techniques, the significance of whole-brain NAA deserves further exploration as a marker of poor prognosis and diffuse tumor spread. Another recently reported MRS technique for detection of tumor infiltration that deserves further study is the use of $CH_2/CH_3$ ratios within the normal brain lipid pool to assay for tumor burden (Fig. 5) [82].

*Magnetic resonance spectroscopy in assessment of treatment response*

Because delayed radiation necrosis is also characterized by the presence of lactate/lipid peaks, the presence of these peaks alone is not useful in the distinction of radiation necrosis from tumor recurrence [83]. Complete absence of NAA and choline peaks or serial MRSI documenting progressive decrease in NAA and choline peaks combined with lactate/lipid peaks should suggest necrosis, particularly when corroborated by a rising ADC and low blood volume. Conversely, a significant increase in choline plus a decrease in NAA over time, with a consequent increase in the choline/NAA ratio or in derived statistics such as the choline/NAA ratio R value, is a sensitive indicator of tumor recurrence when seen in the appropriate anatomic imaging context [77,79,84–86]. Overall, serial MRSI under carefully controlled conditions has been shown to be a useful adjunct to conventional imaging for discrimination of high-grade focal brain tumor recurrence from delayed radiation necrosis in the hands of a few research groups, especially when combined with other imaging data. It is unfortunate that the spatial variation in choline, NAA, lactate, and lipid peaks within an individual tumor is often much greater than the change in these peaks over time. Thus, slight differences between scans in voxel placement or acquisition technique

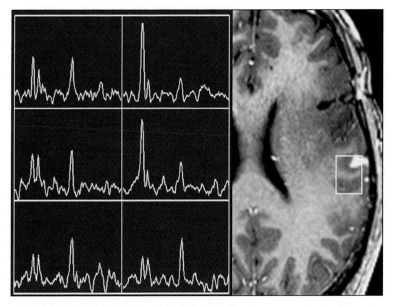

Fig. 5. 2D-MRSI demonstrates high choline/NAA ratio in two voxels within (*top row, middle column*) and immediately adjacent to (*middle row, middle column*) the area of abnormal enhancement, suggesting recurrent anaplastic astrocytoma. Other voxels demonstrate slightly increased choline/NAA ratio consistent with adjacent areas of lower-grade glioma. The rectangle overlayed on the right hand figure illustrates the anatomic location of the voxel from which the spectra were acquired.

can render the assessment of longitudinal change unreliable. Experience has shown that with currently available commercial MRI hardware and software, reliable clinical MRSI requires the direct supervision of each MRS data acquisition by a trained spectroscopist or supertechnologist under direct physician supervision. In the United States, where MRS and MRSI is not reimbursable at present, this requirement imposes a cost burden that has been impossible for most centers to meet and has prevented the establishment of serial MRSI brain tumor monitoring as a practical clinical tool at most centers.

*Magnetic resonance spectroscopy summary*

Selection of an appropriate area of interest and voxel size is critical to produce useful information while avoiding artifacts from partial volume averaging of calvarial marrow fat and susceptibility from bone or metal. Moreover, because the information provided by spectroscopy is generally not specific enough to be useful when only a single time point is available, serial comparison of change in spectra over time is critical for accurate interpretation. This need for serial comparison compounds the data acquisition problem because it requires a high degree of reproducibility in voxel selection over serial scans. As a result, the spectroscopy groups that have had the greatest success using MRS and MRSI in neurooncology have found it necessary to develop significant additional human resources for monitoring data acquisition and processing beyond what is generally available in the routine clinical MR setting. At the present time, MRSI is not reimbursable, so the number of institutions with the financial resources to develop effective spectroscopy laboratories remains small, even among the major academic centers.

## Microvascular imaging in brain tumor: perfusion-weighted imaging MRI and dynamic contrast-enhanced T1 permeability imaging

Much current basic biology research focuses on the interaction of tumor hypoxia, macrophage activation, and glioma gene expression in the transition from normal permeability and blood volume to increased native vessel permeability and volume and finally to frank neoangiogenesis during transformation from low-grade glioma to GBM [87]. In areas in which infiltrative and cellular glioma supplied by native vessels becomes hypoxic, secretion of vasoactive substances (including vascular endothelial growth factor [VEGF], interleukin 8 [IL-8], platelet-derived growth factor [PDGF], and epidermal growth factor receptor [EGFR]) by glioma and host immune cells induces the expression of aquaporins (especially AQP4) and suppresses the expression of endothelial tight junction proteins, resulting in varying degrees of impairment of the blood-brain barrier (BBB) [88]. In GBM, on the other hand, new formation of dense beds of characteristically tortuous and structurally abnormal "corkscrew" neocapillaries produces the extremely high local tissue blood volume. In these neocapillaries, deficiency or absence of basal lamina and pericytes and reduced endothelial expression of occludins and other cell surface proteins result in large endothelial gaps or fenestrations and leaky intercellular tight junctions that together produce the markedly increased capillary permeability [89,90]. These two central features of tumor neovasculature are the focus of the two types of microvascular imaging methods discussed later: dynamic susceptibility T2*-weighted "perfusion" (PMR) techniques used to estimate the volume of the neovascular capillary bed during the first pass of a contrast bolus, and dynamic enhancement T1-weighted "permeability" (T1P) techniques used to estimate impairment of the BBB by monitoring passage of the contrast into the extravascular space during the first pass and early recirculation phases.

### Microvascular hemodynamic imaging: perfusion-weighted imaging MRI

PMR of brain tumors relies on a high pressure injection of a large contrast dose to produce a dynamic decrease in signal intensity on susceptibility (T2*)-weighted images acquired serially throughout the whole brain every 1 to 2 seconds during the injection. The signal change in each voxel is used to compute the relative cerebral blood volume (rCBV) of that voxel, which can then be displayed as a color map or as a graph of the change in signal intensity in a given area over time (time-intensity curve [TIC]). Because clinically available techniques produce relative rather than quantitative blood volume maps, the blood volumes of normal-appearing white and gray matter are used as internal references for visual comparisons and for region-of-interest measurements [91,92]. This methodology works reasonably well, because normal gray matter CBV is approximately 2.7 times that of white matter, a value just above the diagnostic thresholds of 1.5 to 2.5 that have been reported to be most useful for distinguishing high-grade from low-grade glioma. In addition to inspecting the rCBV maps, a reliable interpretation requires inspection of the TIC to detect and account for magnetic susceptibility, motion, bolus timing, and other artifacts. The shape of the TIC provides a rough estimate of capillary permeability that can be very useful in differential diagnosis.

*Perfusion-weighted imaging MRI in preoperative differential diagnosis of intracranial masses*

The rough estimate of permeability derived from the shape of the TIC can provide important clues to the nature of the lesion. Microvessels within tumors of extra-axial and nonglial origin—meningioma, choroid plexus papilloma, metastases, lymphoma, and so forth—do not form a BBB, so a very large fraction of the bolus leaks into the extravascular space during the first pass [93–95]. Because glioma microvessels form a BBB that is impaired but not absent, the TIC returns significantly toward baseline in these tumors, although not as much as in normal brain. The difference between these patterns can contribute significantly to the discrimination of tumor types in cases of peripherally located enhancing tumors when the differential diagnosis includes meningioma and peripheral GBM, and in periventricular enhancing lesions when the differential diagnosis includes choroid plexus papillocarcinoma and GBM (Figs. 6 and 7).

In addition, PMR can aid in distinction of intracranial abscess from cystic glioma by demonstrating an rCBV lower than or equal to the surrounding white matter in abscess [6]. Although a number of reports document that metastases have a variable blood volume that is related to the vascularity of the primary tumor and a range that overlaps with GBM, it is unclear how applicable the data reported in these studies are to rCBV calculated with standard-spin echoplanar technique [96–98]. Thus, pending further study of rCBV in metastasis, PMR is not as useful as DWI and MRS for distinction of abscess from cystic metastasis. In a solitary intra-axial enhancing lesion, however, the combination of significant TIC return to baseline and high rCBV favors glioma. Conversely, low rCBV and very high first-pass contrast leak favors metastasis or lymphoma, especially when correlation with DWI demonstrates high cellularity [9,94]. Finally, if a circumscribed cortical or subcortical lesion has imaging features otherwise suggestive of a circumscribed low-grade glioma but has rCBV maps that demonstrate

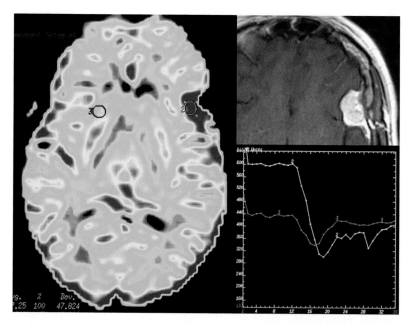

Fig. 6. PMR TIC (*lower right*) and rCBV map (*left*) demonstrate very high microvascular blood volume. The low return to baseline of the lesion TIC (*green curve*) compared with normal brain (*purple curve*) is characteristic of high first-pass leak in an extra-axial lesion without a BBB. In this case, the high permeability also produces prominent enhancement on the delayed post-Gd T1-weighted image (*upper right*) in a pattern strongly suggestive of meningioma, but the distinctive PMR findings illustrated can be very helpful in the differential diagnosis of less classic-appearing lesions.

prominent elevated blood volume equal or greater than cortical gray matter, then the diagnosis of oligodendroglioma should be suspected because the characteristic "chicken-wire" neocapillary architecture found in oligodendroglioma produces a high rCBV regardless of tumor grade. Although quantitative rCBV analysis may address this limitation in future, MRS remains important in these tumors (Fig. 8) [71–74].

*Perfusion-weighted imaging MRI in preoperative tumor grade estimation*

In known or suspected astrocytoma, the strong correlation between the maximum rCBV measured in a tumor and the histologic tumor grade has been extensively documented [99–105]. As noted earlier, the presence of tumor with an rCBV similar to or greater than cortex should strongly suggest the presence of grade IV tumor.

*Perfusion-weighted imaging MRI in operative planning*

Despite the limitations of low spatial resolution, susceptibility artifact, quantitation, and the difficulty of making longitudinal comparisons between

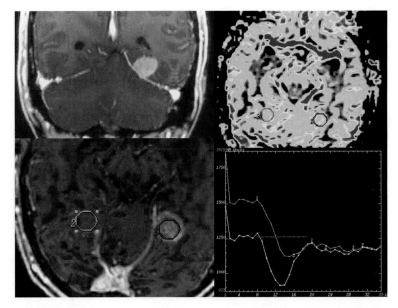

Fig. 7. Comparison of rCBV color map (*upper right*) and TIC (*lower right*) in regions of interest
selected within the dural-based enhancing lesion (*lower left, purple*) and an appropriate region
of interest in the contralateral white matter (*lower left, green*) demonstrate the characteristic
high first-pass leak of a nonglial tumor (TIC) and blood volume only minimally higher than
white matter (TIC and rCBV color map). In combination with the appearance on coronal
post-Gd T1-weighted image (*upper left*), the perfusion imaging strongly suggests dural metastasis, confirmed at biopsy to be from non–small cell lung carcinoma.

echoplanar datasets, maximum rCBV has been demonstrated to be very
helpful in preoperative planning to ensure biopsy, resection, or ablation
of the highest-grade portion of a heterogeneous tumor [105–107].

*Perfusion-weighted imaging MRI in follow-up of therapeutic response*

Several well-designed studies have documented that low rCBV in combination with high ADC is typical of delayed radiation necrosis [28,108]. Early
clinical experience using rCBV to detect tumor recurrence has been promising [109,110]. This application is especially interesting as we enter the age of
antiangiogenic therapy because rCBV has been demonstrated to correlate
with expression of angiogenic factors [102]. It is critical to obtain baseline
preoperative rCBV maps to allow accurate interpretation of changing
rCBV during follow-up, because the vascularity of glioma is very heterogeneous within a single patient's brain and between patients within a given tumor grade [106]. Correlation with steroid dosing during interpretation may
be needed, although to date, technically rigorous reports looking at this subject have reached different conclusions as to whether high-dose steroid administration acutely reduces neovessel CBV in addition to its undisputed

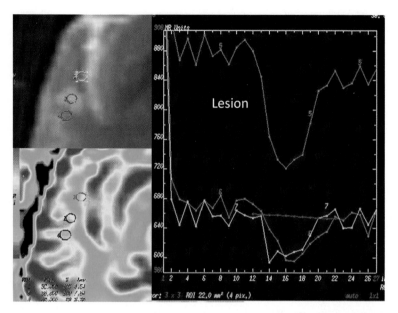

Fig. 8. TIC (*right*) and rCBV color map (*lower left*) demonstrating blood volume more than three times that of normal-appearing white matter in a small non-enhancing circumscribed lesion in the right temporal lobe suggest the diagnosis of oligodendroglioma. The upper TIC curve (*top left*) represents the lesion ROIs and the lower two curves the control ROIs.

effect on permeability [29,111,112]. This controversy will not be trivial to resolve definitively because alteration in permeability has a significant effect on the calculation of CBV (Fig. 9).

## Microvascular permeability imaging: dynamic contrast-enhanced T1 permeability imaging

Low-grade astrocytomas supply their metabolic demand through co-optation of native brain capillaries and are thus limited in the rate of growth and bulk that they can achieve. Neoangiogenesis driven by autologous secretion of VEGF and other cytokines is one of the critical steps in the progression from lower-grade astrocytoma to anaplastic astrocytoma and GBM, enabling the rapid growth of solid tumor that conveys such poor prognosis. Cytokine-mediated abnormality of tight junctions in co-opted brain capillaries produces increased permeability to small molecules and electrolytes, which results in vasogenic edema in low- and high-grade glioma. In addition to permeable tight junctions, GBM neocapillaries have large endothelial gaps that produce a higher permeability to larger molecules, such as the Gd chelates used as MR contrast agents. The familiar enhancement of signal intensity on delayed T1-weighted images is a gross indicator of this abnormal permeability but has not proved to be a reliable

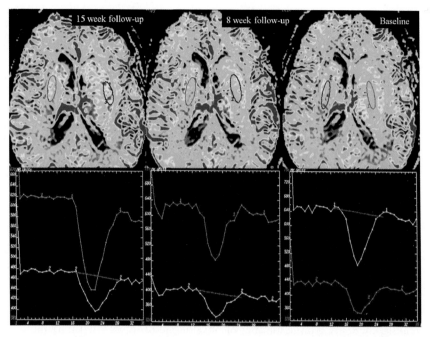

Fig. 9. Serial follow-up (*right to left*) rCBV maps (*top*) and TICs (*below*) demonstrate gradual but accelerating increase in blood volume within a left subinsular recurrent World Health Organization grade III to IV glioma. Although conventional imaging showed no significant change over the same interval, the 15-week follow-up perfusion region-of-interest data demonstrate definite extensive new hypervascularity 2.5 to 3.0 times that of contralateral basal ganglia, strongly suggestive of progressive high-grade recurrence.

predictor of tumor grade [1]. Because the pathophysiologic mechanisms contributing to abnormal permeability in GBM differ from those in lower-grade tumors, quantitation of the degree of abnormal permeability is a rational method of estimating the grade of tumor malignancy.

T1P is essentially a dynamic, semiquantitative adaptation of Gd-enhanced imaging, in which fast-gradient echo–based T1-weighted images of the whole brain continuously from before the contrast bolus arrival until 2 to 3 minutes after injection are used to measure the increase in signal intensity related to leakage of contrast agent from the intravascular compartment into the brain. Because of the lower temporal resolution and longer scan time, T1P is ideal for imaging the steady state leakage of contrast during the first few phases of bolus recirculation, in contrast to PMR, which images exclusively during the first pass. The TIC calculated from T1P can be used to derive a number of parameters related to BBB impairment, the most widely reported of which is the net forward volume transfer constant ($K^{trans}$) from the two-compartment pharmacokinetic modeling equation. Although $K^{trans}$ is related to the slope of the delayed phase of the TIC, corrections for T2* effects, first-pass effects, flow, and surface area are necessary to produce a true estimate. For this and other reasons, a number of different methods yielding related but distinct parameters such as the permeability surface area ($K_{ps}$) and forward transfer constant ($K_1$) are in use in different laboratories. Thus, the author refers to "measures of permeability" in the following text in recognition that most metrics reported in the literature are closely related but not necessarily equivalent to $K^{trans}$. Other metrics derived from T1P data currently under investigation, including relative recirculation [rR] histograms, are closely related to the maximum rate of enhancement during the first pass (max dI/dt), and may therefore reflect a somewhat different feature of microvessel architecture [113–116].

### Dynamic contrast-enhanced T1 permeability imaging in preoperative estimation of tumor grade

As expected from the known correlation of neovessel abnormality with degree of malignancy in a number of models [89], the correlation of increased permeability with increasing tumor grade has been demonstrated to be robust, assuming that a reliable technique is used [113,115–118]. Reports that permeability measures are slightly less predictive of tumor grade than rCBV [118,119] come as no surprise because, in addition to neoangiogenesis, there are a large number of physiologic processes that may increase capillary permeability: local inflammatory response to the tumor, tumor ischemia, release of toxic metabolites, response to corticosteroids, use of immunosuppressant chemotherapeutic agents, and radiation injury, to name a few. As expected, although permeability is independent of blood volume [120], permeability measures are strongly correlated with rCBV in high-grade glioma [121], likely due to coregulation of neoangiogenesis and increased vascular permeability by VEGF and other proangiogenic factors. A large number of articles in press are exploring the utility of different combinations of blood volume and permeability metrics for improved tumor classification.

### Dynamic contrast-enhanced T1 permeability imaging in postoperative therapeutic monitoring

Despite the large number of technique papers and early clinical demonstrations of T1P efficacy in distinction of tumor recurrence from necrosis [114,117], permeability measures have not yet achieved widespread clinical acceptance, largely because (1) the acquisition times are longer than for perfusion imaging, (2) the postprocessing is more complicated, (3) the plethora of metrics reported in the literature has yet to yield to a clear consensus metric, and consequently, (4) postprocessing algorithms in commercial release lag significantly behind perfusion software. Despite these shortcomings, the high sensitivity of T1P to antiangiogenic therapy is accelerating technique development. Future improvements in MR hardware and software

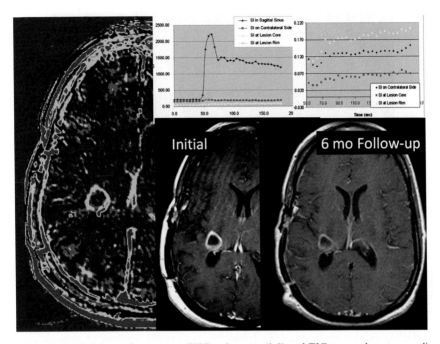

Fig. 10. Endothelial transfer constant (KPS) color map (*left*) and TICs pre and post normalization (*upper middle and upper right, respectively*) demonstrate only minimally increased permeability within the new ring-enhancing lesion (*lower middle*) in this patient post resection, radiation, and chemotherapy for gliosarcoma. The relatively mild increase in permeability suggested radiation necrosis rather than recurrence, as confirmed by the 6-month follow-up postgadolinium T1-weighted image (*lower right*) showing no interval progression. (Postprocessing software courtesy of Timothy Roberts, PhD, Children's Hospital of Philadelphia.)

should allow acquisition at higher temporal and spatial resolutions and of more purely T1-weighted data. These advances, combined with an emergence of academic consensus and the development of standard commercial permeability postprocessing tools, may significantly alter clinical practice in this respect over the next few years (Figs. 10 and 11).

## Summary

Advanced brain tumor MRI evaluation can now routinely produce an impressive array of in vivo data reflecting tumor cellularity, metabolism, invasiveness, neocapillary density, and permeability. Ongoing technical improvements and additional metrics, currently reported in the literature but too preliminary to review here, promise to bring to the clinic further dramatic increases in the quantity and quality of imaging data over the next 5 years. The clinical principles outlined in this article reflect only the most preliminary experience with these new data, but already it is becoming clear that a paradigm shift in neurooncology and neuropathology will be needed

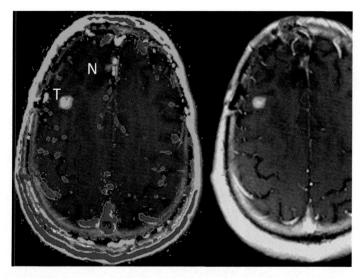

Fig. 11. Endothelial transfer constant (Kps) map superimposed on post-Gd spin-echo T-weighted image (*left*) in a patient who has a right frontal recurrent glioma shows focally elevated permeability similar to systemic scalp capillaries within the area of focal nodular enhancement (T), suggesting high-grade recurrence at this site but not in the area of enhancement at the anterior aspect of the right frontal resection site (N). Six-week follow-up post-Gd T1-weighted image (*right*) demonstrates interval decrease in enhancement at the anterior site (N) consistent with evolving necrosis, but not in the area of suspected recurrence. Although the potential utility of permeability data to aid in the differentiation of recurrent tumor from necrosis has been well established, clinical validation and routine application will require improvements in practicality and reproducibility. This type of data holds promise for distinguishing recurrent tumor from necrosis, but clinical validation and routine application await improvements in postprocessing and display technique. (Postprocessing software courtesy of Timothy Roberts, PhD, Children's Hospital of Philadelphia.)

if we are to make full use of the information available. The primary goal of neuropathologic glioma classification is to provide a clinically meaningful classification of brain tumors based on pathophysiology that will allow reliable prognosis and assessment of the efficacy of new therapies [122]. Already, the MRI data available (to say nothing of positron emission tomography and optical molecular imaging) reflect several independent aspects of brain tumor biology that cannot effectively be integrated into the existing histopathologic classification or used in treatment paradigms designed around that classification. Thus, although technical challenges remain, the greatest current challenge in advanced tumor imaging is the need for a new tumor classification method that can allow better integration of advanced imaging data into brain tumor research and clinical decision making. In essence, what is needed is a significant revision of brain tumor nosology. It is conceivable that a novel tumor classification method encompassing the new, advanced-MRI metrics in addition to nucleoside positron emission tomography data and cellular and molecular microarray data could define novel pathophysiologically relevant subtypes that would better predict brain tumor patient prognoses and responses to targeted chemotherapeutic agents than our current histopathologic grading system. To this end, a number of recent reports have been published evaluating imaging markers by direct comparison with molecular genotype and phenotype [102] and patient outcomes [105,123]. This approach seems likely to become the dominant paradigm in the future.

## References

[1] Ginsberg LE, Fuller GN, Hashmi M, et al. The significance of lack of MR contrast enhancement of supratentorial brain tumors in adults: histopathological evaluation of a series. Surg Neurol 1998;49(4):436–40.

[2] Provenzale J, Mukundan S, Barboriak DP. Diffusion-weighted and perfusion MR imaging for brain tumor characterization and assessment of treatment response. Radiology 2006; 239(3):632–49.

[3] Mardor Y, Pfeffer R, Spiegelmann R, et al. Early detection of response to radiation therapy in patients with brain malignancies using conventional and high b-value diffusion-weighted magnetic resonance imaging. J Clin Oncol 2003;21:1094–100.

[4] Reddy JS, Mishra AM, Behari S, et al. The role of diffusion-weighted imaging in the differential diagnosis of intracranial cystic mass lesions: a report of 147 lesions. Surg Neurol 2006;66(3):246–50.

[5] Mishra AM, Gupta RK, Jaggi RS, et al. Role of diffusion-weighted imaging and in vivo proton magnetic resonance spectroscopy in the differential diagnosis of ring-enhancing intracranial cystic mass lesions. J Comput Assist Tomogr 2004;28(4):540–7.

[6] Erdogan C, Hakyemez B, Yildirim N, et al. Brain abscess and cystic brain tumor: discrimination with dynamic susceptibility contrast perfusion-weighted MRI. J Comput Assist Tomogr 2005;29(5):663–7.

[7] Tsui EY, Leung WH, Chan IH, et al. Tumefactive demyelinating lesions by combined perfusion-weighted and diffusion weighted imaging. Comput Med Imaging Graph 2002;26(5): 343–6.

[8] Guo AC, Cummings TJ, Dash RC, et al. Lymphomas and high-grade astrocytomas: comparison of water diffusibility and histologic characteristics. Radiology 2002;224:177–83.

[9] Calli C, Kitis O, Yunten N, et al. Perfusion and diffusion MR imaging in enhancing malignant cerebral tumors. Eur J Radiol 2006;58(3):394–403.

[10] Okamoto K, Ito J, Ishikawa K, et al. Diffusion-weighted echo-planar MR imaging in differential diagnosis of brain tumors and tumor-like conditions. Eur Radiol 2000;10:1342–50.

[11] Toh CH, Chen YL, Hsieh TC, et al. Glioblastoma multiforme with diffusion-weighted magnetic resonance imaging characteristics mimicking primary lymphoma. Case report. J Neurosurg 2006;105:132–5.

[12] Krabbe K, Gideon P, Wagn P, et al. MR diffusion imaging of human intracranial tumours. Neuroradiology 1997;39(7):483–9.

[13] Kotsenas AL, Roth TC, Manness WK, et al. Abnormal diffusion-weighted MRI in medulloblastoma: does it reflect small cell histology? Pediatr Radiol 1999;29(7):524–6.

[14] Chenevert TL, Stegman LD, Taylor JM, et al. Diffusion magnetic resonance imaging: an early surrogate marker of therapeutic efficacy in brain tumors. J Natl Cancer Inst 2000; 92(24):2029–36.

[15] Chenevert TL, McKeever PE, Ross BD. Monitoring early response of experimental brain tumors to therapy using diffusion magnetic resonance imaging. Clin Cancer Res 1997;3(9): 1457–66.

[16] Filippi CG, Edgar MA, Ulug AM, et al. Appearance of meningiomas on diffusion-weighted images: correlating diffusion constants with histopathologic findings. AJNR Am J Neuroradiol 2001;22(1):65–72.

[17] Hayashida Y, Hirai T, Morishita S, et al. Diffusion-weighted imaging of metastatic brain tumors: comparison with histologic type and tumor cellularity. AJNR Am J Neuroradiol 2006;27(7):1419–25.

[18] Sugahara T, Korogi Y, Kochi M, et al. Usefulness of diffusion-weighted MRI with echoplanar technique in the evaluation of cellularity in gliomas. J Magn Reson Imaging 1999; 9:53–60.

[19] Catalaa I, Henry R, Dillon WP, et al. Perfusion, diffusion and spectroscopy values in newly diagnosed cerebral gliomas. NMR Biomed 2006;19(4):463–75.

[20] Yang D, Korogi Y, Sugahara T, et al. Cerebral gliomas: prospective comparison of multivoxel 2D chemical-shift imaging proton MR spectroscopy, echoplanar perfusion and diffusion-weighted MRI. Neuroradiology 2002;44:656–66.

[21] Bulakbasi N, Kocaoglu M, Ors F, et al. Combination of single-voxel proton MR spectroscopy and apparent diffusion coefficient calculation in the evaluation of common brain tumors. AJNR Am J Neuroradiol 2003;24:225–33.

[22] Castillo M, Smith JK, Kwock L, et al. Apparent diffusion coefficients in the evaluation of high-grade cerebral gliomas. AJNR Am J Neuroradiol 2001;22:60–4.

[23] Mardor Y, Roth Y, Ochershvilli A, et al. Pretreatment prediction of brain tumors' response to radiation therapy using high b-value diffusion-weighted MRI. Neoplasia 2004;6(2):136–42.

[24] Khan RB, Gutin PH, Rai SN, et al. Use of diffusion weighted magnetic resonance imaging in predicting early postoperative outcome of new neurological deficits after brain tumor resection. Neurosurgery 2006;59(1):60–6.

[25] Schaefer PW, Grant PE, Gonzalez RG. Diffusion-weighted MR imaging of the brain. Radiology 2000;217:331–45.

[26] Hein PA, Eskey CJ, Dunn JF, et al. Diffusion-weighted imaging in the follow-up of treated high-grade gliomas: tumor recurrence versus radiation injury. AJNR Am J Neuroradiol 2004;25:201–9.

[27] Chan YL, Yeung DK, Leung SF, et al. Diffusion-weighted magnetic resonance imaging in radiation-induced cerebral necrosis. Apparent diffusion coefficient in lesion components. J Comput Assist Tomogr 2003;27(5):674–80.

[28] Tsui EY, Chan JH, Ramsey RG, et al. Late temporal lobe necrosis in patients with nasopharyngeal carcinoma: evaluation with combined multi-section diffusion weighted and perfusion weighted MR imaging. Eur J Radiol 2001;39(3):133–8.

[29] Bastin ME, Carpenter TK, Armitage PA, et al. Effects of dexamethasone on cerebral perfusion and water diffusion in patients with high-grade glioma. AJNR Am J Neuroradiol 2006;27(2):402–8.

[30] Moffat BA, Chenevert TL, Lawrence TS, et al. Functional diffusion map: a noninvasive MRI biomarker for early stratification of clinical brain tumor response. Proc Natl Acad Sci U S A 2005;102(15):5524–9.

[31] Hamstra DA, Chenevert TL, Moffat BA, et al. Evaluation of the functional diffusion map as an early biomarker of time-to-progression and overall survival in high-grade glioma. Proc Natl Acad Sci U S A 2005;102(46):16759–64.

[32] Inoue T, Ogasawara K, Beppu T, et al. Diffusion tensor imaging for preoperative evaluation of tumor grade in gliomas. Clin Neurol Neurosurg 2005;107(3):174–80.

[33] Field AS, Wu YC, Alexander AL. Principal diffusion direction in peritumoral fiber tracts: color map patterns and directional statistics. Ann N Y Acad Sci 2005;1064: 193–201.

[34] Goebell E, Fiehler J, Ding XQ, et al. Disarrangement of fiber tracts and decline of neuronal density correlate in glioma patients—a combined diffusion tensor imaging and 1H-MR spectroscopy study. AJNR Am J Neuroradiol 2006;27(7):1426–31.

[35] Yu CS, Li KC, Xuan Y, et al. Diffusion tensor tractography in patients with cerebral tumors: a helpful technique for neurosurgical planning and postoperative assessment. Eur J Radiol 2005;56(2):197–204.

[36] Nimsky C, Grummich P, Sorensen AG, et al. Visualization of the pyramidal tract in glioma surgery by integrating diffusion tensor imaging in functional neuronavigation. Zentralbl Neurochir 2005;66(3):133–41.

[37] Lazar M, Alexander AL, Thottakara PJ, et al. White matter reorganization after surgical resection of brain tumors and vascular malformations. AJNR Am J Neuroradiol 2006; 27(6):1258–71.

[38] Schonberg T, Pianka P, Hendler T, et al. Characterization of displaced white matter by brain tumors using combined DTI and fMRI. Neuroimage 2006;30(4):1100–11.

[39] Provenzale JM, McGraw P, Mhatre P, et al. Peritumoral brain regions in gliomas and meningiomas: investigation with isotropic diffusion-weighted MR imaging and diffusion-tensor MR imaging. Radiology 2004;232(2):451–60.

[40] Price SJ, Burnet NG, Donovan T, et al. Diffusion tensor imaging of brain tumours at 3T: a potential tool for assessing white matter tract invasion? Clin Radiol 2003;58: 455–62.

[41] Lu S, Ahn D, Johnson G, et al. Peritumoral diffusion tensor imaging of high-grade gliomas and metastatic brain tumors. AJNR Am J Neuroradiol 2003;24:937–41.

[42] Lu S, Ahn D, Johnson G, et al. Diffusion-tensor MR imaging of intracranial neoplasia and associated peritumoral edema: introduction of the tumor infiltration index. Radiology 2004;232(1):221–8.

[43] Chiang IC, Kuo YT, Lu CY, et al. Distinction between high-grade gliomas and solitary metastases using peritumoral 3-T magnetic resonance spectroscopy, diffusion, and perfusion imagings. Neuroradiology 2004;46:619–27.

[44] Kono K, Inoue Y, Nakayama K, et al. The role of diffusion-weighted imaging in patients with brain tumors. AJNR Am J Neuroradiol 2001;22:1081–8.

[45] Stadnik TW, Chaskis C, Michotte A, et al. Diffusion-weighted MR imaging of intracerebral masses: comparison with conventional MR imaging and histologic findings. AJNR Am J Neuroradiol 2001;22:969–76.

[46] Sundgren PC, Fan X, Weybright P, et al. Differentiation of recurrent brain tumor versus radiation injury using diffusion tensor imaging in patients with new contrast-enhancing lesions. Magn Reson Imaging 2006;24(9):1131–42.

[47] Stieltjes B, Schluter M, Didinger B, et al. Diffusion tensor imaging in primary brain tumors: reproducible quantitative analysis of corpus callosum infiltration and contralateral involvement using a probabilistic mixture model. Neuroimage 2006;31(2):531–42.

[48] Zhou XJ, Engelhard HH, Leeds NE, et al. Studies of glioma infiltration using a fiber coherence index. Magn Reson Med, in press.

[49] van Westen D, Latt J, Englund E, et al. Tumor extension in high-grade gliomas assessed with diffusion magnetic resonance imaging: values and lesion-to-brain ratios of apparent diffusion coefficient and fractional anisotropy. Acta Radiol 2006;47(3):311–9.

[50] Marshall I, Wardlaw J, Cannon J, et al. Reproducibility of metabolite peak areas in 1H MRS of brain. Magn Reson Imaging 1996;14(3):281–92.

[51] Calvar JA. Accurate (1)H tumor spectra quantification from acquisitions without water suppression. Magn Reson Imaging 2006;24(9):1271–9.

[52] Birken DL, Oldendorf WH. N-acetyl-L-aspartic acid: a literature review of a compound prominent in 1H-NMR spectroscopic studies of brain. Neurosci Biobehav Rev 1989; 13(1):23–31.

[53] Moffett JR, Ross B, Arun P, et al. N-acetyl aspartate in the CNS: from neurodiagnostics to neurobiology. Prog Neurobiol 2007;81(2):89–131.

[54] Wyss M, Kaddurah-Daouk R. Creatine and creatinine metabolism. Physiol Rev 2000; 80(3):1107–213.

[55] Christiansen P, Toft P, Larsson HB, et al. The concentration of N-acetyl aspartate, creatine + phosphocreatine, and choline in different parts of the brain in adulthood and senium. Magn Reson Imaging 1993;11(6):799–806.

[56] Brief EE, Whittall KP, Li DK, et al. Proton T1 relaxation times of cerebral metabolites differ within and between regions of normal human brain. NMR Biomed 2003;16(8):503–9.

[57] Degaonkar MN, Pomper MG, Barker PB. Quantitative proton magnetic resonance spectroscopic imaging: regional variations in the corpus callosum and cortical gray matter. J Magn Reson Imaging 2005;22(2):175–9.

[58] Kent C. Regulatory enzymes of phosphatidylcholine biosynthesis: a personal perspective [review]. Biochim Biophys Acta 2005;1733(1):53–66.

[59] Babb SM, Ke Y, Lange N, et al. Oral choline increases choline metabolites in human brain. Psychiatry Res 2004;130(1):1–9.

[60] Cho YD, Choi GH, Lee SP, et al. (1)H-MRS metabolic patterns for distinguishing between meningiomas and other brain tumors. Magn Reson Imaging 2003;21(6):663–72.

[61] Gajewicz W, Papierz W, Szymczak W, et al. The use of proton MRS in the differential diagnosis of brain tumors and tumor like processes. Med Sci Monit 2003;9(9):MT97–T105.

[62] Preul MC, Caramanos Z, Collins DL, et al. Accurate, noninvasive diagnosis of human brain tumors by using proton magnetic resonance spectroscopy. Nat Med 1996;2:323–5.

[63] Del Sole A, Falini A, Ravasi L, et al. Anatomical and biochemical investigation of primary brain tumours [review]. Eur J Nucl Med 2001;28(12):1851–72.

[64] Delorme S, Weber MA. Applications of MRS in the evaluation of focal malignant brain lesions. Cancer Imaging 2006;22(6):95–9.

[65] Lai PH, Ho JT, Chen WL, et al. Brain abscess and necrotic brain tumor: discrimination with proton MR spectroscopy and diffusion-weighted imaging. AJNR Am J Neuroradiol 2002;23(8):1369–77.

[66] Devos A, Lukas L, Suykens JA, et al. Classification of brain tumours using short echo time 1H MR spectra. J Magn Reson 2004;170:164–75.

[67] Li X, Vigneron DB, Cha S, et al. Relationship of MR-derived lactate, mobile lipids, and relative blood volume for gliomas in vivo. AJNR Am J Neuroradiol 2005;26(4):760–9.

[68] Law M, Yang S, Wang H, et al. Glioma grading: sensitivity, specificity, and predictive values of perfusion MR imaging and proton MR spectroscopic imaging compared with conventional MR imaging. AJNR Am J Neuroradiol 2003;24(10):1989–98.

[69] Fayed N, Morales H, Modrego PJ, et al. Contrast/noise ratio on conventional MRI and choline/creatine ratio on proton MRI spectroscopy accurately discriminate low-grade from high-grade cerebral gliomas. Acad Radiol 2006;13(6):728–37.

[70] Chen J, Huang SL, Li T, et al. In vivo research in astrocytoma cell proliferation with 1H-magnetic resonance spectroscopy: correlation with histopathology and immunohistochemistry. Neuroradiology 2006;48(5):312–8.

[71] Jenkinson MD, Smith TS, Joyce K, et al. MRS of oligodendroglial tumors: correlation with histopathology and genetic subtypes. Neurology 2005;64(12):2085–9.

[72] White ML, Zhang Y, Kirby P, et al. Can tumor contrast enhancement be used as a criterion for differentiating tumor grades of oligodendrogliomas? AJNR Am J Neuroradiol 2005;26:784–90.

[73] Lev MH, Ozsunar Y, Henson JW, et al. Glial tumor grading and outcome prediction using dynamic spin-echo MR susceptibility mapping compared with conventional contrast-enhanced MR: confounding effect of elevated rCBV of oligodendrogliomoas [sic]. AJNR Am J Neuroradiol 2004;25:214–21.

[74] Xu M, See SJ, Ng WH, et al. Comparison of magnetic resonance spectroscopy and perfusion-weighted imaging in presurgical grading of oligodendroglial tumors. Neurosurgery 2005;56:919–24.

[75] Chernov M, Hayashi M, Izawa M, et al. Differentiation of the radiation-induced necrosis and tumor recurrence after gamma knife radiosurgery for brain metastases: importance of multi-voxel proton MRS. Minim Invasive Neurosurg 2005;48(4):228–34.

[76] Gajewicz W, Grzelak P, Gorska-Chrzastek M, et al. [The usefulness of fused MRI and SPECT images for the voxel positioning in proton magnetic resonance spectroscopy and planning the biopsy of brain tumors: presentation of the method] [abstract]. Neurol Neurochir Pol 2006;40(4):284–90 [in Polish].

[77] Hall WA, Martin A, Liu H, et al. Improving diagnostic yield in brain biopsy: coupling spectroscopic targeting with real-time needle placement. J Magn Reson Imaging 2001;13(1):12–5.

[78] Payne GS, Leach MO. Applications of magnetic resonance spectroscopy in radiotherapy treatment planning. Br J Radiol 2006;79(Special Issue 1):S16–26.

[79] Graves EE, Nelson SJ, Vigneron DB, et al. A preliminary study of the prognostic value of 1H-spectroscopy in gamma knife radiosurgery of recurrent malignant gliomas. Neurosurgery (Baltimore) 2000;46:319–28.

[80] Graves EE, Pirzkall A, Nelson SJ, et al. Registration of magnetic resonance spectroscopic imaging to computed tomography for radiotherapy treatment planning. Med Phys 2001;28: 2489–96.

[81] Cohen BA, Knopp EA, Rusinek H, et al. Assessing global invasion of newly diagnosed glial tumors with whole-brain proton MR spectroscopy. AJNR Am J Neuroradiol 2005;26(9): 2170–7.

[82] Matulewicz L, Sokol M, Wydmanski J, et al. Could lipid CH2/CH3 analysis by in vivo 1H MRS help in differentiation of tumor recurrence and post-radiation effects? Folia Neuropathol 2006;44(2):116–24.

[83] Chan YL, Yeung DK, Leung SF, et al. Proton magnetic resonance spectroscopy of late delayed radiation-induced injury of the brain. J Magn Reson Imaging 1999; 10(2):130–7.

[84] Graves EE, Nelson SJ, Vigneron DB, et al. Serial proton MR spectroscopic imaging of recurrent malignant gliomas after gamma knife radiosurgery. AJNR Am J Neuroradiol 2001; 2:613–24.

[85] Plotkin M, Eisenacher J, Bruhn H, et al. 123I-IMT SPECT and 1H MR-spectroscopy at 3.0 T in the differential diagnosis of recurrent or residual gliomas: a comparative study. J Neurooncol 2004;70(1):49–58.

[86] Hollingworth W, Medina LS, Lenkinski RE, et al. A systematic literature review of magnetic resonance spectroscopy for the characterization of brain tumors [review]. AJNR Am J Neuroradiol 2006;27(7):1404–11.

[87] Kaur B, Tan C, Brat DJ, et al. Genetic and hypoxic regulation of angiogenesis in gliomas [review]. J Neurooncol 2004;70(2):229–43.

[88] Manoonkitiwongsa PS, Schultz RL, Whitter EF, et al. Contraindications of VEGF-based therapeutic angiogenesis: effects on macrophage density and histology of normal and ischemic brains. Vascul Pharmacol 2006;44(5):316–25.

[89] Liebner S, Fischmann A, Rascher G, et al. Claudin-1 and claudin-5 expression and tight junction morphology are altered in blood vessels of human glioblastoma multiforme. Acta Neuropathol (Berl) 2000;100(3):323–31.

[90] Davies DC. Blood-brain barrier breakdown in septic encephalopathy and brain tumours [review]. J Anat 2002;200(6):639–46.

[91] Nakagawa T, Tanaka R, Takeuchi S, et al. Haemodynamic evaluation of cerebral gliomas using XeCT. Acta Neurochir (Wien) 1998;140(3):223–33.

[92] Muizelaar JP, Fatouros PP, Schroder ML. A new method for quantitative regional cerebral blood volume measurements using computed tomography. Stroke 1997;28(10): 1998–2005.

[93] Yang S, Law M, Zagzag D. Dynamic contrast-enhanced perfusion MR imaging measurements of endothelial permeability: differentiation between atypical and typical meningiomas. AJNR Am J Neuroradiol 2003;24:1554–9.

[94] Hartmann M, Heiland S, Harting I, et al. Distinguishing of primary cerebral lymphoma from high-grade gliomas with perfusion-weighted magnetic resonance imaging. Neurosci Lett 2003;338:119–22.

[95] Rollin N, Guyotat J, Streichenberger N, et al. Clinical relevance of diffusion and perfusion magnetic resonance imaging in assessing intra-axial brain tumors. Neuroradiology 2006; 48(3):150–9.

[96] Essig M, Waschkies M, Wenz F, et al. Assessment of brain metastases with dynamic susceptibility-weighted contrast-enhanced MR imaging: initial results. Radiology 2003;228(1): 193–9.

[97] Kremer S, Grand S, Berger F, et al. Dynamic contrast-enhanced MRI: differentiating melanoma and renal carcinoma metastases from high-grade astrocytomas and other metastases. Neuroradiology 2003;45(1):44–9.

[98] Kremer S, Grand S, Remy C, et al. Contribution of dynamic contrast MR imaging to the differentiation between dural metastasis and meningioma. Neuroradiology 2004;46(8):642–8.

[99] Hakyemez B, Erdogan C, Ercan I, et al. High-grade and low-grade gliomas: differentiation by using perfusion MR imaging. Clin Radiol 2005;60(4):493–502.

[100] Knopp EA, Cha S, Johnson G, et al. Glial neoplasms: dynamic contrast-enhanced T2*-weighted MR imaging. Radiology 1999;211:791–8.

[101] Sugahara T, Korogi Y, Kochi M, et al. Correlation of MR imaging-determined cerebral blood volume maps with histologic and angiographic determination of vascularity of gliomas. AJR Am J Roentgenol 1998;171:1479–86.

[102] Maia AC, Malheiros SM, da Rocha AJ, et al. MR cerebral blood volume maps correlated with vascular endothelial growth factor expression and tumor grade in nonenhancing gliomas. AJNR Am J Neuroradiol 2005;26(4):777–83.

[103] Shin JH, Lee HK, Kwun BD, et al. Using relative cerebral blood flow and volume to evaluate the histopathologic grade of cerebral gliomas: preliminary results. AJR Am J Roentgenol 2002;179(3):783–9.

[104] Aronen HJ, Gazit IE, Louis DN, et al. Cerebral blood volume maps of gliomas: comparison with tumor grade and histologic findings. Radiology 1994;191(1):41–51.

[105] Chaskis C, Stadnik T, Michotte A, et al. Prognostic value of perfusion-weighted imaging in brain glioma: a prospective study. Acta Neurochir (Wien) 2006;148(3):277–85 [comment: 285].

[106] Lupo JM, Cha S, Chang SM, et al. Dynamic susceptibility-weighted perfusion imaging of high-grade gliomas: characterization of spatial heterogeneity. AJNR Am J Neuroradiol 2005;26(6):1446–54.

[107] Maia AC, Malheiros SM, da Rocha AJ, et al. Stereotactic biopsy guidance in adults with supratentorial nonenhancing gliomas: role of perfusion-weighted magnetic resonance imaging. J Neurosurg 2004;101(6):970–6.

[108] Tsui EY, Chan JH, Leung TW, et al. Radionecrosis of the temporal lobe: dynamic susceptibility contrast MRI. Neuroradiology 2000;42(2):149–52.

[109] Siegal T, Rubinstein R, Tzuk-Shina T, et al. Utility of relative cerebral blood volume mapping derived from perfusion magnetic resonance imaging in the routine follow up of brain tumors. J Neurosurg 1997;86(1):22–7.

[110] Sugahara T, Korogi Y, Tomiguchi S, et al. Posttherapeutic intraaxial brain tumor: the value of perfusion-sensitive contrast-enhanced MR imaging for differentiating tumor recurrence from nonneoplastic contrast-enhancing tissue. AJNR Am J Neuroradiol 2000;21(5): 901–9.

[111] Ostergaard L, Hochberg FH, Rabinov JD, et al. Early changes measured by magnetic resonance imaging in cerebral blood flow, blood volume, and blood-brain barrier permeability following dexamethasone treatment in patients with brain tumors. J Neurosurg 1999;90(2): 300–5.

[112] Wilkinson ID, Jellineck DA, Levy D, et al. Dexamethasone and enhancing solitary cerebral mass lesions: alterations in perfusion and blood-tumor barrier kinetics shown by magnetic resonance imaging. Neurosurgery 2006;58(4):640–6.

[113] Roberts HC, Roberts TP, Ley S, et al. Quantitative estimation of microvascular permeability in human brain tumors: correlation of dynamic Gd-DTPA-enhanced MR imaging with histopathologic grading. Acad Radiol 2002;9(Suppl 1):S151–5.

[114] Hazle JD, Jackson EF, Schomer DF, et al. Dynamic imaging of intracranial lesions using fast spin-echo imaging: differentiation of brain tumors and treatment effects. J Magn Reson Imaging 1997;7(6):1084–93.

[115] Uematsu H, Maeda M, Sadato N, et al. Vascular permeability: quantitative measurement with double-echo dynamic MR imaging—theory and clinical application. Radiology 2000; 214:912–7.

[116] Roberts HC, Roberts TPL, Brasch RC, et al. Quantitative measurement of microvascular permeability in human brain tumors achieved using dynamic contrast-enhanced MR imaging: correlation with histologic grade. AJNR Am J Neuroradiol 2000;21:891–9.

[117] Provenzale JM, Wang GR, Brenner T, et al. Comparison of permeability in high-grade and low-grade brain tumors using dynamic susceptibility contrast MR imaging. AJR Am J Roentgenol 2002;178:711–6.

[118] Law M, Yang S, Babb JS, et al. Comparison of cerebral blood volume and vascular permeability from dynamic susceptibility contrast enhanced perfusion MR imaging with glioma grade. AJNR Am J Neuroradiol 2003;25:746–55.

[119] Law M, Young R, Babb J, et al. Comparing perfusion metrics obtained from a single compartment versus pharmacokinetic modeling methods using dynamic susceptibility contrast-enhanced perfusion MR imaging with glioma grade. AJNR Am J Neuroradiol 2006;27(9): 1975–82.

[120] Jackson A, Kassner A, Annesley-Williams D, et al. Abnormalities in the recirculation phase of contrast agent bolus passage in cerebral gliomas: comparison with relative blood volume and tumor grade. AJNR Am J Neuroradiol 2002;23(1):7–14.

[121] Provenzale JM, York G, Moya MG, et al. Correlation of relative permeability and relative cerebral blood volume in high-grade cerebral neoplasms. AJR Am J Roentgenol 2006; 187(4):1036–42.

[122] Preusser M, Haberler C, Hainfellner JA. Malignant glioma: neuropathology and neurobiology [review]. Wien Med Wochenschr 2006;156(11–12):332–7.

[123] Law M, Oh S, Babb JS, et al. Low-grade gliomas: dynamic susceptibility-weighted contrast-enhanced perfusion MR imaging—prediction of patient clinical response. Radiology 2006; 238(2):658–67.

ELSEVIER
SAUNDERS

NEUROLOGIC
CLINICS

Neurol Clin 25 (2007) 975–1003

# Advances in Brain Tumor Surgery

Ashok R. Asthagiri, MD[a],*, Nader Pouratian, MD, PhD[b],
Jonathan Sherman, MD[b], Galal Ahmed, MD[b],
Mark E. Shaffrey, MD[b]

[a]*National Institutes of Health/NINDS, Bethesda, MD, USA*
[b]*Department of Neurological Surgery, University of Virginia, P.O. Box 800212,
Charlottesville, VA 22908-0212, USA*

There is perhaps no more daunting challenge in all of medicine than the management of patients diagnosed with a brain tumor. Wielding what now would seem elementary neurosurgical concepts in antisepsis, anesthesia, and preoperative localization, Rickman Godlee operated on a 25-year-old Scottish farmer who presented with focal motor seizures and progressive hemiparesis in November 1884. The patient underwent surgical resection of an oligodendroglioma, clinically localized to the region of cortical substance near the upper third of the rolandic fissure, but eventually succumbed to complications of meningitis 28 days later. Although an undesirable outcome, the operation highlighted the new belief of brain tumor vulnerability and ushered the field forward into the modern age of brain tumor surgery.

Contemporaneous with early success in the treatment of intracranial extra-axial masses, such as meningiomas and schwannomas, surgeons were met with equilibrating results from surgical management of intrinsic brain tumors. Only in the past 20 to 30 years have we witnessed significant improvements in microneurosurgical strategies and techniques that have revolutionized the management of primary glial neoplasms and help shed the dogma of their unresectability [1]. Microneurosurgical techniques, however, with the use of the operating microscope alone, have limitations in the definition of the boundaries of glial neoplasms and of the localization of eloquent cerebral cortex and subcortical white matter.

Important technologic adjuncts have come to the forefront over the past 15 years that have allowed neurosurgeons to enhance volumetric resections and open surgical corridors to lesions in eloquent cortices while curtailing

---

\* Corresponding author.
*E-mail address:* asthagiria@ninds.nih.gov (A.R. Asthagiri).

surgical morbidity and improving survival. These recent surgical developments have centered on identification of eloquent cortex through preoperative functional imaging, awake craniotomy, and cortical stimulation; fusing
preoperative structural data with real-time surgical anatomy via frameless
neuronavigation systems; and real-time image-based guidance of tumor resection with intraoperative MRI (iMRI). Another area within neuro-oncology displaying significant change has been the development of surgical
methods to deliver local adjunctive radiotherapy and chemotherapy, historically restricted to the extraoperative treatment armamentarium. Before de-
lineating the usefulness of these advances, this article reviews a fundamental
query: the putative benefit of maximal resection in the treatment of gliomas.

## Low-grade gliomas

The World Health Organization classification of low-grade gliomas en-
compasses several grade I and II tumors with heterogeneous clinical, pathologic, and molecular features [2]. Chief among these are grade II diffuse
astrocytomas, oligdendrogliomas, and oligoastrocytomas, all of which
have malignant potential and together represent approximately 20% of gliomas [3]. The prognostic effect of extent of resection in surgery for
low-grade gliomas, as it relates to clinical outcome, has not been evaluated
specifically in any randomized study. Thus, all available management strategies are satisfactory treatment options, yet none is supported by enough
high-quality evidence to be considered a treatment standard.

Most authorities agree that surgery or biopsy at the time of initial detection, rather than at the time of disease progression, is an appropriate initial
step along the management pathway. Risks associated with delaying diagnosis include progression to a higher level of malignancy, interval tumor growth,
and potential development of an irreversible neurologic deficit [4]. Furthermore, establishment of tumor histology, pathologic grade, and genotype carry
increasingly important prognostic and therapeutic implications [5].

Historically, it was common for patients who had low-grade gliomas to
be diagnosed only after signs of increased intracranial pressure were manifested because of the size of the lesions. With the increasing availability of
MRI, patients now typically are diagnosed after presenting with a single seizure when other neurologic signs are minimal or absent. The metamorphosis
in the clinical presentation of patients harboring low-grade gliomas resulting
from improved diagnostic imaging has only fed the controversy between cytoreductive surgery and biopsy alone. There is evidence that radical resection may improve symptom control, particularly with regard to seizures
[6]. The anecdotal experience of many surgeons is that partial resections often results in an exacerbation of edema and worsening of symptoms,
whereas complete resections are associated with less postoperative edema
and improved symptom palliation.

Cytoreductive surgery has the additional advantage of providing more tumor specimen for histopathologic analysis over biopsy alone. The larger sample size decreases the likelihood of underestimating tumor grade or missing regions of tumor that may display more characteristic features of the biology and behavior of the tumor (ie, sampling error). With a greater amount of tumor available, genetic analysis and tissue donation for research also may be possible. Additional theoretic advantages of cytoreductive surgery include decreasing the risk for genetic progression of the remaining tumor cells and improving the effect of adjuvant radiotherapy. Nonetheless, these purported advantages have been questioned extensively [7,8].

Recurrence and malignant progression are major causes of morbidity and mortality in patients initially diagnosed with low-grade gliomas, but the impact of radical surgical therapy in altering this course of events is controversial. A study by Recht and colleagues [9] comparing delayed therapy to immediate treatment found that the rates of and times to malignant progression were not affected by the timing of intervention. Steiger and colleagues showed an improvement in 38-month progression-free survival for patients undergoing gross total resection versus those who had partial resection or biopsy, but this difference was not statistically significant ($P = .09$) [10]. Berger and colleagues [11] reported evidence that a greater extent of resection and smaller residual tumor volume significantly prolong the time to recurrence and reduce the malignant transformation rate.

More recently, Keles and colleagues [4] performed a critical review of the literature pertaining to low-grade gliomas of the cerebral hemisphere in adults. This was a systematic review of 30 series addressing extent of surgical resection and outcome to determine whether or not treatment-related guidelines could be established. Although each series had design or methodology flaws, an increasing number of retrospective uncontrolled studies did support extensive resections over biopsy (Table 1). Hitherto, there has been a void in class I evidence supporting or refuting radical tumor removal. The potential advantages of maximal resection in terms of diagnosis, symptom control, and cytoreduction, however, have led to its common recommendation, especially with large tumors that cause neurologic deficits.

## High-grade gliomas

The optimal management for patients who have malignant gliomas also continues to be controversial, despite decades of intense clinical and basic science investigation and debate. The majority of studies have shown a survival advantage for patients who undergo radical tumor resection [1,12–15]. The concern regarding these studies is that in the absence of prospective randomized data, significant selection bias may have occurred [16]. The actual difference between survival in patients treated with biopsy, as opposed to radical resection plus adjunctive therapy, may not be as profound as might be assumed from cursory review of retrospective data.

Table 1
Breakdown of studies showing a positive trend toward the number of studies in which extensive resection is favored over time

Studies in which the prognostic effect of extent of resection on survival was assessed using statistical analysis

| Prognostic effect | Authors and year (no. of patients) | | | |
|---|---|---|---|---|
| | 1985 and before | 1986–1990 | 1991–1995 | 1996–2000 |
| Statistics favor more extensive resections | Laws Jr et al, 1984 (461) | Soffietti et al, 1989 (85) | Ito et al, 1994 (87) | Bahary et al, 1996 (63) |
| | | North et al, 1990 (77) | Nicolato et al, 1995 (74) | Karim et al, 1996 (343) |
| | | | Philippon et al, 1993 (179) | Piepmeier et al, 1996 (55) |
| | | | Shaw et al, 1994 (71) | Scerrati et al, 1996 (131) |
| | | | Rajan et al, 1994 (82) | Leighton et al, 1997 (167) |
| | | | Janny et al, 1994 (32) | Lote et al, 1997 (97) |
| | | | | Jeremic et al, 1998 (37) |
| | | | | Peraud et al, 1998 (75) |
| | | | | van Veelen et al, 1998 (90) |
| Statistics do not favor any resection group | | Piepmeier 1987 (60) | Eyre et al, 1993 (54) | Lote et al, 1997 (379) |
| | | Medberry et al, 1988 (50) | Miralbell et al, 1993 (49) | Rudoler et al, 1998 (30) |
| | | Shaw et al, 1989 (126) | Shibamoto et al, 1993 (101) | Bauman et al, 1999 (401) |
| | | Shaw et al, 1989 (49) | Singer, 1995 (43) | |
| | | Whitton and Bloom 1990 (88) | | |

*Reproduced from* Keles GE, Lamborn KR, Berger MS. Low-grade hemispheric gliomas in adults: a critical review of extent of resection as a factor influencing outcome. J Neurosurg. 2001;95(5):735–45; with permission.

In 1991, Quigley and Maroon [17] analyzed all surgical series published in English with at least 75 patients treated for supratentorial malignant gliomas. Twenty surgical series, with a total of 5691 patients, were included in the meta-analysis. Twenty-one percent of patients underwent gross total resection, based solely on a neurosurgeon's intraoperative impression rather than objective postoperative neuroimaging. In general, more radical cytoreduction was associated with improved median survival. Eight of sixteen series showed improved survival with more aggressive surgery, although half of these could not display statistical significance with subsequent multivariate analysis. The relatively modest effect of surgery was confounded by the impact of other fixed prognostic factors on survival, most notably patient age, histology, and preoperative Karnofsky performance status (KPS) scores. A surgeon's assessment of extent of resection, which is subject to reporting bias, and the inability to detect microscopic tumor adds serious limitations to the extrapolation of data found in these series.

Contemporaneously, Nazzaro and Neuwelt [18] systematically reviewed the same topic and noted that most publications failed to compensate for the important effects of patient age, performance status, and tumor location. They observed that craniotomy and biopsy techniques had improved markedly in recent years and that the use of corticosteroids had a major impact on nonsurgical management of increased intracranial pressure. The investigators reviewed the limitations of CT and magnetic resonance (MR) scanning in delimiting the extent of tumor and surgeons'uo; "impression" of the extent of resection. Many of the reports included in the review, unfortunately, did not report details of radiation, chemotherapy, and reoperation adequately, all of which have a potential impact on survival. In analyzing each study with regards to the hierarchy of strength of study design (randomized controlled trials to uncontrolled case series), most were along the weaker end of the spectrum and often entirely lacked statistical analysis. Despite these limitations, the investigators concluded that patients who underwent aggressive surgical resection in the absence of chemotherapy and radiation clearly did better than patients who did not, although benefits of debulking in patients undergoing postoperative adjuvant therapy remained unproved.

Lacroix and colleagues [14] retrospectively reviewed 416 patients who had glioblastoma whose tumors were debulked between 1993 and 1999 at the MD Anderson Cancer Center. This represented the initial surgery for 233 patients, the remainder having had biopsy or initial cytoreductive surgery elsewhere. The criteria for undergoing debulking were not specified, but only 9% of tumors were in the basal ganglia, thalamus, insula, or posterior fossa. Preoperative and postoperative MRIs underwent quantitative analysis for tumor volume. Approximately half of the operations yielded over a 98% reduction in tumor burden. Multivariate analysis of tumor location, preoperative tumor volume, presence of mass effect, and initial versus repeat surgery for recurrence did not reveal a statistically significant impact on survival. Resection of greater than 89% of preoperative tumor volume was necessary to demonstrate improved survival after surgery. The benefit was augmented with increasing extent of resection. A resection greater than 98% was associated with signfiicant survival advantage at univariate and multivariate analyses (median survival 13 months after surgery versus 8.8 months if <98%). Survival benefit from these extensive resections was demonstrable in patients undergoing initial surgery and those undergoing repeat surgery for recurrence. The investigators concluded that a gross total resection should be performed whenever possible, although not at the expense of neurologic function (which was not analyzed in this report) [14].

The Glioma Outcomes Project represents a contemporary analysis of the management of malignant gliomas. This observational database of 788 patients from multiple sites over a 4-year period (1997–2001) was used to evaluate the influence of resection, as opposed to biopsy, on patient outcome as measured by the length of survival. This study provided class II evidence to support resection (compared with biopsy) as a strong prognostic factor [20]. In a more recent retrospective analysis of factors influencing survival in 340 patients who had newly diagnosed glioblastoma multiforme, radical surgery was ranked second in its power as prognostic factor [21].

Scott and colleagues identified 15 long-term survivors of glioblastoma (> 36 months) in a Canadian provincial cancer registry and matched them to controls based on age, gender, and year of diagnosis [22]. Patients were classified as undergoing gross total resection or less than gross total resection. Long-term survivors were more likely to have had gross total tumor resection based on a surgeon's assessment (40% versus 14%). Other studies of long-term survivors, although uncontrolled, also suggest that patients who have aggressive resections are overly represented among long-term survivors [23–25].

The past decade has seen widespread acceptance of the principle that impact on quality of life may be as important as impact on survival. Until recently, the literature on this topic was limited to retrospective reports by Ammirati and colleagues and Ciric and colleagues [12,26], who noted that patients undergoing gross total tumor resection experienced postoperative improvements in KPS score and survival not seen in patients undergoing subtotal tumor resection and that postresection patients usually were neurologically stable (55%) or improved (41%) [12]. The best data on the effect of surgery on quality of life in malignant glioma come from a study of 65 glioblastomas treated surgically between 1995 and 1998 with preoperative MR scanning, use of the operating microscope, and in most cases neuronavigation [27]. All patients underwent attempted resection, with the extent of resection based on early postoperative enhanced CT scan. Pre- and postoperative (day 7) KPS and neurologic functional status were assessed. Four of five patients who had KPS scores that deteriorated greater than 20 points had severe systemic complications. Patients who had tumors in eloquent cortex dropped a median of 6.5 points, whereas patients who had tumors in silent cortex rose a median of 5 points. Patients who had at least 75% reduction in tumor volume displayed a marginal improvement in KPS, whereas those having lesser amounts of tumor removed declined 7.3 points. Of note, the subtotal tumor resections generally were in eloquent cortex. The subset of patients undergoing gross total resection generally was found to have significant functional improvement.

The debate regarding the need for maximal resection in high-grade gliomas continues, but in certain circumstances, there can be no question regarding surgical approach. Patient who have a large frontopolar or temporal tip mass with substantial mass effect or herniation require debulking; patients who have tumor in the heart of eloquent cortex, in whom resection would produce aphasia or substantial permanent hemiparesis, should undergo biopsy. Many cases fall into neither category, however. In the absence of class I data, no firm conclusions regarding the benefit of aggressive resection for these malignant gliomas can be drawn. Nonetheless, the magnitude of this benefit—at most a few months on average—is small. Continued technologic improvements may make resections safer in terms of sparing eloquent cortex, but their role in improving survival substantially is yet to be delineated [28].

## Brain mapping

Historically, adjacency to eloquent cortices, including language and motor cortices, predetermined that many brain tumors were inoperable. Now, with advances in preoperative and intraoperative brain mapping techniques, surgeons reliably can predict the localization of brain function and thereby operate on brain tumors once believed inoperable, maximize the resection of pathologic tissue, and minimize iatrogenic damage during neurosurgical resections. Although intraoperative brain mapping, in particular electrocortical stimulation mapping (ESM), has been an integral part of neurosurgical procedures for decades, recent reports of its beneficial impact on outcomes of brain tumor surgery have increased its use and applications [29,30]. Moreover, surgeons increasingly are using subcortical stimulation mapping to identify functional white matter tracts to be spared during surgery, theoretically making brain tumor surgery even safer. Although advances in intraoperative brain mapping have allowed surgeons to resect tumors more aggressively during surgery, advances in preoperative mapping have revolutionized the neurosurgical approach to brain tumors. By providing a preoperative noninvasive assessment of brain function, preoperative brain mapping techniques, in particular functional MRI (fMRI) and magnetic source imaging (MSI), have empowered surgeons to operate on patients who had brain tumors whom they may not have considered eligible for surgical resection in the past.

### Intraoperative brain mapping

### Evoked potentials

Measurement of somatosensory evoked potentials (SSEPs) can provide accurate and rapid localization of the central sulcus in patients under local or general anesthesia [31]. A phase reversal of the evoked potentials recorded between cortical electrodes corresponds to the site of the central sulcus. Early reports confirmed the reliability and accuracy of SSEPs, relative to the gold standard (stimulation mapping, described later) [31,32]. The application of SSEPs for brain tumors surgery is limited, however, compared with the versatility and reliability of stimulation mapping.

*Cortical and subcortical stimulation mapping*

Cortical and subcortical stimulation are used to map the brain intraoperatively by activating the tissue of interest (motor mapping) or by inducing temporary, reversible dysfunction that interrupts function (language mapping). Technologic advances have made ESM easier to implement and a more routine part of neurosurgery. Advances in neuroanesthesia have made awake craniotomies increasingly tolerable and safe [19,33,34]. Moreover, for motor mapping, patients now can remain asleep throughout surgery with motor responses detected using electromyography.

ESM has emerged as the gold standard for neurosurgical brain mapping because the effects of direct cortical stimulation mimic the effects of resection. Foerster [35] first used ESM to map motor and sensory cortices more than 70 years ago. Penfield and Roberts [36] later demonstrated that ESM can be used to map language cortices. In the first comprehensive study of the reliability of ESM, Haglund and colleagues [37] reported that resection of cortical tissue greater than 1 cm away from essential language sites was associated with 100% language recovery whereas resection of cortices within 1 cm of these sites was associated with long-term language deficits. In more recent series, surgeons actively stimulate the margins of the resection cavity throughout the resective procedure. Further reports confirm that ESM not only is predictive of postoperative outcomes but also is also task specific, allowing surgeons to investigate multiple cognitive functional intraoperatively. For example, in bilingual patients, stimulation of some cortical areas may disrupt processing of only one language [38,39].

To quantify the contribution of ESM to the efficacy and safety of glioma surgery, Duffau and colleagues [29] compared a retrospective series of 100 patients operated on without intraoperative mapping (between 1985 and 1996) and a prospective series of 122 patients operated on with the use of ESM (between 1996 and 2003). Although the latter group had an increased mean duration of surgery (5 versus 3 hours), it had a significantly lower rate of severe permanent deficits (6.5% versus 17%), a higher rate of gross total and subtotal resections (25% and 51% versus 6% and 37%, respectively), and a survival advantage [29]. The definition of "operability" changed significantly between the two series: the percent of tumors operated on within eloquent cortices increased from 35% to 62%. These advantages associated with the routine use of ESM for the resection of brain tumors increasingly are important in light of mounting evidence that extent of resection improve outcomes (see previous discussion). Despite its advantages, ESM has potential drawbacks, the most important of which are the induction of after-discharge (or seizure) activity, long mapping times, and limited spatial resolution.

Stimulation of subcortical white matter tracts increasingly has become an important adjunct to intraoperative mapping, allowing surgeons to spare these descending pathways and predict postoperative morbidity. Keles and colleagues [40] retrospectively analyzed 294 patients who were operated on for perirolandic gliomas. Patients in whom subcortical motor tracts were identified (149 patients, 51%) were significantly more likely to experience temporary (28% versus 13%) and permanent (7% versus 2%) motor deficits compared with patients in whom subcortical motor pathways could not be identified [40]. Duffau and colleagues [41] reported that subcortical stimulation mapping was useful in minimizing permanent language deficits in patients who had dominant hemisphere gliomas and maximizing tumor resection. Based on these findings, the investigators advocate routinely alternating tumor resection with stimulation mapping to avoid interrupting descending pathways.

Cortical stimulation mapping also can be done by implanting strips or grids of subdural electrodes. Although this offers a well-controlled environment in which to map a patient's brain, this requires a second surgery for the implantation procedure, limits the resolution of cortical mapping to 1-cm increments (based on the spacing of electrodes in implanted grids), precludes the opportunity to perform subcortical mapping, and exposes patients to potential infections associated with externalized electrode leads. Consequently, intraoperative mapping is preferred.

*Optical imaging of intrinsic signals*

Intraoperative optical imaging of intrinsic signals (iOIS) maps the brain by detecting cortical reflectance changes that are related to perfusion-related responses that are coupled to neuronal activity. iOIS offers potential advantages over the current gold standard, ESM, including spatial resolution as high as 200 μm, resulting in a more detailed functional map, thereby allowing more extensive resection and a more rapid assessment than ESM of large areas of cortex. Optical maps are created by using a highly sensitive charge-coupled device camera to detect changes in cortical light reflectance, on a pixel-by-pixel basis, between a resting and an activated state (for example, while performing an object naming task).

Optical responses first were reported in humans by Haglund and colleagues [42] during after-discharge activity, in motor cortex during tongue movement, and in Broca's and Wernicke's areas during visual object naming exercises. Optical maps are correlated spatially with maps derived using electrophysiologic techniques (ESM) but offer higher spatial resolution than these other techniques [42–45]. Ninety-eight percent of sites deemed active by ESM demonstrate optical changes. This indicates that those areas identified by ESM as essential for a specific task consistently demonstrate optical activity [46]. The high sensitivity of iOIS brain mapping allows surgeons to resect tissues not deemed active by iOIS aggressively. Optical maps extend beyond the regions indicated by ESM, however, detecting all areas that are active during a task rather than just those that are "essential." Areas that demonstrate optical signals, therefore, must be interrogated further with ESM to determine whether or not they must be preserved. Combining iOIS with ESM potentially decreases the total time of intraoperative mapping (as opposed to ESM alone) when mapping several functions.

The limitations of iOIS as an intraoperative tool arise from the fact that maps are based on the coupled perfusion response. It long has been assumed that neurovascular coupling is tight. Although many studies conclude that brain tumors alter perfusion responses significantly [47–49], others have not found a deleterious effect [50,51]. In cases where decreased response magnitudes are noted, the observed decrease in primary motor cortex activation may be the result of several factors, including decreased number of functional neurons in the motor strip, the effect of compression of eloquent cortices, tumor-mediated changes in local cerebral hemodynamics, and changes in global perfusion resulting from the presence of a neoplasm [47].

*Preoperative brain mapping*

Preoperative brain mapping offers the opportunity to map multiple tasks before surgery in a repeated fashion. Moreover, by providing a preoperative assessment of the localization of brain function, preoperative brain mapping enables surgeons to offer surgery to patients who have brain tumors whom they otherwise may not have considered for surgery (Fig. 1). These preoperative maps help determine the need for intraoperative mapping, the best approach (or corridor) to tumor resection that would spare eloquent cortices, and the limits of resection before taking patients to surgery. Moreover, they hold the potential of reducing intraoperative mapping time if accurate and reliable preoperative maps can be generated; preoperative maps can help direct the intraoperative selection of stimulation sites for more efficient intraoperative mapping. Attempts have been made to integrate preoperative maps with frameless stereotactic navigation systems [52,53]. Because of "brain shift," or the herniation or collapse of the brain after craniotomy and dural reflection, however, preoperative maps cannot be relied on solely for functional localization, thereby reserving a place for intraoperative mapping (structural and functional).

Positron emission tomography (PET) was the first tomographic modality used for preoperative functional brain mapping [54]. Because of the accessibility and increased spatial resolution of other modalities that do not require the use of radioisotopes, PET largely has been replaced by fMRI and MSI.

*Functional MRI*

fMRI has become the predominant functional neuroimaging technique since its original report [55]. Like iOIS, blood-oxygen-level dependent–fMRI is a functional neuroimaging technique that maps the brain by detecting perfusion-related changes that are coupled to neuronal activity (see Fig. 1). fMRI has become increasingly sensitive and reliable with recent technologic advances, including increasing MR field strengths, better sequence design and selection, improved task design and selection, and superior analysis techniques (see, for example, the report of Roessler and colleagues [56]). Increasing field strength provides a greater dynamic range

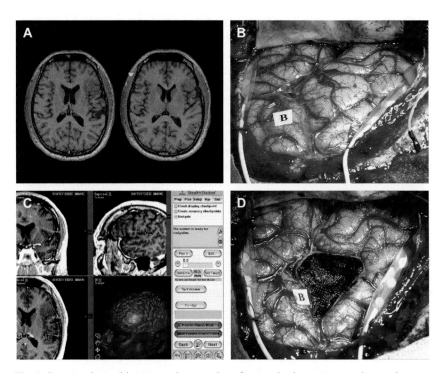

Fig. 1. Preoperative and intraoperative mapping of expressive language areas in a patient presenting with progressive seizures and a left inferior frontal tumor. (*A*) Preoperative fMRI mapping cortical areas activated during an object-naming task. Activated areas (*represented in red*) are posterior to the tumor allowing the surgeon to proceed with resection. (*B*) Intraoperative ESM identified a single cortical area that when stimulated consistently induces aphasia (labeled "B") (*C*) Using intraoperative neuronavigation, the surgeon can identify the location of the essential language site (indicated by green crosshair), confirming the accuracy of the preoperative fMRI map. The tumor, as indicated by the preoperative fMRI, is anterior to the language area. (*D*) Based on the preoperative fMRI map and intraoperative ESM, the surgeon is able to perform a gross total resection of the tumor, sparing critical language areas, without postoperative language deficit. (*Courtesy of* Dr. Jeff Elias, Charlottesville, VA.)

of data collection and, ultimately, a greater signal-to-noise ratio (SNR) and contrast-to-noise ratio [57]. Increasing field strength also provides greater spatial resolution for preoperative brain mapping, which enhances the technique's sensitivity, particularly where small differences in localization of function are crucial to the clinical decision or outcome. Finally, higher field strengths allow more rapid imaging, which is particularly important in clinical populations that may not tolerate prolonged imaging sessions in the bore of the MR scanner. Higher field strengths also introduce challenges, in particular that of significantly increased susceptibility artifacts, especially near the air-filled sinuses, which can interfere with the identification of temporal lobe language sites.

FitzGerald and colleagues [58] studied the correlation of fMRI with ESM in patients who had glioma using multiple language tasks. They required that "activation from only one of the tasks [was] required to touch the language tag" for a positive match to be identified, reporting high sensitivity (percent of positive ESM sites, which colocalized with fMRI activations, ranging from 81%–92%) but low specificity (0%–53%), meaning that many, if not all, ESM sites negative for language overlapped with fMRI activations [58]. Pouratian and colleagues [59] similarly reported the sensitivity and specificity of fMRI activations during expressive linguistic tasks of up to 100% and 66.7%, respectively, in the frontal lobe and during comprehension linguistic tasks up to 96.2% and 69.8%, respectively, in the parietal/temporal lobes. As with iOIS, the low specificity likely is the result of activation of nonessential cortices. Based on these results, preoperative fMRI can direct surgeons to areas of interest to determine whether or not activated cortices are essential or nonessential, obviating mapping the entirety of the exposed cortex (see Fig. 1). In contrast, Roux and colleagues [52] reported that fMRI has poor sensitivity (22%–57%) but excellent specificity (approximately 97%). The differences in results likely are attributable to multiple factors, including task design and postacquisition analysis techniques. Despite the inconsistencies, one pattern that has emerged is that the reliability of preoperative fMRI maps is enhanced by mapping multiple cognitive tasks preoperatively [52,59].

Although several studies have quantified the sensitivity and specificity of fMRI activations relative to electrophysiologic maps [52,60–65], the relationship between fMRI maps and clinical outcomes remains uncharacterized. Like iOIS, fMRI is plagued by the question of whether or not perfusion-related responses are affected adversely by the adjacent tumor (see previous discussion). As long-term outcomes ultimately are the most important variable in clinical neurosurgery, outcomes studies, like that of Haglund and colleagues [37] that characterized clinical outcomes postoperatively relative to stimulation-based maps, are needed to define the best approach to clinical fMRI mapping.

*Magnetoencephalography and magnetic source imaging*

Magnetoencephalography (MEG) is the detection of minute magnetic fields produced by the brain's electrical activity. Although in its earliest manifestation, MEG was done with a single detector, the introduction of whole-scalp MEG instruments revolutionized the role and contribution of MEG to the field of neurosurgery. MSI represents the fusion of multichannel MEG and MRI, in which the source localization of MEG signals is coregistered with anatomic MRI. Rather than defining extent of activation, MEG/MSI approximates the center of gravity of activation. This estimation depends on post-acquisition analysis, which is challenging because of the lack of a unique solution. Multiple models (each with unique assumptions) are used, therefore, to localize the magnetic source (see other reports for a full discussion) [66,67]. Like other mapping techniques, MSI maps are generated by comparing activity during a resting state with that detected during a specific task (eg, finger tapping for mapping motor cortex). Ultimately, task selection for MSI mapping depends on the location of the tumor and the area targeted for mapping.

Like fMRI, MSI correlates well with intraoperative maps [67,68]. Schiff-bauer and colleagues [67] compared MSI with intraoperative maps of somatosensory and motor cortex in 224 patients (the largest quantitative comparison to date), reporting a mean 2-D difference of 12.5 mm between somatosensory maps derived by MSI and ESM (range 1.5–30.3 mm). Although not a precise colocalization, MSI was helpful for preoperative assessment and planning. Moreover, MSI can be used to identify the 25% to 46% of patients who have gliomas who are at risk for neurologic deficit from surgical intervention because of the presence of functional active tissue within or at the border of tumor [69–71]. This information can be used in a systematic manner for determining which patients can be referred for surgical debulking: patients who have MSI in or within 5 mm of the tumor margin are considered high-risk for neurologic deficit; those who have source localizations between 6 and 10 mm of the tumor margin are slated for subtotal resection; and those who have localizations greater than 10 mm are deemed candidates for gross total resection [70].

As the causes of the mapping signals are different in MEG/MSI and fMRI, the maps generated often are different. MSI may be more accurate than fMRI for mapping the central sulcus, presumably because of activation of nonprimary cortices with the latter methodology [72]. Still, other institutions have found that combining fMRI and MEG for preoperative evaluation and intraoperative guidance is a superior technique. Using this strategy, Grummich and colleagues [71] limited transient postoperative language deficits to 5.6% of the 124 patients they included in their series, with no patients experiencing permanent deficits.

*Diffusion tensor imaging*

Diffusion-tensor imaging (DTI) is an MRI technique of creating probabilistic maps of white matter pathways based on voxel anisotropy or the preferential direction of diffusion of water. The major white matter bundles traversing each voxel determine the direction of diffusion, allowing extrapolation of white matter tracts. This has become an increasingly important modality for the planning of glioma surgery; DTI can identify white matter pathways that should be spared during surgery to ensure that functional cortices (identified by other techniques) are not disconnected from their respective projection areas (Fig. 2) [73]. Kamada and coworkers [74] verified that preoperative cortical and subcortical maps generated by a combination of fMRI, MSI, and DTI are predictive and can be confirmed by intraoperative cortical and subcortical stimulation mapping. Such maps potentially can be useful for planning surgical approaches and extent of resection, especially with the development of new techniques in DTI.

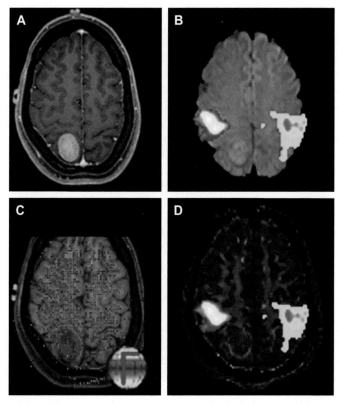

Fig. 2. Combining fMRI with DTI to guide brain tumor resection. (*A*) Gadolinium-enhanced T1 axial MRI revealing a right parietal meningioma, presumably immediately posterior to the central sulcus. (*B*) fMRI map demonstrates activations (colored blobs) in pre- and postcentral gyri during finger tapping tasks. (*C*) Diffusion-tensor map illustrates a color-coded scheme to delineate the preferential direction of diffusion of water at each voxel, presumably analogous to the direction of the predominant white matter pathway at each voxel. As indicated by the legend, voxels with white matter pathways predominantly in the lateral direction are red/pink; those with pathways predominantly in the anterior posterior direction are green (with few voxels with such a representation in the selected slice); and those with pathways predominantly in the superior-inferior direction are green. (*D*) DTI and fMRI maps then can be fused for intraoperative guidance. (*Courtesy of* Dr. Lubdha Shah, Charlottesville, VA.)

## Neuronavigation and intraoperative MRI

The applicability of brain mapping techniques to tumor surgery is unquestionable. Contemporaneous to the growing interest in expanding the clinical usefulness of brain mapping techniques, others have focused their efforts in increasing the efficacy and safety of surgery, especially in noneloquent regions, through development of tools that aide surgeons'uo; comprehension of the distorted anatomy. Techniques that improve surgeons'uo; orientation within the intracranial cavity at the time of surgery and assist in determining the margins of tumor tissue should, in theory, allow improved volumetric resections.

*Neuronavigation*

In the past, surgeons have relied on their own 3-D extrapolation of preoperative imaging studies, knowledge of pertinent neuroanatomy, and intraoperative visual and tactile evaluation to guide their resection. The introduction of image guidance for stereotactic localization and intraoperative assistance can be credited to Spiegel and colleagues [75]. In 1947, they obtained ventriculographic images with a rigid frame attached to the patient's head. Correlation of reference marks on the frame with the neuroanatomic relationship between cerebral structures and the ventricles obtained from the imaging enabled them to localize lesions within the brain. The "encephalatome," as it was termed, soon was followed by the development of other stereotactic frames, including those compatible with improving diagnostic imaging technology. The introduction of CT and MRI into clinical practice in the 1970s and 1980s revolutionized the perioperative management of patients and also allowed stereotactic biopsies to be performed with increasing accuracy and precision.

Although this frame-based stereotaxy represented an improvement over surgeons'uo; conceptualized view in most cases, it made open surgical approaches to tumors cumbersome for neurosurgeons and the application of the frame uncomfortable for patients undergoing a biopsy. In 1986, as computer software and hardware became more robust and affordable, the idea of frameless navigation using concepts of acoustic triangulation was introduced by Roberts and coworkers [76]. The current frameless stereotactic neuronavigation devices used by most neurosurgeons use optical/light-emitting diode (LED) triangulation or low-frequency electromagnetic fields to determine the location of the pointer/instrument within the operative field. Preoperative CT and MRI scans are obtained with fiducial markers, and these are calibrated with the affixed reference array at the time of surgery. This allows surgeons to refer intraoperatively to preoperative images in several planes of view simultaneously and render 3-D reconstructions that ease the conceptualization of regional anatomic relationships. The usefulness of neuronavigation may be highlighted in the resection of low-grade gliomas, where preoperative imaging may clearly may depict pathology, but intraoperative findings are too miniscule to differentiate by simple visual or tactile evaluation by a surgeon. Most neurosurgeons believe that neuronavigational systems are easy to use and helpful in the resection of glial tumors [77]. The accuracy of these systems also has allowed the majority of biopsies to be performed without the use of stereotactic frames, making biopsies less cumbersome, less painful, and more time efficient.

Despite the advances in neuronavigational systems, intraoperative stereotactic localization of potentially functional cerebral cortex is unreliable because the presence of tumor may distort the normal cortical anatomy

[78]. The combination of cortical mapping and neuronavigation for resection of intracranial lesions is reported favorably. Stapleton and colleagues [79] used both techniques to facilitate the removal of lesions in eloquent locations in 16 pediatric patients. The investigators reported one postoperative neurologic deficit, which was transient in nature. Half of the lesions in this series were glial neoplasms. Lumenta and colleagues [80] described a series of 40 patients who underwent resection of deep-seated intracerebral lesions using neuronavigation and cortical mapping. Complete resections were possible in all but three patients. Permanent neurologic deficits were present in two patients only. Twenty-one of these patients had glial neoplasms. Meyer and coworkers [78] reported a series of 65 consecutive patients who underwent intraoperative cortical/subcortial mapping and frameless stereotactic resection of glial tumors located in functional tissue. More than 50% of patients had a greater than 90% reduction in tumor volume based on postoperative MRI. Seventy-four percent of patients developed intraoperative deficits but 71% recovered to a modified Rankin grade of 0 or 1 by 3 months postoperatively. Forty-five of these patients had grade III or IV infiltrating glial neoplasms. There was no operative mortality.

*Intraoperative MRI*

The accuracy of preoperative MRI as an intraoperative guide decreases as cerebrospinal fluid is lost, tumor is removed, and brain edema accumulates. This discrepancy, which may be up to 1 cm in most neurosurgical cranial procedures, is termed, "brain shift" [81,82]. The collapse of tumor resection cavities and intraparenchymal changes are difficult to model [83]. Brain shift is a continuous and dynamic process that evolves differently in distinct brain regions and is one of the greatest criticisms of using frameless neuronavigation as the sole guide for resection of tumors that are large or located in a dependent position. With the advent of open MR systems, the applicability of real-time MRI as an intraoperative tool became realized.

There are several types of intraoperative MR systems, and they differ based on field strength (low and high), surgeons'uo; access to patients ease of use, and time efficiency in image acquisition [84]. In most low-field systems, except the GE double donut, surgery is performed outside the 5-gauss line where standard operative equipment and microscope can be used [85]. Surgery is halted and patients are brought within the magnet for image acquisition. This process tends to lengthen the operative time and disrupts the flow of the operation. When the double donut is used, surgery is performed within the magnet itself without the need to move patient or magnet and allows surgeons to acquire images easily (each plane within 60 to 120 seconds) [84]. Surgeons who use the double donut take images throughout the procedure, whereas those using systems where patients must be brought into the scanner tend to take images less frequently. The GE double-donut system, however, creates a somewhat restricted surgical field and requires specific MR-compatible instruments, microscope, and anesthesia equipment.

Also in use are high-field systems made by Phillips (at the University of Minnesota, National Institutes of Health), the 1.5-T Magnex system (at the University of Calgary), and the Siemens 1.5-T imager. Within the past 2 years, a 3-T high-field system installed at the University of Minnesota has been used and reported on [86]. These systems provide superior-quality images and allow surgeons to use MRI-incompatible equipment outside the 5-gauss line. High-field systems improve SNR and provide standard diagnostic MR capabilities, including MR spectroscopy, MR angiography, MR venography, diffusion-weighted imaging, and functional imaging [87,88]. The high-field imager allows shorter examination times but its primary drawback is the significant financial and structural investment in comparison to their low-field system counterparts. Each of these systems requires transportation of patient or magnet to obtain images. Although in the Phillips and Siemens systems patients are transported into the scanner, in the Calgary system it is the scanner that is brought around patients [89].

The first interventional unit was installed in Boston in 1994. Since that time, selected centers have used MRI in interventional and operative forums and report the extent of tumor resection can be monitored with significantly improved accuracy [89–96]. The largest single center experience includes more than 900 neurosurgical procedures performed at the Brigham and Women's Hospital from 1995 to 2004. Black and colleagues [97] report that in more than one third of cases, a surgeon's judgment of no residual tumor was incorrect, leading to the possibility of further resection. In a series of 16 brain tumor patients, Nimsky and colleagues [82] reported that the real-time updating of the neuronavigational system with iMRI data was associated with high accuracy and added only 15 minutes to operation time. Complete tumor removal was achieved in 14 patients. In 2000, Wirtz and colleagues [98] reported on 97 procedures for supratentorial glioma treatment that were analyzed with respect to iMRI results and postoperative outcomes. For high-grade gliomas, the percentage of cases in which residual tumor was identified was reduced from 62% intraoperatively to 33% postoperatively, which was paralleled by a significant increase in survival times for patients who did not have residual tumor. The mean progression-free interval was 3.4 months for patients who had residual glioblastoma multiforme compared with 6.2 months for patients who did not have residual tumor.

At this time, each available iMRI system is a prototype. The balancing of expense, SNR and resolution, ease of access during surgery, and time efficiency has made the development of the ideal system difficult. It would be one that provides rapid high-quality multiplanar images with maximal access to patients in a variety of surgical positions without requiring new surgical equipment or instruments. The authors are confident that the shortcomings are temporary and that the discretionary use of iMRI will help this technology find a suitable niche in brain tumor surgery.

**Advances in surgical adjunctive therapy**

Despite these advances in tumor resection surgery, malignant gliomas remain among the most rapidly fatal neoplasms. Unlike the treatment of systemic cancer, effective systemic treatment of malignant gliomas must reach widely infiltrating tumor cells, many protected by an intact blood-brain barrier. The challenge of crossing this barrier while minimizing systemic toxicity has led researchers to explore the role of interstitial treatment options. The concurrent expansion along this frontier provides a biologic modality that may augment the usefulness of resection in the surgical treatment of these lesions. Intuitively, molecular approaches have garnered significant hope for the effective local treatment of residual microinvasive tumor cells. The most extensively studied and used of these treatment modalities include interstitial therapeutics via sustained release polymers, convection-enhanced delivery (CED), brachytherapy, and gene therapy (the latter is not presented in this discussion).

*Sustained release polymers*

Interstitial chemotherapy via sustained release polymers requires a polymer-drug combination that delivers the chemotherapeutic agent directly to a resection cavity immediately after surgical resection of a malignant glioma. The polymer provides a controlled release of the drug from a biodegradable matrix. Of the various chemotherapeutic agents that could be used as a possible treatment agent, carmustine (BCNU) is the only Food and Drug Administration (FDA)–approved drug for current use with a sustained release polymer. The polymer-BCNU combination is marketed as Gliadel and is approved for use in patients who have recurrent (1996) or newly diagnosed (2003) glioblastomas [99].

BCNU is an alkylating agent that traditionally is used for treatment of malignant gliomas via intravenous perfusion. A variety of systemic toxicities, however, characterize the medication and include delayed hematopoietic depression and cytotoxic effects on the lungs, kidney, liver, and central nervous system [100]. Furthermore, BCNU penetrates approximately only 2 mm through local brain tissue through the ependymal surface, limiting the intracranial volume of distribution via cerebrospinal fluid [101]. Several polymer-BCNU systems initially were studied in xenograft models and the polyanhydride [(poly(bis(p-carboxyphenoxy)-propane) (PCPP–sebacic acid (SA) (PCPP-SA) polymer was found nontoxic and biocompatible [102]. Subsequent studies investigated interstitial chemotherapy of malignant gliomas in xenograft models and displayed a sustained delivery of BCNU for approximately 5 days after treatment and a significant delay in tumor growth [103,104].

As is standard for a dose-escalation trial, human clinical trials started at much lower doses of BCNU than those used with laboratory animals. A multi-institutional phase I–II clinical trial found 3.85% BCNU, the intermediate dose, to be the safest and potentially the most effective dose [105]. A phase III subsequently was conducted in 27 centers and included 222 patients who had recurrent malignant gliomas. The patients were randomized into groups that received the polymer with BCNU or the polymer alone. The study displayed a statistically significant increase in 6-month survival with 64% in the BCNU-polymer group and 44% in the polymer alone group [106]. The FDA subsequently approved the BCNU-polymer implant as Gliadel for use in patients who have recurrent malignant glioma.

Theoretically, treatments that are effective at recurrence should be equally effective, if not more effective, at initial presentation. Based on this theory, a phase I and phase III study subsequently were performed to test the BCNU-polymer implant in patients who had newly diagnosed malignant glioma. Valtonen and colleagues [107] performed the initial phase III trial, in which 32 patients were divided randomly into a BCNU-polymer group and a placebo group. The study displayed a median survival of 58.1 weeks in the BCNU-polymer group and a median survival of 39.9 weeks in the placebo group ($P = .008$). In addition, 25% of the former and 6% of the latter were alive after 3 years. A second phase III study was conducted by the European Association of Neurological Surgeons and showed similar efficacy. This study included 240 patients and displayed a median survival of 14 months in the BCNU-polymer group as compared with 11.6 months in the placebo group [108]. Based on the aforementioned clinical trials, the FDA subsequently approved the use of Gliadel of the initial treatment of glioblastoma.

A variety of interstitial chemotherapy trials are underway with the goal of improving drug delivery and effectiveness. As discussed previously, human clinical trials of BCNU started with lower doses than those tolerated by laboratory animals. Subsequent dose escalation trials in rats and primates displayed increased efficacy with a concentration of 20% BCNU. Tissue concentrations of significant concentration also were found up to 2 cm from the polymer site up to 30 days after surgery implantation [109]. A human phase I study displayed the maximum tolerated dose at 20% BCNU leading to a current phase III trial [110]. In addition to BCNU, a variety of chemotherapeutic agents are being combined with polymer preparations and tested in dose escalation studies. These agents include Taxol, campothecin, carboplatin, and 4-hydroperoxycyclophosphamide [110–113]. In addition to chemotherapeutic agents, other medications, such as minocycline, a angiogenic inhibitor; 5-iodo-2'-deoxyuridine (IUdR), a radiosensitizer; and interferon, an immunomodulator, currently are under clinical investigation [114–116]. Finally, BCNU-polymer implants are being investigated in combination with other treatment modalities, such as resistance modulators (eg, $O^6$-benzylguanine) and immunotherapy [117,118].

## Convection-enhanced delivery

The delivery method of therapeutic agents into the intracranial interstitial cavity must provide regional specificity, a quantifiable volume of distribution, and a uniform concentration in the region of interest. The primary goal of such a delivery technique is to provide an accurate therapeutic dosage of the selected drug while decreasing the risk for toxic or subtherapeutic concentrations. CED is a drug-delivery method currently investigated to provide such drug-delivery goals [119].

CED is a direct drug transfer technique via a bulk flow mechanism. In this method, a syringe pump provides a small pressure gradient through intracranial catheters to direct a drug to a specific target site [120]. CED provides a greater volume of distribution of the drug than simple diffusion procedures. Real-time in vivo imaging using a low-molecular-weight tracer displays a linear relationship between volume of infusion and volume of distribution. Such a tracer allows for effective monitoring of drug delivery, as seen in in vivo models [121].

In addition to analyzing volume of distribution, design and appropriate placement of the infusion catheter are important for accurate and effective drug delivery. A primary design goal for these catheters is to prevent reflux of a potentially cytotoxic agent and subsequent leakage at the surface of the brain. Such a catheter allows for a high infusion rate, as previous designs correlated increased infusion rate with an increased rate of reflux. The placement of the catheters also is vital to the precise delivery of a drug to a specific location at a uniform concentration [122]. CED typically is studied after tumor resection. The primary region of interest for drug infusion involves brain parenchyma directly adjacent to the tumor cavity without actually infusing the drug into the cavity itself. In addition, the catheters should not be too close to the subarachnoid space or to the ventricle to prevent diffusion of the drug into the cerebrospinal fluid. Stereotaxy is a method by which these catheters are placed accurately into the appropriate locations around the tumor resection cavity (Fig. 3).

The technique of CED currently is under clinical investigation using a variety of therapeutic agents. These agents include chemotherapeutic drugs, toxins derived from bacteria, and radioisotope-labeled monoclonal antibodies. Phase I–III clinical trials currently are focusing on patients who have recurrent high-grade gliomas. Lidar and colleagues [123] performed a phase I–II clinical study in such a patient population and delivered paclitaxel to patients over a maximum of 5 days. The primary complication that reduced the number of treatment cycles was chemical meningitis. This complication was presumed secondary to leakage of paclitaxel into the subarachnoid space. Overall, the treatment showed an antitumor response in 11 of 15 patients. Additional chemotherapeutic studies have been conducted in intracranial brain tumor xenograft models with promising results and include such medications as carboplatin, gemcitabine, topotecan, and doxorubicin [124,125].

The two primary bacterial toxins currently in clinical trial include *Pseudomonas* exotoxin (PE) and diphtheria toxin. PE has been coupled to cytokines interleukin (IL)-4 and IL-13, the receptors of which are overexpressed

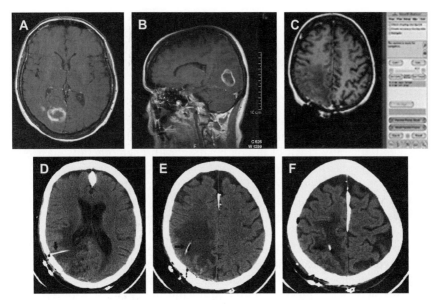

Fig. 3. Stereotactic placement of intracranial catheters for the purpose of CED. Preoperative axial (*A*) and sagittal (*B*) MRI of a right occipital glioblastoma. After surgical resection of the glioblastoma, intracranial catheters are placed in a second operation. (*C*) Frameless stereotaxy is used to place these catheters accurately around the resection cavity. (*D–F*) Postoperative CT images of the three catheters placed for CED.

in brain tumors. Three phase I clinical trials displayed the safety and tolerability of IL-4 PE via CED [126–128]. Three phase I studies analyzed a recombinant mutated PE linked to IL-13, so named IL-13–PE38QQR or cintredekin besudotox. These studies assessed the optimization of catheter placement (IL-13–PEI-103), intraparenchymal infusate distribution (IL-13–PEI-105), and the maximum tolerated infusate toxicity (IL-13–PEI-002). The studies included a total of 51 patients, in whom intratumoral infusion was generally well tolerated. Although not designed to show efficacy, some improvement in survival was noted. A phase III trial, known as the PRECISE trial, recently concluded, in which 288 patients were treated with IL-13 PE via CED or BCNU wafers. The data from this study currently are being analyzed [129]. A modified diphtheria toxin, CRM107, currently is in clinical trials in combination with transferrin, the receptor for which is present on all rapidly dividing cells. Thirty-three patients who had high-grade gliomas were included in a phase II multi-institutional trial. The data from this trial remain unpublished but displayed some evidence of improved survival [130].

In addition to the therapeutic agents discussed previously, radioisotopes can be targeted to deliver focal radiation to malignant gliomas. Phase I and phase II trials have concluded in which 51 patients were treated with a [131]I-labeled chimeric monoclonal antibody (Cotara). Single photon emission CT scanning revealed increased drug distribution correlated with increased length of survival. Minimal exposure to surrounding brain parenchyma also was noted. Such issues as delivery rate, ideal catheter placement, and catheter effect on the surrounding tissue currently are under investigation [131].

*Interstitial brachytherapy*

Radiation therapy is a standard adjunct in the treatment of malignant gliomas. After initial resection of these tumors, patients treated with external beam radiotherapy (EBRT) in combination with chemotherapy have improved local control and survival [132]. Current EBRT techniques limit fractionation to a total dose of 60 Gy to limit radiation to the normal brain parenchyma. Interstitial brachytherapy attempts to limit toxicity to this normal tissue while maximizing the radiation dose delivered to tumor cells.

The GliaSite Radiation Therapy System (RTS) is a treatment modality that provides intracavitary low-dose-rate brachytherapy [133]. GliaSite RTS involves the placement of an inflatable balloon into a resection cavity at the time of surgery. Low-dose-rate brachytherapy is provided by inflating the balloon with an aqueous solution of organically bound $^{125}$I. Initial studies analyzed the role of GliaSite RTS with recurrent glioblastoma multiforme. Tatter and colleagues performed a multi-institutional trial of 21 patients who had recurrent malignant gliomas treated with postresection GliaSite RTS. The trial supports the finding that this treatment modality can effectively deliver the prescribed dose of radiation needed [133]. Subsequently, two retrospective reviews have been published and both suggest a modest survival benefit after treatment. Johns Hopkins University assessed 24 patients, whereas a multi-institutional study assessed 95 patients, and after treatment of recurrent disease, the patients displayed a median survival of 9.1 months and 9.0 months, respectively [134,135]. RTS currently is being studied as part of the initial treatment for patients who have glioblastoma multiforme [136].

**Summary**

Advances in the fields of molecular and translational research, oncology, and surgery have emboldened the medical community to believe that the majority of intrinsic brain tumors, once perceived "invulnerable," may possess an Achilles heel. The combination of intraoperative imaging and brain mapping provides a powerful means to attempt extensive resections of tumors in a relatively safe manner. The judicious use of appropriate resources based on the level of intraoperative guidance that will be required and an understanding of the relative usefulness and limitations of each modality will limit the superfluous use of these advanced neurosurgical techniques. Intraoperative neuroimaging is not a replacement for surgical experience and a thorough knowledge of regional anatomy but provides another tool by which neurosurgeons can reduce the risk associated with surgical treatment of brain tumors. Despite advances in functional brain mapping that have enabled operating immediately adjacent to eloquent regions of brain with increased confidence, no surgical method will be able to treat the infiltrating lesion admixed with critical functional regions of cortex or the distant microscopic satellite lesions present after a seemingly extensive resection. It is continued research into the delivery of an efficacious chemobiologic agent that will allow treatment of these elusive problems in the management of primary brain tumors.

## References

[1] Winger MJ, Macdonald DR, Cairncross JG. Supratentorial anaplastic gliomas in adults. The prognostic importance of extent of resection and prior low-grade glioma. J Neurosurg 1989;71(4):487–93.

[2] World Health Organization classification of tumors: pathology and genetics of tumours of nervous system. In: Kleihues P, Cavenee WK, editors. Lyon: IARC Press; 2000.

[3] CBTRUS. Statistical report: primary brain tumors in the United States, 1998–2002. Hinsdale (IL): Central Brain Tumor Registry of the United States; 2005.

[4] Keles GE, Lamborn KR, Berger MS. Low-grade hemispheric gliomas in adults: a critical review of extent of resection as a factor influencing outcome. J Neurosurg 2001;95(5): 735–45.

[5] Norden AD, Wen PY. Glioma therapy in adults. Neurologist 2006;12(6):279–92.

[6] Keles GE, Aldape K, Berger MS. Low-grade gliomas: astrocytoma, oligodendroglioma and mixed gliomas. In: Winn HR, Youmans JR, editors. Youmans neurological surgery. 5th edition. Philadelphia: Saunders; 2004. p. 950–68.

[7] Lunsford LD, Somaza S, Kondziolka D, et al. Survival after stereotactic biopsy and irradiation of cerebral nonanaplastic, nonpilocytic astrocytoma. J Neurosurg 1995;82(4):523–9.

[8] Kondziolka D, Lunsford LD. The role of stereotactic biopsy in the management of gliomas. J Neurooncol 1999;42(3):205–13.

[9] Recht LD, Lew R, Smith TW. Suspected low-grade glioma: is deferring treatment safe? Ann Neurol 1992;31(4):431–6.

[10] Steiger HJ, Markwalder RV, Seiler RW, et al. Early prognosis of supratentorial grade 2 astrocytomas in adult patients after resection or stereotactic biopsy. An analysis of 50 cases operated on between 1984 and 1988. Acta Neurochir (Wien) 1990;106(3–4):99–105.

[11] Berger MS, Deliganis AV, Dobbins J, et al. The effect of extent of resection on recurrence in patients with low grade cerebral hemisphere gliomas. Cancer 1994;74(6):1784–91.

[12] Ammirati M, Vick N, Liao YL, et al. Effect of the extent of surgical resection on survival and quality of life in patients with supratentorial glioblastomas and anaplastic astrocytomas. Neurosurgery 1987;21(2):201–6.

[13] Devaux BC, O'Fallon JR, Kelly PJ. Resection, biopsy, and survival in malignant glial neoplasms. A retrospective study of clinical parameters, therapy, and outcome. J Neurosurg 1993;78(5):767–75.

[14] Lacroix M, Abi-Said D, Fourney DR, et al. A multivariate analysis of 416 patients with glioblastoma multiforme: prognosis, extent of resection, and survival. J Neurosurg 2001; 95(2):190–8.

[15] Nitta T, Sato K. Prognostic implications of the extent of surgical resection in patients with intracranial malignant gliomas. Cancer 1995;75(11):2727–31.

[16] Hess KR. Extent of resection as a prognostic variable in the treatment of gliomas. J Neurooncol 1999;42(3):227–31.

[17] Quigley MR, Maroon JC. The relationship between survival and the extent of the resection in patients with supratentorial malignant gliomas. Neurosurgery 1991;29(3):385–8 [discussion: 388–9].

[18] Nazzaro JM, Neuwelt EA. The role of surgery in the management of supratentorial intermediate and high-grade astrocytomas in adults. J Neurosurg 1990;73(3):331–44.

[19] Bulsara KR, Johnson J, Villavicencio AT. Improvements in brain tumor surgery: the modern history of awake craniotomies. Neurosurg Focus 2005;18(4):1–3.

[20] Laws ER, Parney IF, Huang W, et al. Survival following surgery and prognostic factors for recently diagnosed malignant glioma: data from the glioma outcomes project. J Neurosurg 2003;99(3):467–73.

[21] Mineo JF, Bordron A, Baroncini M, et al. Prognosis factors of survival time in patients with glioblastoma multiforme: a multivariate analysis of 340 patients. Acta Neurochir (Wien) 2007;149(3):245–53.

[22] Scott JN, Rewcastle NB, Brasher PM, et al. Long-term glioblastoma multiforme survivors: a population-based study. Can J Neurol Sci 1998;25(3):197–201.

[23] Vertosick FT Jr, Selker RG. Long-term survival after the diagnosis of malignant glioma: a series of 22 patients surviving more than 4 years after diagnosis. Surg Neurol 1992; 38(5):359–63.

[24] Salcman M, Scholtz H, Kaplan RS, et al. Long-term survival in patients with malignant astrocytoma. Neurosurgery 1994;34(2):213–9 [discussion: 219–20].

[25] Chandler KL, Prados MD, Malec M, et al. Long-term survival in patients with glioblastoma multiforme. Neurosurgery 1993;32(5):716–20 [discussion: 720].

[26] Ciric I, Ammirati M, Vick N, et al. Supratentorial gliomas: surgical considerations and immediate postoperative results. Gross total resection versus partial resection. Neurosurgery 1987;21(1):21–6.

[27] Muhlbauer M, Gebhart E, Pfisterer W, et al. Microsurgery for glioblastoma preserves short-term quality of life both in functionally impaired and independent patients. Wien Klin Wochenschr 2002;114(19–20):866–73.

[28] Schiff D, Shaffrey ME. Role of resection for newly diagnosed malignant gliomas. Expert Rev Anticancer Ther 2003;3(5):621–30.

[29] Duffau H, Lopes M, Arthuis F, et al. Contribution of intraoperative electrical stimulations in surgery of low grade gliomas: a comparative study between two series without (1985-96) and with (1996–2003) functional mapping in the same institution. J Neurol Neurosurg Psychiatry 2005;76(6):845–51.

[30] Reithmeier T, Krammer M, Gumprecht H, et al. Neuronavigation combined with electrophysiological monitoring for surgery of lesions in eloquent brain areas in 42 cases: a retrospective comparison of the neurological outcome and the quality of resection with a control group with similar lesions. Minim Invasive Neurosurg 2003;46(2):65–71.

[31] Wood CC, Spencer DD, Allison T, et al. Localization of human sensorimotor cortex during surgery by cortical surface recording of somatosensory evoked potentials. J Neurosurg 1988;68(1):99–111.

[32] Sutherling WW, Crandall PH, Darcey TM, et al. The magnetic and electric fields agree with intracranial localizations of somatosensory cortex. Neurology 1988;38(11):1705–14.

[33] Picht T, Kombos T, Gramm HJ, et al. Multimodal protocol for awake craniotomy in language cortex tumour surgery. Acta Neurochir (Wien) 2006;148(2):127–37.

[34] Huncke K, Van De Wiele B, Fried I, et al. The asleep-awake-asleep anesthetic technique for intraoperative language mapping. Neurosurgery 1998;42(6):1312–6.

[35] Foerster O. The cerebral cortex of man. Lancet 1931;109:309–12.

[36] Penfield W, Roberts L. Speech and brain mechanisms. Princeton (NJ): Princeton University; 1959.

[37] Haglund MM, Berger MS, Shamseldin M, et al. Cortical localization of temporal lobe language sites in patients with gliomas. Neurosurgery 1994;34(4):567–76 [discussion: 576].

[38] Walker JA, Quinones-Hinojosa A, Berger MS. Intraoperative speech mapping in 17 bilingual patients undergoing resection of a mass lesion. Neurosurgery 2004;54(1):113–7 [discussion: 118].

[39] Roux FE, Lubrano V, Lauwers-Cances V, et al. Intra-operative mapping of cortical areas involved in reading in mono- and bilingual patients. Brain 2004;127(Pt 8):1796–810.

[40] Keles GE, Lundin DA, Lamborn KR, et al. Intraoperative subcortical stimulation mapping for hemispherical perirolandic gliomas located within or adjacent to the descending motor pathways: evaluation of morbidity and assessment of functional outcome in 294 patients. J Neurosurg 2004;100(3):369–75.

[41] Duffau H, Capelle L, Sichez N, et al. Intraoperative mapping of the subcortical language pathways using direct stimulations. An anatomo-functional study. Brain 2002;125(Pt 1): 199–214.

[42] Haglund MM, Ojemann GA, Hochman DW. Optical imaging of epileptiform and functional activity in human cerebral cortex. Nature 1992;358(6388):668–71.

[43] Toga AW, Cannestra AF, Black KL. The temporal/spatial evolution of optical signals in human cortex. Cerebral Cortex 1995;5(6):561–5.

[44] Cannestra AF, Bookheimer SY, Pouratian N, et al. Temporal and topographical characterization of language cortices using intraoperative optical intrinsic signals. Neuroimage 2000;12:41–54.

[45] Pouratian N, Bookheimer SY, O'Farrell AM, et al. Optical imaging of bilingual cortical representations: case report. J Neurosurg 2000;93:686–91.

[46] Pouratian N, Martin NA, Cannestra AF, et al. Intraoperative sensorimotor and language mapping using optical intrinsic signal imaging: comparison with electrophysiologic techniques and fMRI in 40 patients. Paper presented at: 2000 American Association of neurological surgeons annual meeting. San Francisco, California, April 8–13, 2000.

[47] Krings T, Topper R, Willmes K, et al. Activation in primary and secondary motor areas in patients with CNS neoplasms and weakness. Neurology 2002;58(3):381–90.

[48] Holodny AI, Schulder M, Liu WC, et al. The effect of brain tumors on BOLD functional MR imaging activation in the adjacent motor cortex: implications for image-guided neurosurgery. AJNR Am J Neuroradiol 2000;21:1415–22.

[49] Schreiber A, Hubbe U, Ziyeh S, et al. The influence of gliomas and nonglial space-occupying lesions on blood-oxygen-level-dependent contrast enhancement. AJNR Am J Neuroradiol 2000;21:1055–63.

[50] Schlosser R, Husche S, Gawehn J, et al. Characterization of BOLD-fMRI signal during a verbal fluency paradigm in patients with intracerebral tumors affecting the frontal lobe. Magn Reson Imaging 2002;20:7–16.

[51] Righini A, de Divitiis O, Prinster A, et al. Functional MRI: primary motor cortex localization in patients with brain tumors. J Comput Assist Tomogr 1996;20(5):702–8.

[52] Roux FE, Boulanouar K, Lotterie JA, et al. Language functional magnetic resonance imaging in preoperative assessment of language areas: correlation with direct cortical stimulation. Neurosurgery 2003;52(6):1335–45 [discussion: 1345–7].

[53] Nimsky C, Ganslandt O, Buchfelder M, et al. Intraoperative visualization for resection of gliomas: the role of functional neuronavigation and intraoperative 1.5 T MRI. Neurol Res 2006;28(5):482–7.

[54] Fox PT, Mintun MA, Raichle ME, et al. Mapping human visual cortex with positron emission tomography. Nature 1986;323(6091):806–9.

[55] Belliveau JW, Kennedy DN Jr, McKinstry RC, et al. Functional mapping of the human visual cortex by magnetic resonance imaging. Science 1991;254(5032):716–9.

[56] Roessler K, Donat M, Lanzenberger R, et al. Evaluation of preoperative high magnetic field motor functional MRI (3 Tesla) in glioma patients by navigated electrocortical stimulation and postoperative outcome. J Neurol Neurosurg Psychiatry 2005;76(8):1152–7.

[57] Kruger G, Kastrup A, Glover GH. Neuroimaging at 1.5 T and 3.0 T: comparison of oxygenation-sensitive magnetic resonance imaging. Magn Reson Med 2001;45(4):595–604.

[58] FitzGerald DB, Cosgrove GR, Ronner S, et al. Location of language in the cortex: a comparison between functional MR imaging and electrocortical stimulation. AJNR Am J Neuroradiol 1997;18:1529–39.

[59] Pouratian N, Bookheimer SY, Rex DE, et al. Utility of preoperative functional magnetic resonance imaging for identifying language cortices in patients with vascular malformations. J Neurosurg 2002;97(1):21–32.

[60] Mueller WM, Yetkin FZ, Hammeke TA, et al. Functional magnetic resonance imaging mapping of the motor cortex in patients with cerebral tumors. Neurosurgery 1996;39(3): 515–20 [discussion: 520–1].

[61] Roux FE, Boulanouar K, Ranjeva JP, et al. Usefulness of motor functional MRI correlated to cortical mapping in Rolandic low-grade astrocytomas. Acta Neurochir (Wien) 1999; 141(1):71–9.

[62] Lurito JT, Lowe MJ, Sartorius C, et al. Comparison of fMRI and intraoperative direct cortical stimulation in localization of receptive language areas. J Comput Assist Tomogr 2000;24(1):99–105.

[63] Majos A, Tybor K, Stefanczyk L, et al. Cortical mapping by functional magnetic resonance imaging in patients with brain tumors. Eur Radiol 2005;15(6):1148–58.

[64] Pouratian N, Sicotte N, Rex D, et al. Spatial/temporal correlation of BOLD and optical intrinsic signals in humans. Magn Reson Med 2002;47(4):766–76.

[65] Lehericy S, Duffau H, Cornu P, et al. Correspondence between functional magnetic resonance imaging somatotopy and individual brain anatomy of the central region: comparison with intraoperative stimulation in patients with brain tumors. J Neurosurg 2000; 92(4):589–98.

[66] Makela JP, Forss N, Jaaskelainen J, et al. Magnetoencephalography in neurosurgery. Neurosurgery 2006;59(3):493–510 [discussion: 510–1].

[67] Schiffbauer H, Berger MS, Ferrari P, et al. Preoperative magnetic source imaging for brain tumor surgery: a quantitative comparison with intraoperative sensory and motor mapping. J Neurosurg 2002;97(6):1333–42.

[68] Gallen CC, Schwartz BJ, Bucholz RD, et al. Presurgical localization of functional cortex using magnetic source imaging. J Neurosurg 1995;82(6):988–94.

[69] Schiffbauer H, Ferrari P, Rowley HA, et al. Functional activity within brain tumors: a magnetic source imaging study. Neurosurgery 2001;49(6):1313–20 [discussion: 1320–1].

[70] Ganslandt O, Buchfelder M, Hastreiter P, et al. Magnetic source imaging supports clinical decision making in glioma patients. Clin Neurol Neurosurg 2004;107(1):20–6.

[71] Grummich P, Nimsky C, Pauli E, et al. Combining fMRI and MEG increases the reliability of presurgical language localization: a clinical study on the difference between and congruence of both modalities. Neuroimage 2006;32(4):1793–803.

[72] Korvenoja A, Kirveskari E, Aronen HJ, et al. Sensorimotor cortex localization: comparison of magnetoencephalography, functional MR imaging, and intraoperative cortical mapping. Radiology 2006;241(1):213–22.

[73] Berman JI, Berger MS, Mukherjee P, et al. Diffusion-tensor imaging-guided tracking of fibers of the pyramidal tract combined with intraoperative cortical stimulation mapping in patients with gliomas. J Neurosurg 2004;101(1):66–72.

[74] Kamada K, Todo T, Masutani Y, et al. Visualization of the frontotemporal language fibers by tractography combined with functional magnetic resonance imaging and magnetoencephalography. J Neurosurg 2007;106(1):90–8.

[75] Spiegel E, Wycis H, Marks M, et al. Stereotaxic apparatus for operations on the human brain. Science 1947;106:349–50.

[76] Roberts DW, Strohbehn JW, Hatch JF, et al. A frameless stereotaxic integration of computerized tomographic imaging and the operating microscope. J Neurosurg 1986; 65(4):545–9.

[77] McDermott M. Intracranial gliomas. In: Barnett GH, Roberts DW, Maciunas RJ, editors. Image-guided neurosurgery: clinical applications of surgical navigation. St. Louis (MO): Quality Medical Pub.; 1998. p. 77–86.

[78] Meyer FB, Bates LM, Goerss SJ, et al. Awake craniotomy for aggressive resection of primary gliomas located in eloquent brain. Mayo Clin Proc 2001;76(7):677–87.

[79] Stapleton SR, Kiriakopoulos E, Mikulis D, et al. Combined utility of functional MRI, cortical mapping, and frameless stereotaxy in the resection of lesions in eloquent areas of brain in children. Pediatr Neurosurg 1997;26(2):68–82.

[80] Lumenta CB, Gumprecht HK, Leonardi MA, et al. Three-dimensional computer-assisted stereotactic-guided microneurosurgery combined with cortical mapping of the motor area by direct electrostimulation. Minim Invasive Neurosurg 1997;40(2):50–4.

[81] Maurer CR Jr, Hill DL, Martin AJ, et al. Investigation of intraoperative brain deformation using a 1.5-T interventional MR system: preliminary results. Ieee Transactions on Medical Imaging 1998;17(5):817–25.

[82] Nimsky C, Ganslandt O, Hastreiter P, et al. Intraoperative compensation for brain shift. Surg Neurol 2001;56(6):357–64 [discussion: 364–5].

[83] Nabavi A, Black PM, Gering DT, et al. Serial intraoperative magnetic resonance imaging of brain shift. Neurosurgery 2001;48(4):787–97 [discussion: 797–8].

[84] Albayrak B, Samdani AF, Black PM. Intra-operative magnetic resonance imaging in neurosurgery. Acta Neurochir (Wien) 2004;146(6):543–56, [discussion: 557].

[85] Fahlbusch R, Ganslandt O, Buchfelder M, et al. Intraoperative magnetic resonance imaging during transsphenoidal surgery. J Neurosurg 2001;95(3):381–90.

[86] Truwit CL, Hall WA. Intraoperative magnetic resonance imaging-guided neurosurgery at 3-T. Neurosurgery Apr 2006;58(4 Suppl 2):ONS-338-345 [discussion: ONS-345–6].

[87] Tummala RP, Chu RM, Liu H, et al. Optimizing brain tumor resection. High-field interventional MR imaging. Neuroimaging Clin N Am 2001;11(4):673–83.

[88] Lewin JS, Metzger A, Selman WR. Intraoperative magnetic resonance image guidance in neurosurgery. J Magn Reson Imaging 2000;12(4):512–24.

[89] Sutherland GR, Kaibara T, Louw D, et al. A mobile high-field magnetic resonance system for neurosurgery. J Neurosurg 1999;91(5):804–13.

[90] Hall WA, Liu H, Maxwell RE, et al. Influence of 1.5-Tesla intraoperative MR imaging on surgical decision making. Acta Neurochir 2003;85(Suppl):29–37.

[91] McPherson CM, Bohinski RJ, Dagnew E, et al. Tumor resection in a shared-resource magnetic resonance operating room: experience at the University of Cincinnati. Acta Neurochir 2003;85(Suppl):39–44.

[92] Jolesz FA, Blumenfeld SM. Interventional use of magnetic resonance imaging. Magn Reson Q 1994;10(2):85–96.

[93] Black PM, Moriarty T, Alexander E 3rd, et al. Development and implementation of intraoperative magnetic resonance imaging and its neurosurgical applications. Neurosurgery 1997;41(4):831–42 [discussion: 842–5].

[94] Lipson AC, Gargollo PC, Black PM. Intraoperative magnetic resonance imaging: considerations for the operating room of the future. J Clin Neurosci 2001;8(4):305–10.

[95] Kanner AA, Vogelbaum MA, Mayberg MR, et al. Intracranial navigation by using low-field intraoperative magnetic resonance imaging: preliminary experience. J Neurosurg 2002;97(5):1115–24.

[96] Schulder M, Sernas TJ, Carmel PW. Cranial surgery and navigation with a compact intraoperative MRI system. Acta Neurochir 2003;85(Suppl):79–86.

[97] Black PM, Alexander E 3rd, Martin C, et al. Craniotomy for tumor treatment in an intraoperative magnetic resonance imaging unit. Neurosurgery 1999;45(3):423–31, [discussion: 431–3].

[98] Wirtz CR, Knauth M, Staubert A, et al. Clinical evaluation and follow-up results for intraoperative magnetic resonance imaging in neurosurgery. Neurosurgery 2000;46(5): 1112–20 [discussion: 1120–2].

[99] Lawson HC, Sampath P, Bohan E, et al. Interstitial chemotherapy for malignant gliomas: the Johns Hopkins experience. J Neurooncol 2006;83(1):61–7.

[100] Wang CC, Li J, Teo CS, et al. The delivery of BCNU to brain tumors. J Control Release 1999;61(1–2):21–41.

[101] Blasberg RG, Patlak C, Fenstermacher JD. Intrathecal chemotherapy: brain tissue profiles after ventriculocisternal perfusion. J Pharmacol Exp Ther 1975;195(1):73–83.

[102] Tamargo RJ, Epstein JI, Reinhard CS, et al. Brain biocompatibility of a biodegradable, controlled-release polymer in rats. J Biomed Mater Res 1989;23(2):253–66.

[103] Tamargo RJ, Myseros JS, Epstein JI, et al. Interstitial chemotherapy of the 9L gliosarcoma: controlled release polymers for drug delivery in the brain. Cancer Res 1993;53(2):329–33.

[104] Yang MB, Tamargo RJ, Brem H. Controlled delivery of 1,3-bis (2-chloroethyl)-1-nitrosourea from ethylene-vinyl acetate copolymer. Cancer Res 1989;49(18):5103–7.

[105] Brem H, Mahaley MS Jr, Vick NA, et al. Interstitial chemotherapy with drug polymer implants for the treatment of recurrent gliomas. J Neurosurg 1991;74(3):441–6.

[106] Brem H, Piantadosi S, Burger PC, et al. Placebo-controlled trial of safety and efficacy of intraoperative controlled delivery by biodegradable polymers of chemotherapy for recurrent gliomas. The Polymer-brain tumor treatment group. Lancet 1995;345(8956):1008–12.

[107] Valtonen S, Timonen U, Toivanen P, et al. Interstitial chemotherapy with carmustine-loaded polymers for high-grade gliomas: a randomized double-blind study. Neurosurgery 1997;41(1):44–8 [discussion: 48–9].

[108] Westphal M, Hilt DC, Bortey E, et al. A phase 3 trial of local chemotherapy with biodegradable carmustine (BCNU) wafers (Gliadel wafers) in patients with primary malignant glioma. Neurooncol 2003;5(2):79–88.

[109] Sipos EP, Tyler B, Piantadosi S, et al. Optimizing interstitial delivery of BCNU from controlled release polymers for the treatment of brain tumors. Cancer Chemother Pharmacol 1997;39(5):383–9.

[110] Olivi A, Ewend MG, Utsuki T, et al. Interstitial delivery of carboplatin via biodegradable polymers is effective against experimental glioma in the rat. Cancer Chemother Pharmacol 1996;39(1–2):90–6.

[111] Walter KA, Cahan MA, Gur A, et al. Interstitial taxol delivered from a biodegradable polymer implant against experimental malignant glioma. Cancer Res 1994;54(8):2207–12.

[112] Weingart JD, Thompson RC, Tyler B, et al. Local delivery of the topoisomerase I inhibitor camptothecin sodium prolongs survival in the rat intracranial 9L gliosarcoma model. Int J Cancer 1995;62(5):605–9.

[113] Judy KD, Olivi A, Buahin KG, et al. Effectiveness of controlled release of a cyclophosphamide derivative with polymers against rat gliomas. J Neurosurg 1995;82(3):481–6.

[114] Weingart JD, Sipos EP, Brem H. The role of minocycline in the treatment of intracranial 9L glioma. J Neurosurg 1995;82(4):635–40.

[115] Williams JA, Dillehay LE, Tabassi K, et al. Implantable biodegradable polymers for IUdR radiosensitization of experimental human malignant glioma. J Neurooncol 1997;32(3): 181–92.

[116] Wiranowska M, Ransohoff J, Weingart JD, et al. Interferon-containing controlled-release polymers for localized cerebral immunotherapy. J Interferon Cytokine Res 1998;18(6): 377–85.

[117] Rhines LD, Sampath P, Dolan ME, et al. O6-benzylguanine potentiates the antitumor effect of locally delivered carmustine against an intracranial rat glioma. Cancer Res 2000; 60(22):6307–10.

[118] Sampath P, Hanes J, DiMeco F, et al. Paracrine immunotherapy with interleukin-2 and local chemotherapy is synergistic in the treatment of experimental brain tumors. Cancer Res 1999;59(9):2107–14.

[119] Nguyen TT, Pannu YS, Sung C, et al. Convective distribution of macromolecules in the primate brain demonstrated using computerized tomography and magnetic resonance imaging. J Neurosurg 2003;98(3):584–90.

[120] Bobo RH, Laske DW, Akbasak A, et al. Convection-enhanced delivery of macromolecules in the brain. Proc Natl Acad Sci U S A 1994;91(6):2076–80.

[121] Croteau D, Walbridge S, Morrison PF, et al. Real-time in vivo imaging of the convective distribution of a low-molecular-weight tracer. J Neurosurg 2005;102(1):90–7.

[122] Krauze MT, Saito R, Noble C, et al. Reflux-free cannula for convection-enhanced high-speed delivery of therapeutic agents. J Neurosurg 2005;103(5):923–9.

[123] Lidar Z, Mardor Y, Jonas T, et al. Convection-enhanced delivery of paclitaxel for the treatment of recurrent malignant glioma: a phase I/II clinical study. J Neurosurg 2004; 100(3):472–9.

[124] Degen JW, Walbridge S, Vortmeyer AO, et al. Safety and efficacy of convection-enhanced delivery of gemcitabine or carboplatin in a malignant glioma model in rats. J Neurosurg 2003;99(5):893–8.

[125] Yamashita Y, Krauze MT, Kawaguchi T, et al. Convection-enhanced delivery of a topoisomerase I inhibitor (nanoliposomal topotecan) and a topoisomerase II inhibitor (pegylated liposomal doxorubicin) in intracranial brain tumor xenografts. Neurooncol 2007;9(1):20–8.

[126] Weber F, Asher A, Bucholz R, et al. Safety, tolerability, and tumor response of IL4-Pseudomonas exotoxin (NBI-3001) in patients with recurrent malignant glioma. J Neurooncol 2003;64(1–2):125–37.

[127] Rainov NG, Heidecke V. Long term survival in a patient with recurrent malignant glioma treated with intratumoral infusion of an IL4-targeted toxin (NBI-3001). J Neurooncol 2004;66(1–2):197–201.

[128] Rand RW, Kreitman RJ, Patronas N, et al. Intratumoral administration of recombinant circularly permuted interleukin-4-Pseudomonas exotoxin in patients with high-grade glioma. Clin Cancer Res 2000;6(6):2157–65.

[129] Kunwar S, Prados MD, Chang SM, et al. Direct intracerebral delivery of cintredekin besudotox (IL13-PE38QQR) in recurrent malignant glioma: a report by the Cintredekin Besudotox Intraparenchymal Study Group. J Clin Oncol 2007;25(7):837–44.

[130] Vandergrift WA, Patel SJ, Nicholas JS, et al. Convection-enhanced delivery of immunotoxins and radioisotopes for treatment of malignant gliomas. Neurosurg Focus 2006;20(4):1–8.

[131] Patel SJ, Shapiro WR, Laske DW, et al. Safety and feasibility of convection-enhanced delivery of Cotara for the treatment of malignant glioma: initial experience in 51 patients. Neurosurgery 2005;56(6):1243–52 [discussion: 1252–3].

[132] Walker MD, Green SB, Byar DP, et al. Randomized comparisons of radiotherapy and nitrosoureas for the treatment of malignant glioma after surgery. N Engl J Med 1980; 303(23):1323–9.

[133] Tatter SB, Shaw EG, Rosenblum ML, et al. An inflatable balloon catheter and liquid 125I radiation source (GliaSite radiation therapy system) for treatment of recurrent malignant glioma: multicenter safety and feasibility trial. J Neurosurg 2003;99(2):297–303.

[134] Chan TA, Weingart JD, Parisi M, et al. Treatment of recurrent glioblastoma multiforme with GliaSite brachytherapy. Int J Radiat Oncol Biol Phys 2005;62(4):1133–9.

[135] Gabayan AJ, Green SB, Sanan A, et al. GliaSite brachytherapy for treatment of recurrent malignant gliomas: a retrospective multi-institutional analysis. Neurosurgery 2006;58(4): 701–9 [discussion: 701–9].

[136] Welsh J, Sanan A, Gabayan AJ, et al. GLIASite brachytherapy boost as part of initial treatment of glioblastoma multiforme: a retrospective multi-institutional pilot study. Int J Radiat Oncol Biol Phys 2007;68(1):159–65.

ELSEVIER
SAUNDERS

NEUROLOGIC
CLINICS

Neurol Clin 25 (2007) 1005–1033

# Advances in Radiation Therapy for Brain Tumors

Volker W. Stieber, MD[a],*, Minesh P. Mehta, MD[b]

[a]*Department of Radiation Oncology, Wake Forest University School of Medicine, Medical Center Boulevard, Winston-Salem, NC 27157-1030, USA*
[b]*Department of Human Oncology, University of Wisconsin, Madison, WI 53792, USA*

## General concepts of radiation therapy

*Definitive radiation therapy for brain tumors*

Radiation therapy plays a primary role in the management of most malignant and many benign primary central nervous system (CNS) tumors. It is used frequently in the management of patients who have various CNS neoplasms (Box 1), often postoperatively as adjunctive therapy to decrease local failure; to delay tumor progression and prolong survival (as in malignant glioma); as a curative treatment for diseases such as primitive neuroectodermal tumors and germ cell tumors; or as a therapy that halts further tumor growth, as in schwannoma, meningioma, pituitary tumors, and craniopharyngioma, thereby avoiding serious neurologic sequelae. Often, the primary rationale for using radiation therapy for pituitary tumors is to alter function (ie, diminish endocrine overproduction). Table 1 [1–9] provides a referenced overview of the most common primary CNS tumors, accompanied by International Commission on Radiation Units and Measurements (ICRU) definitions of treatment volumes for initial and (when applicable) boost fields, general dosing guidelines, and outcome end points.

*Palliative and emergency radiation therapy for brain tumors*

Radiation therapy is also frequently used for palliation. It is the primary modality for the treatment of brain metastases [10,11]. Many patients treated with medical therapy and radiation therapy experience improvement in their performance status. Radiation therapy dosing schedules for the

* Corresponding author.
*E-mail address:* vwstieber@novanhealth.org (V.W. Stieber).

doi:10.1016/j.ncl.2007.07.005

---

**Box 1. Brain tumors with a defined or possible role for radiation therapy**

- Low-grade astrocytoma
- Anaplastic astrocytoma (AA)
- Glioblastoma multiforme (GBM)
- Low-grade oligodendroglioma
- Anaplastic oligodendroglioma
- Mixed gliomas
- Ependymoma
- Primitive neuroectodermal tumors
- Primary CNS lymphoma
- Meningioma
- Vestibular and other schwannoma
- Craniopharyngioma
- Pituitary tumors
- CNS germ cell tumors
- Pilocytic astrocytoma
- Ganglioglioma
- Hemangioblastoma
- Hemangiopericytoma
- Sarcoma
- Choroid plexus carcinoma

---

emergency treatment of patients should take into account the initial response to steroids, the extent of extracranial disease, and the primary diagnosis and its anticipated response to systemic therapy. Two randomized trials comparing radiation therapy with or without surgical resection in the management of a solitary brain metastasis have documented a survival advantage with the addition of surgery, over radiation alone [12,13] (although a third randomized trial was negative) [14]. No level I evidence demonstrates any survival benefit from operating on patients who have multiple metastases. However, patients who have severe neurologic symptoms from one or more dominant metastases who are unresponsive to medical therapy may benefit from a craniotomy. An improvement in the patient's performance status can then be followed by external beam radiation therapy. Acute leukemic brain infiltration is a rare, potentially fatal, presentation also treated with whole-brain radiation therapy. Patients who have malignant glioma who require emergency treatment are treated typically with surgical debulking and steroid therapy. Patients with a poor performance status who are unable to undergo surgical debulking may be treated with a short course of whole-brain radiation similar to that used for brain metastases.

## Technology of radiation therapy

Ionizing radiation is a mainstay of the treatment of several intracranial tumors. Numerous tools exist to deliver a specific dose of radiation to a specific target with a specific intent. The three most commonly used types of radiation in the treatment of tumors are photons, electrons, and particles (eg, protons). Electrons are rarely used because they have poor penetration through the cranium; they are not discussed further here. By far, the most commonly used are photons; these are generated most often using a linear accelerator. This machine accelerates electrons to strike a target, resulting in the release of a focused beam of photons [15]. After linear accelerators, Cobalt-60 is the second most commonly used source of photon radiation in this particular clinical setting. Protons are the most commonly used particles, also generated in accelerators. Very few dedicated clinical proton facilities exist in the world, mainly because of cost [16]. Photons and particles are delivered as focused beams aimed at the tumor from varying angles.

Absorbed dose is measured in Gray (1 Gy = 100 cGy; 1 cGy = 1 rad in old nomenclature). Dose is prescribed at a percent isodose line, which is the line encompassing the target on a two-dimensional (2D) image along which the delivered dose is the same at every point (in three dimensions, the term "isodose surface" is used) and referenced to the dose at a particular point, often the geometric center of the target.

Radiation therapy can be delivered in multiple treatments ("fractions") or in a single treatment. Radiosurgery specifically refers to the delivery of a large single dose of radiation given in a highly focused manner to a well-delineated target using stereotactic targeting, which is expected to result in the same biologic effect as a course of several weeks of fractionated radiation therapy [17]. Stereotactic treatment uses a specialized method of targeting, whereby the target lesion is referenced not to the patient but to a reproducible Cartesian coordinate system. This method of targeting is used when a very high degree of accuracy and precision is required because the coordinate system is affixed (usually invasively) to the patient. The Leksell and Brown-Roberts-Wells (BRW) neurosurgical head frames are the most common examples; they immobilize the patient's head and provide the reference coordinate system required for targeting. In general, any type of treatment can be delivered stereotactically. Practically speaking, stereotactic delivery is useful when extremely tight margins of error are necessary because critical normal structures are extremely close to a well-demarcated target and would otherwise receive excessive dose.

Three-dimensional (3D) conformal radiation therapy refers to a specialized situation where the volumetric distribution of the desired dose (isodose surface) accurately mimics the shape of the target. Fractionated radiation therapy and radiosurgery may be delivered in this fashion. Intensity-modulated radiation therapy (IMRT) is a subset of 3D conformal radiation therapy; the intensity of the photon flux within the treatment field or fields is

Table 1
Suggested definitions of International Commission on Radiation Units and Measurements volumes by diagnosis, based on MRI and dose ranges (in Gy) delivered to those volumes

| Diagnosis | Definition of initial treatment field (CTV) | Usual dose to CTV | Definition of final field (to GTV) | Usual dose to GTV | Dose to craniospinal axis (if indicated) | MS | DFS5 | OS1 | OS5 | LC5 | Reference |
|---|---|---|---|---|---|---|---|---|---|---|---|
| WHO grade I glioma | n/a | n/a | Enhancing tumor (T1 + C) 1.0-cm margin | 45.0–50.4 Gy | n/a | — | 95% | — | 95% | — | [1] |
| WHO grade II glioma | Enhancing tumor (T1 + C; Edema (T2/FLAIR) 2.0-cm margin | 45 Gy | Enhancing tumor (T1 + C) 2.0-cm margin | 50.4–54.0 Gy | n/a | — | 37%–50% | — | 58%–73% | — | [62–64] |
| WHO grade III glioma | Enhancing tumor (T1 + C); Edema (T2/FLAIR) 2.0-cm margin | 45.0–50.4 Gy | Enhancing tumor (T1 + C) 2.0-cm margin | 59.4 Gy | Leptomeningeal spread on MRI: 30.0–39.6 Gy; Bulky disease: 55.8–59.4 Gy | 17.5–58.6 mo | — | — | 38% | — | [2,3,60] |
| WHO grade IV glioma | Enhancing tumor (T1 + C); Edema (T2/FLAIR) 2.0-cm margin | 45.0–50.4 Gy | Enhancing tumor (T1 + C) 2.0-cm margin | 59.4–64.8 Gy | Leptomeningeal spread on MRI: 30.0–39.6 Gy; Bulky disease: 55.8–59.4 Gy | 17.5–17.1 mo | — | 28%–70% | 0%–14% | — | [21] |
| Meningioma, benign/ atypical | n/a | n/a | Enhancing tumor (T1 + C) 1.0-cm margin | 52.2–64.8 Gy | n/a | — | 48%–89% | — | 58%–85% | — | [90,101,103] |

| Tumor | Initial target volume | Initial dose | Boost target volume | Boost dose | CSF/special dosing | | | | | | Reference |
|---|---|---|---|---|---|---|---|---|---|---|---|
| Meningioma, malignant | Enhancing tumor (T1 + C); Edema (T2/FLAIR) 2.0-cm margin | 45.0–50.4 Gy | Enhancing tumor (T1 + C) 2.0-cm margin | 55.8–59.4 Gy | n/a | 1.5 y | — | — | — | — | [4] |
| Pituitary adenoma | n/a | n/a | Enhancing tumor (T1 + C) 0.7- to 1.0-cm margin | 45.0–50.4 Gy (nonfunctioning) 45.0–54.0 Gy (functioning) | n/a | — | — | — | — | 90%–95% (33%–95% biochemical control) | [115] |
| Ependymoma | Enhancing tumor (T1 + C); Edema (T2/FLAIR) 2.0-cm margin | 45.0 Gy | Enhancing tumor (T1 + C) 2.0-cm margin | 50.4–55.8 Gy | Negative CSF: 30.0 Gy; Positive CSF: 36.0 Gy; Gross leptomeningeal spread on MRI: 39.6 Gy; Bulky disease: 54.0 Gy | — | — | 67%–100% | — | 95%–100% | [5] |
| Chordoma, chondrosarcoma | Enhancing tumor (T1 + C); Tumor bed 2.0-cm margin | 50.4 Gy | Enhancing tumor (T1 + C) 2.0-cm margin | 59.4–70.2 Gy | n/a | — | — | 36%–72% | 75%–80% | 40%–75% | [5] |

(continued on next page)

Table 1 (*continued*)

| Diagnosis | Definition of initial treatment field (CTV) | Usual dose to CTV | Definition of final field (to GTV) | Usual dose to GTV | Dose to craniospinal axis (if indicated) | MS | DFS$_5$ | OS$_1$ | OS$_5$ | LC$_5$ | Reference |
|---|---|---|---|---|---|---|---|---|---|---|---|
| Central neurocytoma | n/a | n/a | FLAIR changes 1.0-cm margin | 50.4–55.8 Gy | n/a | — | — | — | 98% | 98% | [6,7] |
| Brain metastases | Whole brain | 30.0–37.5 Gy (adjuvant 40.0–50.4 Gy) | n/a | n/a | n/a | 3.8–7.1 mo | — | 12%–32% | — | — | [8,20] |
| Leukemic brain infiltration | Whole brain | 24.0–30.0 Gy in 1.8- to 3.0-Gy fractions | n/a | n/a | 18.0 Gy | 9 mo | — | — | — | — | [9] |

The numbers in subscript denote years.

*Abbreviations:* CSF, cerebrospinal fluid; CTV, clinical target volume; DFS, disease-free survival; FLAIR, fluid-attenuated inversion recovery; GTV, gross tumor volume; LC, local control; MS, median survival; n/a, not applicable; OS, overall survival; WHO, World Health Organization; + C, with contrast.

modulated, resulting in a nonuniform dose-distribution, with exquisite conformality around the target and avoidance of critical structures. A similar effect can be achieved with protons by varying the depth of the Bragg peak, the point in the tissues at which these particles deposit most of their therapeutic energy.

The basic rationale for using conformal delivery is to spare adjacent normal tissue from receiving unnecessary dose. The use of IMRT in the treatment of CNS tumors also has theoretic benefits [18]. Improved dose distribution can reduce dose to the many dose-limiting organs at risk (OAR) within the cranium, including the optic chiasm, the optic nerves and globes, the brain stem, the inner ear, the area postrema, and the uninvolved normal brain, especially the optic cortex and temporal lobes [19]. Reducing dose to the area postrema may reduce the incidence of treatment-related nausea [19]. If conventional treatment planning results in unacceptable dose delivery (dose per fraction, total dose, or both) to uninvolved OAR, the use of IMRT should be considered. This decision must include an honest assessment of the patient's expected lifespan because late toxicities usually do not manifest until 6 months after treatment [20,21]. Also, because most primary CNS malignancies recur locally, IMRT may be used to improve dose delivery to target volumes; an example would be concomitant boost therapy for World Health Organization (WHO) grade IV gliomas [22,23]. The late effects of IMRT, which theoretically may expose more normal tissue to lower doses, are not yet known and work is underway to model these responses biologically [24].

Image-guided radiation therapy (IGRT) is the newest development in radiation delivery systems. The treatment of intracranial lesions is based on 3D volumetric data sets (CT and MR imaging), which delineate the target for the computer-aided planning and simulation of treatment before the actual treatment takes place. True IGRT acquires another 3D volumetric data set at the time of treatment delivery, ideally using the treatment machine itself, to confirm that the target is localized correctly with respect to the radiation beams [25]. (Some devices only obtain orthogonal 2D images, which makes positional corrections difficult). This data set is useful when dealing with targets that may have shifted between treatment simulation and treatment delivery; this scenario rarely applies to intracranial lesions.

Thus, a wide array of terms can be used, such as "fractionated stereotactic IMRT" or "image-guided radiosurgery," which are not to be confused with the trade names of different devices using different technologic approaches to achieve a similar goal, often used to advertise to equipment buyers and the general public. The authors provide a brief survey of the most commonly used commercial devices in the treatment of brain tumors. The Leksell gamma knife (Elekta, Stockholm, Sweden), in its traditional configuration, uses 201 stationary cobalt sources to deliver a single, focused, ellipsoid sphere of radiation dose with a reproducibility of 0.1 mm. The newest configuration of the device (Perfexion) uses fewer sources to achieve a higher degree of conformality than previously possible. Modified linear accelerators, often collectively referred to as "linac radiosurgery," achieve similar precision and dose-distribution. The Cyberknife (Accuray, Sunnyvale, California) is a small linear accelerator mounted on a robotic arm that can focus a single photon beam of fixed shape at a tumor from a wide variety of angles; this system incorporates orthogonal imaging for 2D IGRT [26]. The Synergy and Axesse (Elekta, Stockholm, Sweden) represent a standard medical linear accelerator mounted on a rotating gantry, which, in combination with a moving table, can deliver a photon beam that can be shaped and its flux modulated; this system incorporates CT for 3D IGRT [25]. The Trilogy (Varian, Palo Alto, California) is a standard medical linear accelerator rotating on a fixed axis, which, in combination with a moving table, can deliver a photon beam that can be shaped and its flux modulated; this system incorporates orthogonal imaging for 2D IGRT, and also kilovoltage cone-beam CT for 3D IGRT. The Novalis (BrainLAB, Feldkirchen, Germany) is similar to the Trilogy in execution. Helical tomotherapy consists of a 6-MeV linear accelerator mounted on a ring gantry that rotates around a patient who is continually translated through the ring, resulting in helical fan beam radiation delivery with adjustable beam thickness (TomoTherapy, Inc., Madison, Wisconsin) [27]. CT detectors on the gantry opposite the linear accelerator allow IGRT delivery. Proton beam facilities (Optivus Technology, Inc., San Bernardino, California; and Ion Beam Applications, Louvain-la-Neuve, Belgium) consist of a very large, gantry-mounted, single-beam delivery system and a mobile patient table for delivering a focused particle beam from a wide variety of angles.

*Volume definition, treatment planning, and dose prescription*

Most commercial treatment-planning systems perform dose calculations from CT data sets. Registration of MR scan data sets with the treatment planning CT scan is essential for accurate definition of the tumor and the surrounding OAR. All diagnostic information, but particularly MR scans (including T2 and fluid-attenuated inversion recovery [FLAIR] images) and CT scans, and clinical and surgical findings, should be combined to define the tumor volume and OAR. Functional and metabolic imaging studies may provide additional information for radiation therapy treatment planning [28–31]. Functional MR scans, which image cerebral blood flow, can show regions of normal brain function (eg, motor strip and expressive and receptive language areas) [32]. Magnetoencephalography (MEG) provides similar functional information [33]. Using multivoxel 3D MR spectroscopy (MRS), the choline-to-$N$-acetylaspartate ratio or index (CNI) appears to be sensitive and specific at differentiating tumor from normal tissue [34]. [$^{11}$C]-methionine positron emission tomography (PET) imaging may help in better defining the extent of low-grade gliomas [35].

Treatment-planning volumes are based on reports 50 and 62 of the ICRU [36,37]. Gross tumor volume (GTV) represents grossly visible disease (ie, the enhancing component on a T1-weighted MR scan) [36,37]. The clinical target volume (CTV) is subclinical microscopic tumor extent (ie, seen as T2-weighted changes on MR scans) and is often better visualized as FLAIR abnormality [36]. In the CNS, the planning target volume, also referred to as the dosimetric margin, accounts for physiologic variations, such as (potential) fluctuations in tumor position from cerebral edema that may occur over the course of treatment, and the set-up margin, taking into account uncertainties in patient-to-beam positioning. OAR are critical normal structures whose relative radiation sensitivity and proximity to the CTV may significantly influence the prescribed dose and the treatment planning strategy. It is especially important to limit the risk of late toxicities by respecting the dose-tolerances of normal structures when patients are expected to survive for 6 months or longer beyond treatment.

## Treatment

### Glioblastoma multiforme

Of all treatment modalities, radiation therapy has the greatest impact on survival in GBM, followed by temozolomide chemotherapy and then surgical resection [38–41]. One large retrospective analysis, one prospective trial, and the Radiation Therapy Oncology Group (RTOG) recursive partitioning analysis (RPA) classification system analysis demonstrated that a more extensive resection predicts longer median survival [21,41,42]. However, fewer than one half of GBM patients are able to undergo gross total resection (GTR) at presentation [43].

After radiation therapy (with BCNU chemotherapy) for newly diagnosed GBM, median survival times range from 7.1 to 17.5 months [21]. Moderate radiation dose-escalation has shown a survival benefit [44–47]. The European Organization for Research and Treatment of Cancer (EORTC) has published a phase III study demonstrating significantly improved survival with the addition of concomitant and sequential temozolomide to radiation therapy [40]. The 2-year survival rate was 26.5% with radiation therapy plus temozolomide, and 10.4% with radiation therapy alone [48].

In most biologic systems, radiation exhibits stochastic properties. In cell culture systems, when survival curves as a function of dose are generated, a dose-dependant response, with an initial "shoulder" and subsequent slope, is clearly identified. These cell-survival curves are best described by a linear-quadratic function. In the human context, these clinical dose-response curves are characterized by a sigmoidal shape, with low doses initially producing a relatively flat response curve, but demonstrating an upward response-inflection after a certain threshold dose, beyond which the response slope is large for a small change in dose; at much higher doses, the curve flattens, resulting in lower incremental gain. For malignant brain tumors such as glioblastoma, traditional therapeutic trials have explored the

0- to 60-Gy dose range, hyperfractionation trials have explored doses up to 80 Gy, and brachytherapy trials have reached 100 to 120 Gy. Although the dose-response phenomenon across this large range has not been evaluated prospectively, a review of the composite data from various clinical trials and institutional experiences (Table 2) suggests a shallow dose-response effect. Although no-dose versus high-dose studies have shown a survival benefit, clinical trials seeking to identify survival differences between dose-schedules of modest dose variation (eg, 60–80 Gy) have not produced statistically meaningful results.

Escalating radiation therapy dose can be biologically modeled. A biologic model taking into account repair and dose rate may be used to calculate a biologically effective dose (BED) for varying treatment times and prescription doses [49–51]. This model is useful when comparing different radiation schema. For example, the standard dose for GBM is 60 Gy in 30 daily fractions given 5 days per week. Brachytherapy would deliver 60 Gy as a continuous dose over 5 days. Radiosurgery might give 20 Gy in one treatment over 20 minutes. One can generate the BED for the alternative schedules and then back-calculate it to a normalized tumor dose at 2 Gy per fraction. The same can be modeled for normal brain injury. Investigators at the University of Cambridge [52] have extracted biologic data from clinical data to develop a mathematic model using pathologic and radiation biology concepts. Their data suggest that the therapeutic window is quite narrow because brain injury (necrosis) predominates at doses well below an acceptable cure rate. Retrospective studies show that 90% of recurrences occur within 2 cm of the enhancing edge of the original tumor, and multifocal disease is rare [45,53,54]. Because the main pattern of failure is local, an improvement in local control might result in an improvement in survival.

Various strategies to escalate radiation dose focally have been attempted in phase III studies, notably stereotactic radiosurgery (SRS) and brachytherapy [46,47]. Neither approach has yielded a significant improvement in survival or local control. RTOG 0023, a phase I study of accelerated radiation

Table 2
Local control is a function of dose for glioblastoma multiforme

| Dose (Gy) | MS (wk) | 25% survival | $P$ |
|---|---|---|---|
| 0 | 18 | N/A | N/A |
| <45 | 14 | N/A | ns |
| 50 | 28 | 52 | <0.001 |
| 55 | 36 | 57 | <0.001 |
| 60 | 42 | 68 | <0.001 |

Median survival increases from 14 weeks at less than 45 Gy to 42 weeks at 60 Gy. In GBM, local failure results in rapid death; therefore, improved survival with increased dose suggests improved local control.

*Abbreviations:* MS, median survival; N/A, not applicable; ns, not significant; 25% Survival, 25th percentile survival.

therapy using weekly stereotactic conformal boosts for GBM, did not show a survival benefit overall, but patients who had undergone a GTR showed a trend toward improved median survival (17 versus 12 months), implying that focal strategies might work in well-selected patients. Therefore, a more appropriate strategy to reduce the risk of local failure may be to escalate dose to microscopic residual disease after a GTR. This procedure has been done using GliaSite brachytherapy, which is able to deliver a focal boost of radiation therapy to microscopic disease after maximum resection [55,56]. It uses a balloon catheter intracavitary system as a spherically shaped volumetric radiation source (4–35 mL) designed to fill the resection cavity, allowing the dose to be defined precisely and reproduced easily. A recently launched trial sought to determine the maximum tolerated dose of GliaSite brachytherapy with external beam radiation therapy in the treatment of newly diagnosed GBM [57]. Eighty percent of the patients treated in this study were in RPA class IV. The median time of survival for patients who had no residual tumor was double (20.2 months) that of those who had residual tumor (9.1 months), almost reaching statistical significance ($P = .0584$).

Studies using radiation modifiers in conjunction with radiation therapy to overcome the hypoxia present in malignant gliomas have generally shown disappointing results. Several agents, such as hydroxyurea, halogenated pyrimidines (S-phase sensitizers), tirapazamine (a cytotoxic agent that is significantly more toxic to hypoxic than to normoxic cells), perfluorocarbons (oxygen-carrying hypoxic sensitizers), misonidazole (hypoxic sensitizer), motexafin gadolinium (a redox modulator), carbogen and nicotinamide (to modulate vascular tension to reduce hypoxia), RSR-13 (a hypoxic sensitizer), and so forth, have been tested in phase II-III trials, without convincing evidence for superiority.

The EORTC trial did show significant benefit with the use of daily temozolomide, and a post hoc analysis suggested that maximum benefit was achieved in the subgroup of patients who had promoter region methylation of the *MGMT* gene involved in repairing the cytotoxic lesion produced by temozolomide [40]. In a recent study, the authors demonstrated that temozolomide, in fact, enhances the radiation responsiveness of malignant glioma cell lines lacking MGMT expression; concurrent temozolomide-radiation in MGMT-negative GBM cells results in decreased repair of DNA double-strand breaks; further, the use of the MGMT inhibitor O-6 benzylguanine led to enhancement of the antitumor activity of temozolomide-radiation in MGMT-expressing GBM cells, thereby providing a mechanistic approach to future clinical trial development based on MGMT status [58].

Therefore, the current recommendation for GBM remains the use of 60-Gy radiation therapy dose, in 1.8 to 2 Gy per fraction, to the contrast-enhancing tumor volume, plus an appropriately defined margin, and, based on the EORTC trial, this dose is given concomitantly with temozolomide, which putatively acts as a radiosensitizer in this context (Table 3).

Table 3
Outcomes after treatment of newly diagnosed glioblastoma multiforme

| RPA class[a] | Treatment | Median survival (mo) | 1-y survival (%) | 2-y survival (%) | 3-y survival (%) | 5-y survival (%) | Reference |
|---|---|---|---|---|---|---|---|
| RPA III | RT | 15.0 | — | 20.0 | — | — | [48] |
| | RT + BCNU | 17.1 | 70.0 | 30.0 | 20.0 | 14.0 | [21,38] |
| | RT + temozolomide | 21.4 | — | 43.4 | — | — | [48] |
| RPA IV | RT | 13.0 | — | — | 11.0 | — | [48] |
| | RT + BCNU | 11.2 | 46.0 | 17.0 | 7.0 | 4.0 | [21,38] |
| | RT + temozolomide | 16.3 | — | 27.9 | — | — | [48] |
| RPA V/VI | RT | 9.0 | — | 6.0 | — | — | [48] |
| | RT + BCNU | 7.5 | 28.0 | 5.0 | 1.0 | 0.0 | [21,38] |
| | RT + temozolomide | 10.3 | — | 16.5 | — | — | [48] |

*Abbreviation:* RT, radiation therapy.

[a] Class III, age under 50 and Karnofsky Performance Score (KPS) 90% to 100%; class IV, age under 50 and KPS less than 90%, or age over 50 with surgical resection and good neurologic function; class V, age 50 or older and KPS 70% to 100%, either surgical resection and neurologic function that inhibits the ability to work, or biopsy only, followed by at least 54.4 Gy RT; class VI , age over 50 with abnormal mental status and KPS less than 70%, or age 50 or older, KPS 70% to 100%, biopsy only, receiving less than 54.4 Gy RT.

## Anaplastic gliomas

Anaplastic gliomas constitute approximately 25% of high-grade gliomas in adults. They generally occur during young to middle adulthood. Anaplastic gliomas, comprising AA, anaplastic oligodendrogliomas, and anaplastic mixed oligoastrocytomas, correspond to WHO grade III. Overall, patients who have AA have a median survival of approximately 3 years following diagnosis. Patients who have anaplastic oligodendroglioma have a better prognosis, particularly those with tumor characterized by loss of heterozygosity of 1p and 19q, for whom median survival is approximately 7 years. The prognosis for patients who have a mixed tumor, anaplastic oligoastrocytoma, varies, depending on the dominant histologic cell type.

Radiation therapy is an integral part of the standard of care for these patients. Level 1 data are not convincing that the addition of chemotherapy or radiosensitizers prolongs survival in patients who have AA. Two recent phase III trials, RTOG 94-02 [59,60] and EORTC 26,951 [61], demonstrated that the early addition of porcarbazine, CCNU, and vincristine (PCV) did not result in a better outcome compared with radiation therapy alone. RTOG 9404 randomized AA patients to conventional radiation therapy with or without bromodeoxyuridine (BUdR) plus adjuvant PCV [59,60].

The study was closed before full accrual, based on an interim analysis that predicted no survival advantage for the bromodeoxyuridine (BUdR) arm. The radiation dose delivered in both trials was 59.4 Gy in 33 fractions at 1.8 Gy per fraction. Temozolomide has shown activity in patients who have recurrent AA, but level I evidence for a survival benefit in newly diagnosed AA does not exist; RTOG 9813, a phase III trial designed to compare temozolomide to BCNU, closed in 2007 because of failure to complete accruals. Therefore, the current standard of care for patients who have anaplastic gliomas is maximal surgical resection followed by postoperative radiation therapy to dose of 59.4 Gy in 33 fractions; the use of chemotherapy, although very common, is based on less than level 1 evidence.

*Low-grade glioma*

Level I evidence clearly demonstrates the benefit of radiation therapy in delaying time to progression in patients who have low-grade glioma. However, radiation therapy has never been demonstrated to improve overall survival in phase III studies. Thus, debate continues as to whether these patients should be observed until progression or treated at time of diagnosis. One randomized controlled trial of immediate radiation therapy versus observation following surgery has been conducted successfully. EORTC 22,845 was a prospective, multi-institutional trial initiated in 1986 that randomized 311 patients to observation or immediate radiation therapy after surgery [62]. The 5-year survival rate was no different between the two arms: 63% in the radiation therapy arm and 66% in the observation arm. The time-to-progression was 4.8 years for immediate radiation therapy versus 3.4 years for observation ($P = .02$). The 5-year progression-free survival rate was 44% for the radiation therapy arm and 37% for the observation arm ($P = .02$). The interpretation of the investigators was that, because immediate radiation therapy did not improve survival over observation, radiation therapy could be deferred until disease progression.

Two prospective phase III randomized trials attempted to answer the question of the optimum dose of radiation therapy. EORTC 22,844 was a prospective randomized study of low- versus high-dose radiation therapy [63]. Patients were randomized to either 4500 cGy in 25 fractions or 5940 cGy in 33 fractions. With a median follow-up time of more than 6 years, the 5-year overall survival rates (58% versus 59%, low-dose versus high-dose) and progression-free survival rates (47% versus 50%, low-dose versus high-dose) were not significantly different. The second phase III trial to evaluate radiation dose was an Intergroup trial that randomized 211 patients to local radiation therapy with either 5040 cGy or 6480 cGy [64]. The median follow-up time was 6.5 years. Five-year survival did not differ between the two arms: 72% for the low-dose versus 64% for the high-dose group. The median survival for the entire patient cohort was 9.25 years. Data on treatment failure with respect to radiation field were available on 65 of 114 patients with disease progression. Ninety-two percent of failures occurred within the radiation field, 3% failed outside the field but within 2 cm of it, and 5% failed outside the field and beyond 2 cm.

Based on the adverse prognostic factors identified in these studies [64,65], RTOG 9802 randomized unfavorable patients (age 40 and older who had subtotal resection or biopsy) to standard-dose radiation therapy (54 Gy in 30 fractions) plus or minus six cycles of standard dose PCV [66]. Favorable patients (age under 40 who underwent GTR) were observed. The unfavorable group showed no significant difference in overall survival. Progression-free survival at 2 and 5 years was 73% and 39%, respectively, with radiation therapy alone versus 72% and 61%, respectively, with radiation therapy and PCV ($P = .38$). For the favorable patients, overall survival at 2 and 5 years was 99% and 94%, respectively. Progression-free survival at 2 and 5 years was 82% and 50%. The results of all published phase III trials are summarized in Table 4.

*Quality of life outcomes in low-grade glioma*

Given the relatively long survival of patients who have low-grade gliomas, and retrospective data suggesting a decline in cognitive function after radiation therapy in patients who have low-grade glioma, the EORTC and Intergroup trials included companion studies evaluating quality of life outcomes [67–70]. The EORTC study suffered from poor compliance, with fewer than 50% of patients completing at least one questionnaire. Thus, data were insufficient to compare baseline preradiation scores to posttreatment scores. Comparisons between the high- and low-dose radiation therapy arms were made for two time points: (1) from the completion of radiation therapy to 6 months and (2) from 7 to 15 months after radiation therapy was completed. In the initial postradiation therapy 6-month interval, the high-dose–arm patients reported lower levels of functioning and

Table 4
Dose-response of unfavorable low-grade gliomas to radiation in randomized trials

| Treatment | $OS_2$ | $OS_5$ | MOST (y) | $PFS_2$ | $PFS_5$ | MPFST | Study |
|-----------|--------|--------|----------|---------|---------|-------|-------|
| Observation | — | — | — | — | — | 3.4 | EORTC 22,845 |
| Observation (F) | 99% | 94% | n/a | 82% | 50% | n/a | RTOG 9802 |
| 4500 | — | 58% | 6.0 | — | 47% | 5.0 | EORTC 22,844 |
| 5040 | — | 72% | ~9.8 | — | n/a | 5.5 | Intergroup |
| 5400 | — | 68% | 7.2 | — | 55% | 5.3 | EORTC 22,845 |
| 5400 (UF) | 87% | 61% | NR | 73% | 39% | 4.0 | RTOG 9802 |
| 5400 + PCV (UF) | 86% | 70% | 6.0 | 72% | 61% | 6.0 | RTOG 9802 |
| 5940 | — | 59% | ~7.0 | — | 50% | 5.0 | EORTC 22,844 |
| 6480 | — | 64% | ~8.4 | — | n/a | 5.5 | Intergroup |

Blank fields indicate data are not available.

*Abbreviations:* F, favorable; MOST, median overall survival time; MPFST, median progression-free survival time; n/a, not available; $OS_x$, overall survival at x years; $PFS_x$, progression-free survival at x years; UF, unfavorable (see text for definitions).

more symptoms than patients in the low-dose arm. In the 7- to 15-month post-RT interval, statistically significant differences favoring the low-dose arm were observed in leisure time activity and emotional functioning. This quality of life study, in general, did not reveal any major differences between the high- and low-dose arms, nor between early and late radiation therapy.

In its companion study, the Intergroup trial assessed cognitive function, as measured by the Folstein Mini-Mental Status Examination (MMSE) [68,70,71]. The MMSE has a range of 0 to 30 with "normal" for this study being from 27 to 30 and "abnormal" from 0 to 26. A change from baseline of three or more points was considered a priori to be clinically significant. Patients' MMSE scores were obtained at baseline and at all subsequent scheduled follow-up visits. In patients who did not have tumor progression, significant deterioration from baseline occurred at years 1, 2, and 5 in 8%, 5%, and 5% of patients, respectively. Patients who had abnormal baseline MMSE scores were as likely to have a clinically significant improvement in MMSE score as a decrease, following radiation therapy. Changes in MMSE were not predicted by radiation therapy dose, technique, age, sex, tumor size, or presence of seizures. These data suggest that patients who have pre-existing neurologic deficits related to their tumor may benefit from early radiation therapy.

*Visual pathway glioma*

Visual pathway gliomas are typically diagnosed before age 10 and represent 1% to 5% of all pediatric brain tumors [72–74]. Bilateral optic nerve involvement is more common in patients who have neurofibromatosis type I [75–78]. Almost 90% of patients may experience some degree of visual dysfunction [74]. In general, patients who have visual pathway gliomas do not die from the local effects of their tumors, and cause-specific survival rates approach 100%. Therefore, the multidisciplinary management of visual pathway gliomas emphasizes minimizing treatment sequelae. Surgical excision with clear margins results in excellent local control, but does not spare vision [79]. Radiation therapy (typically 45 Gy in 25 fractions at 1.8 Gy per fraction [80,81]) results in 10-year survival rates ranging from 40% to 93%, but at significant potential cost to young children [82–87]. Risks may include endocrine disorders, neurodevelopmental disorders, and second malignancy. Chemotherapy may be used to delay progression [88].

*Meningioma*

After GTR, the factors that predict for meningioma recurrence include subtotal resection, optic sheath location, four or more mitoses per high power field, male gender, age under 40, and microscopic brain invasion [89,90]. Five- and ten-year progression-free survival rates are 88% and

75% for patients who have a GTR versus 61% and 39% for patients who do not have a GTR [90]. The 5-year recurrence rates after resection for benign, atypical, and brain-invasive meningiomas are 12%, 41%, and 56%, respectively [91]. Location is often the critical factor in the decision to offer resection because some lesions are in a location prohibiting a safe operation that will yield a GTR [90,92,93]. Optic nerve sheath meningiomas require especially thoughtful management because complete resection is not possible in two thirds of cases [94]. Therefore, most investigators now recommend fractionated radiation therapy for definitive management of these lesions [95,96].

Fractionated daily radiation therapy is regarded by many (but not universally accepted) as the standard of care for subtotally resected meningiomas, those recurrent after resection, medically inoperable cases, tumors in unresectable locations, and those with atypical or malignant histology (WHO grade II-III) [94,97–104]. Definitive radiation therapy is also considered by some as an acceptable alternative to resection. For benign meningiomas, doses at or above 5000 to 5300 cGy in conventional fractionation are required for durable control [101,103,104]. Most investigators recommend higher doses for higher histologic grades [102,104,105]. Stable or improved visual fields and visual acuity can be expected in 95% to 100% of cases treated with definitive radiation therapy [95,100,106,107]. Local control rates for benign meningiomas that are unresected or subtotally resected and then treated with radiation therapy are equivalent to those for lesions treated with resection alone. An overview of local control and disease-specific survival rates is seen in Table 5.

Radiosurgery has been used for well-circumscribed WHO grade I meningiomas [108]. It is not considered definitive therapy for WHO grade II or higher-grade lesions because of the high risk of failure outside the treated volume [109]. Local control rates are similar to those with GTR, subtotal resection followed by radiation therapy, or definitive radiation therapy [109,110]. Most investigators advocate doses of 11 to 18 Gy at the isodose prescription line encompassing the tumor volume (marginal dose) [108,110–114].

*Pituitary tumors*

The management of pituitary tumors is complex and should be multidisciplinary [115]. The goals are to accomplish the following without producing hypopituitarism or injury to adjacent structures: define the extent of tumor, evaluate hormone deficits or excesses, remove or destroy tumor masses, control hypersecretion, and correct endocrine deficiencies. Excellent control can be achieved for patients who have pituitary adenomas. Appropriate treatment depends on the size of the tumor and the need for rapid amelioration of signs and symptoms that have resulted from excess hormone production. Pretreatment studies should include MRI-based imaging, a comprehensive

Table 5
Meningiomas: incidence, histopathologic findings, treatment and outcomes by World Health Organization grade

| | WHO grade I/benign | WHO grade II/atypical | WHO grade III/malignant |
|---|---|---|---|
| Incidence | 81% | 15% | 12% |
| Necrosis | – | focal | extensive |
| Brain invasion | – | –/+ | + |
| Metastases | – | – | + |
| Mitotic index | <4/10 HPF | 4–10/10 HPF | ≥20/10 HPF |
| Anaplasia | – | – | + |
| Nuclear atypia | – | – | + |
| Recommended doses for fractionated radiation therapy (subtotal resection or definitive therapy) | ≥5220 cGy in 29 fx | 5400–5940 cGy in 27–33 fx | 60 Gy in 30 fx |
| Recommended dose for radiosurgery | 12–18 Gy | 16–24 Gy | 18–24 Gy |
| 5-Year local with surgery alone | 88% | 59% | 0%–44% |
| 5-Year local control with radiation therapy or radiosurgery (subtotal resection or definitive therapy) | 88%–96% | 33%–68% | 0% |
| 5-Year disease-specific survival | 88%–94% | 34%–76% | 0%–5% |
| Median survival | n/a | 10.6 years | 1.5 years |

*Abbreviations:* +, present; –, absent; fx, fractions; HPF, high-power fields; n/a, not available.

endocrinologic testing, and formal visual field testing. A suggested decision-making tree is shown in Fig. 1.

The management recommendations for this group of tumors lacks level 1 evidence. After complete resection of a benign adenoma and no adjuvant treatment, 68% of patients will have long-term local control [116]. The treatment for large tumors presenting with mass effect is resection, potentially followed by radiation therapy or radiosurgery. Although radiation therapy alone is effective in selected cases, surgical decompression plus postoperative irradiation provides better results, particularly in patients who have moderately advanced visual field deficits. With very large invasive tumors, reliance should be primarily on radiation therapy because complete resection is usually not possible and attempted radical removal is associated with a high mortality and morbidity. However, subtotal resection may be required as an urgent debulking measure if vision is severely compromised.

The efficacy of external beam radiation therapy and SRS in managing pituitary tumors is well documented in retrospective institutional series. Primary radiation therapy is potentially effective for control of the mass

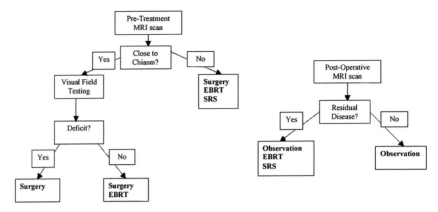

Fig. 1. Decision tree for the management of pituitary tumors. Medical management is not illustrated in this flow diagram. SRS, stereotactic radiosurgery. (*Courtesy of* Volker W. Stieber, MD, Winston-Salem, NC.)

effect of larger tumors; in general, however, it is preferable to decompress the chiasm and then irradiate. External radiation therapy is also used in the treatment of tumors that are recurrent after primary surgery [117]. SRS has become an important adjunct, but also lacks categoric evidence. The goal of radiosurgical management is control of tumor growth and hormone hypersecretion. Uncommonly used forms of radiation therapy include proton and α-particle radiation therapy and implantation of radioactive sources ($^{90}$Y or $^{198}$Au). Like radiosurgery, these modalities also deliver large doses to highly restricted volumes within the pituitary gland; thus, their application is limited to small, essentially intrasellar tumors.

Pituitary adenomas show dose-response rates that depend on tumor type. Nonfunctioning tumors are usually controlled (stable disease) with 45 to 50.4 Gy of conventionally fractionated external beam radiation therapy, or SRS delivering 20 to 25 Gy, with control rates in the 95% range. Functioning tumors require slightly higher doses, typically 50 to 54 Gy of conventionally fractionated external beam radiation therapy, or SRS delivering 25 to 30 Gy. Control rates are slightly lower than for nonfunctioning tumors [118–137]. A summary of dosing guidelines is shown in Table 6.

Table 6
Radiation therapy and radiosurgery treatment guidelines for pituitary tumors

| | External beam radiation therapy (1.8 Gy/fraction) | Radiosurgery (optic chiasm dose ≤9 Gy) | Local tumor control | Biochemical control |
|---|---|---|---|---|
| Nonfunctioning tumors | 45.0–50.4 Gy | 12.0–24.0 Gy to margin | 95% | n/a |
| Functioning tumors | 45.0–54.0 Gy | 25.0–30.0 Gy to margin | 90%–95% | 33%–95% |

*Abbreviation:* n/a, not applicable.

*Craniopharyngioma*

Because radical resection is associated with a high rate of visual loss and impaired hormone function requiring replacement therapy, many investigators recommend less radical surgery (subtotal resection or biopsy) followed by radiation therapy After incomplete resection followed by irradiation, treatment-related toxicity also includes impairment of hormone function, but the interval between treatment and onset of the disorder is much longer and less severe [138]. Impairment of vision is reported in less than 10% of patients treated with incomplete resection followed by irradiation, compared with up to 20% after complete resection [139]. If the diagnosis can be made radiographically with reasonable accuracy, and surgical intervention is not required to reverse mass effect, radiation therapy may be considered as the primary modality. Fractionated radiation therapy to a median dose of 52.2 Gy results in 10-year local control rates of 84% to 100%, compared with 42% with surgery alone, with the caveat that these are non-randomized data [140,141]. Because radiation therapy is also effective as salvage therapy, overall survival appears similar, at approximately 85% at 10 years. A growing body of evidence suggests that radiosurgery alone could be considered. With doses in the range of 10 to 12 Gy, the actuarial 10-year survival rate is 91%, but the progression-free survival rate is only 54% (at 10 years) [142].

**Complications of radiation therapy**

Suggested definitions of, and doses typically prescribed to, ICRU volumes are provided in Table 1, arranged by histologic diagnosis. Late complications from radiation therapy depend on the region irradiated and the structures in the surrounding area that receive significant dose. In the dose range of 45 to 60 Gy, used most commonly when treating CNS tumors, the probability of causing serious late toxicity is relatively low. Without compromising therapeutic dose to the GTV, attempts should be made to limit OAR dose as follows: optic chiasm (54 Gy); optic nerves (60 Gy); optic globes including retina (50 Gy); brainstem (54 Gy); pituitary gland (50 Gy); and spinal cord (50 Gy) [23].

Damage to the lacrimal gland, with dry eye and corneal damage, and cataract formation occur most commonly with doses exceeding 35 Gy [143]. The incidence of symptomatic radiation necrosis of brain parenchyma is expected to be 2.5% at 5040 cGy and 5% at 6480 cGy [64]. Damage to the optic chiasm and nerves is, in fact, rare and dose dependent, usually seen in patients treated with 2 Gy fractions or higher, demonstrating a combined incidence of injury of 0.3% below 2 Gy versus 4% at 2 Gy or higher. At 10 years, patients treated with daily doses of 180 cGy to 45 Gy can expect no risk of visual impairment from therapy, and most recent series report no symptomatic visual injury below 55 Gy [144]. In pediatric patients, doses as low as 18 Gy have been implicated in neurocognitive deficits, and recent data suggest that the sensitivity of stem cells in the hippocampus responsible for neurogenesis, serving memory functions, may indeed be as low as 5 Gy, and this remains an active area of investigation [145–147].

With single-fraction radiosurgery, injury to the optic apparatus is highly dose dependent. Chiasm dose should not exceed 9 to 10 Gy [148,149]. A dose response appears evident, with a 27% incidence of optic neuropathy at doses between 10 and 15 Gy, a 78% incidence above 14 Gy, and little or no incidence below 10 Gy [148,150]. The cranial nerves traversing the cavernous sinus are relatively radioresistant, with a reported 13% incidence (8% permanent) of neuropathy at single doses up to 40 Gy [151].

Secondary malignancies are a rare but known late complication of radiation therapy. The most common secondary intracranial tumors are meningiomas [152]. Literature review encompassing several decades and thousands of patient-years estimates the risk of secondary malignancies after fractionated radiation therapy at 1.35% at 10 years and 1.9% at 20 years, with a calculated risk of approximately 0.04% at doses between 4500 and 5040 cGy [153,154]. Among children with primary brain tumors who receive definitive radiation therapy, disability is related to age under 3 at the time of treatment and tumor extension to the hypothalamus; their incidence of second intracranial malignancy is 1.6% [155].

## Future directions

At the time of treatment planning, dose-function histogram analysis can display the relative function of a structure versus dose and may provide additional data needed to obtain or evaluate desired heterogeneous dose distributions. Using IMRT, the dose could be conformed either directly or inversely proportional to the biologic properties of a target or normal tissues, depending on what information the corresponding functional imaging set represents for a particular structure. Late effects of IMRT, which theoretically may expose more normal tissue to lower doses, are not yet known, and work is underway to model these responses biologically [24].

Additional imaging studies, may reflect the biologic characteristics of CNS tumors, such as metabolism, proliferation, oxygenation, and blood flow, and the function of surrounding normal brain to these include MRS, functional MRI, PET, and single photon emission tomography scans. Integration of such biologic data into the treatment planning process may allow further optimization of dose, based on biologic parameters [28,29,156]. For example, 3D MRS may be used to assess the CNI and is thought to represent infiltrative malignant glioma more accurately than conventional MRI [157–162]. Comparison of volumes of microscopic tumor infiltration, as defined by T2 changes on conventional MRI versus the CNI as determined by 3D MRS, demonstrate a median increase of 14% in volume size with the addition of the latter modality [156]. Given that the volume extensions using 3D MRS are typically immediately adjacent to the treatment volumes as defined by conventional MRI, the failure of highly focal dose-escalation strategies using brachytherapy or SRS may well be due to undertreatment of adjacent microscopic disease. [$^{11}$C]-methionine PET imaging may be useful to define the extent of low-grade gliomas better [35]. Functional MRI scans can show regions of normal brain function [32] (eg, motor and expressive and receptive language areas); MEG [33] provides similar functional information. Integrating MEG data into treatment planning with IMRT implementation may allow further sparing of the normal functional regions of the brain [33].

After completion of radiation therapy, accurate evaluation of MRI changes may be difficult because necrosis and tumor progression often have similar appearances (ie, enhancement on T1-weighted MR images with increase in surrounding edema), which is especially problematic in the setting of dose escalation [22]. Differentiating treatment-related new contrast enhancement from tumor progression, although difficult [57], is important, because early posttreatment MRI-based tumor progression appears to predict median survival [163]. Three-dimensional MRS may be useful in differentiating between necrosis and viable tumor [164–169].

## Summary

Radiation therapy is used postoperatively as adjunctive therapy to decrease local failure, to delay tumor progression and prolong survival; as a curative treatment; as a therapy that halts further tumor growth; to alter function; and for palliation. The most commonly used form is photon therapy. Radiation therapy can be delivered in multiple fractions or as single-dose radiosurgery. Registration of MRI scan data sets with the treatment-planning CT scan is essential for accurate definition of the tumor and surrounding OAR. Integrating additional imaging studies that reflect the biologic characteristics of CNS tumors is an area of active research. Conformal treatment delivery is used to spare adjacent normal tissue from receiving unnecessary dose. In the dose range used when treating CNS tumors, the probability of causing serious late toxicity is relatively low, and secondary malignancies are rare.

## References

[1] Brown PD, Buckner JC, O'Fallon JR, et al. Adult patients with supratentorial pilocytic astrocytomas: a prospective multicenter clinical trial. Int J Radiat Oncol Biol Phys 2004;58: 1153–60.

[2] Scott CB, Scarantino C, Urtasun R, et al. Validation and predictive power of Radiation Therapy Oncology Group (RTOG) recursive partitioning analysis classes for malignant glioma patients: a report using RTOG 90-06. Int J Radiat Oncol Biol Phys 1998;40:51–5.

[3] Tortosa A, Vinolas N, Villa S, et al. Prognostic implication of clinical, radiologic, and pathologic features in patients with anaplastic gliomas. Cancer 2003;97:1063–71.

[4] Perry A, Scheithauer BW, Stafford SL, et al. "Malignancy" in meningiomas: a clinicopathologic study of 116 patients, with grading implications. Cancer 1999;85:2046–56.

[5] Stieber V, Tatter S, Shaw EG. Primary spinal tumors. In: Schiff D, editor. Principles of neuro-oncology. 1st edition. New York: McGraw-Hill Professional Publishing; 2005. p. 501–31.

[6] Rades D, Fehlauer F, Schild S, et al. [Treatment for central neurocytoma: a meta-analysis based on the data of 358 patients]. Strahlenther Onkol 2003;179:213–8 [in German].

[7] Rades D, Fehlauer F, Lamszus K, et al. Well-differentiated neurocytoma: what is the best available treatment? Neuro Oncol 2005;7:77–83.

[8] Gaspar L, Scott C, Rotman M, et al. Recursive partitioning analysis (RPA) of prognostic factors in three Radiation Therapy Oncology Group (RTOG) brain metastases trials. Int J Radiat Oncol Biol Phys 1997;37:745–51.

[9] Sanders KE, Ha CS, Cortes-Franco JE, et al. The role of craniospinal irradiation in adults with a central nervous system recurrence of leukemia. Cancer 2004;100:2176–80.

[10] Hazuka MB, Burleson WD, Stroud DN, et al. Multiple brain metastases are associated with poor survival in patients treated with surgery and radiotherapy. J Clin Oncol 1993;11: 369–73.

[11] Patchell RA. The management of brain metastases. Cancer Treat Rev 2003;29:533–40.

[12] Patchell RA, Tibbs PA, Walsh JW, et al. A randomized trial of surgery in the treatment of single metastases to the brain. N Engl J Med 1990;322:494–500.

[13] Vecht CJ, Haaxma-Reiche H, Noordijk EM, et al. Treatment of single brain metastasis: radiotherapy alone or combined with neurosurgery? Ann Neurol 1993;33:583–90.

[14] Mintz AH, Kestle J, Rathbone MP, et al. A randomized trial to assess the efficacy of surgery in addition to radiotherapy in patients with a single cerebral metastasis. Cancer 1996;78: 1470–6.

[15] Thwaites DI, Tuohy JB. Back to the future: the history and development of the clinical linear accelerator. Phys Med Biol 2006;51:R343–62.

[16] Schulz-Ertner D, Jakel O, Schlegel W. Radiation therapy with charged particles. Semin Radiat Oncol 2006;16:249–59.

[17] Leksell L. Stereotactic radiosurgery. J Neurol Neurosurg Psychiatry 1983;46:797–803.

[18] Deye, J, Abrams, J, Coleman, N. The National Cancer Institute guidelines for the use of intensity-modulated radiation therapy in clinical trials. Bethesday (MD): National Cancer Institute; 2005.

[19] Miller AD, Leslie RA. The area postrema and vomiting. Front Neuroendocrinol 1994;15: 301–20.

[20] Gaspar LE, Scott C, Murray K, et al. Validation of the RTOG recursive partitioning analysis (RPA) classification for brain metastases. Int J Radiat Oncol Biol Phys 2000;47: 1001–6.

[21] Shaw EG, Seiferheld W, Scott C, et al. Reexamining the Radiation Therapy Oncology Group (RTOG) recursive partitioning analysis (RPA) for glioblastoma multiforme (GBM) patients. Int J Radiat Oncol Biol Phys 2003;57:S135–6.

[22] Stieber V, Tatter S, Lovato J, et al. A phase I dose escalating study of intensity modulated radiation therapy (IMRT) for the treatment of glioblastoma multiforme (GBM). Int J Radiat Oncol Biol Phys 2004;(Suppl 1):261.

[23] Stieber VW, Munley M. Central nervous system tumors. In: Mundt AJ, Roeske JC, editors. Intensity-modulated radiation therapy: a clinical perspective. 1st edition. Ontario (CA): BC Decker, Inc.; 2005. p. 231–41.

[24] Niemierko A. Reporting and analyzing dose distributions: a concept of equivalent uniform dose. Med Phys 1997;24:103–10.

[25] Jaffray DA, Siewerdsen JH, Wong JW, et al. Flat-panel cone-beam computed tomography for image-guided radiation therapy. Int J Radiat Oncol Biol Phys 2002;53:1337–49.

[26] Adler JR Jr, Murphy MJ, Chang SD, et al. Image-guided robotic radiosurgery. Neurosurgery 1999;44:1299–306.

[27] Mackie TR, Balog J, Ruchala K, et al. Tomotherapy. Semin Radiat Oncol 1999;9:108–17.

[28] Munley MT, Kearns WT, Hinson WH, et al. Bioanatomic IMRT treatment planning with dose function histograms. Int J Radiat Oncol Biol Phys 2002;54:126.

[29] Pirzkall A, Larson DA, McKnight TR, et al. MR-spectroscopy results in improved target delineation for high-grade gliomas. Int J Radiat Oncol Biol Phys 2000;48:115.

[30] Carson PL, Giger M, Welch MJ, et al. Biomedical Imaging Research Opportunities Workshop: report and recommendations. Radiology 2003;229:328–39.

[31] Morris DE, Bourland JD, Rosenman JG, et al. Three-dimensional conformal radiation treatment planning and delivery for low- and intermediate-grade gliomas. Semin Radiat Oncol 2001;11:124–37.

[32] Ricci PE, Dungan DH. Imaging of low- and intermediate-grade gliomas. Semin Radiat Oncol 2001;11:103–12.

[33] Babiloni F, Mattia D, Babiloni C, et al. Multimodal integration of EEG, MEG and fMRI data for the solution of the neuroimage puzzle. Magn Reson Imaging 2004;22:1471–6.

[34] McKnight TR, dem Bussche MH, Vigneron DB, et al. Histopathological validation of a three-dimensional magnetic resonance spectroscopy index as a predictor of tumor presence. J Neurosurg 2002;97:794–802.

[35] Nuutinen J, Sonninen P, Lehikoinen P, et al. Radiotherapy treatment planning and long-term follow-up with [C-11] methionine PET in patients with low-grade astrocytoma. Int J Radiat Oncol Biol Phys 2000;48:43–52.

[36] International Commission on Radiation Units and Measurements, Inc. ICRU Report 50, Prescribing, recording, and reporting photon beam therapy. 50. Bethesda, (MD): Nuclear Technology Publishing; 1993.

[37] International Commission on Radiation Units and Measurements, Inc. ICRU Report 62: Prescribing, recording and reporting photon beam therapy (Supplement to ICRU Report 50). Wambersie A, Landberg T. Journal of the ICRU 62. Bethesda, (MD): Nuclear Technology Publishing; 1999.

[38] Curran WJ Jr, Scott CB, Horton J, et al. Recursive partitioning analysis of prognostic factors in three Radiation Therapy Oncology Group malignant glioma trials. J Natl Cancer Inst 1993;85:704–10.

[39] Walker MD, Alexander E Jr, Hunt WE, et al. Evaluation of BCNU and/or radiotherapy in the treatment of anaplastic gliomas. A cooperative clinical trial. J Neurosurg 1978;49: 333–43.

[40] Stupp R, Mason WP, van den Bent MJ, et al. Radiotherapy plus concomitant and adjuvant temozolomide for glioblastoma. N Engl J Med 2005;352:987–96.

[41] Lacroix M, Abi-Said D, Fourney DR, et al. A multivariate analysis of 416 patients with glioblastoma multiforme: prognosis, extent of resection, and survival. J Neurosurg 2001; 95:190–8.

[42] Vuorinen V, Hinkka S, Farkkila M, et al. Debulking or biopsy of malignant glioma in elderly people–a randomised study. Acta Neurochir (Wien) 2003;145:5–10.

[43] Chang SM, Parney IF, Huang W, et al. Patterns of care for adults with newly diagnosed malignant glioma. JAMA 2005;293:557–64.

[44] Walker MD, Strike TA, Sheline GE. An analysis of dose-effect relationship in the radiotherapy of malignant gliomas. Int J Radiat Oncol Biol Phys 1979;5:1725–31.

[45] Lee SW, Fraass BA, Marsh LH, et al. Patterns of failure following high-dose 3-D conformal radiotherapy for high-grade astrocytomas: a quantitative dosimetric study. Int J Radiat Oncol Biol Phys 1999;43:79–88.

[46] Selker RG, Shapiro WR, Burger P, et al. The Brain Tumor Cooperative Group NIH Trial 87-01: a randomized comparison of surgery, external radiotherapy, and carmustine versus surgery, interstitial radiotherapy boost, external radiation therapy, and carmustine. Neurosurgery 2002;51:343–55.

[47] Souhami L, Seiferheld W, Brachman D, et al. Randomized comparison of stereotactic radiosurgery followed by conventional radiotherapy with carmustine to conventional radiotherapy with carmustine for patients with glioblastoma multiforme: report of Radiation Therapy Oncology Group 93-05 protocol. Int J Radiat Oncol Biol Phys 2004; 60:853–60.

[48] Mirimanoff RO, Gorlia T, Mason W, et al. Radiotherapy and temozolomide for newly diagnosed glioblastoma: recursive partitioning analysis of the EORTC 26981/22981-NCIC CE3 phase III randomized trial. J Clin Oncol 2006;24:2563–9.

[49] Fowler JF. Brief summary of radiobiological principles in fractionated radiotherapy. Semin Radiat Oncol 1992;2:16–21.

[50] Nilsson P, Thames HD, Joiner MC. A generalized formulation of the 'incomplete-repair' model for cell survival and tissue response to fractionated low dose-rate irradiation. Int J Radiat Biol 1990;57:127–42.

[51] Thames HD. An 'incomplete-repair' model for survival after fractionated and continuous irradiations. Int J Radiat Biol Relat Stud Phys Chem Med 1985;47:319–39.

[52] Burnet NG, Jena R, Jefferies SJ, et al. Mathematical modelling of survival of glioblastoma patients suggests a role for radiotherapy dose escalation and predicts poorer outcome after delay to start treatment. Clin Oncol (R Coll Radiol) 2006;18:93–103.

[53] Chan JL, Lee SW, Fraass BA, et al. Survival and failure patterns of high-grade gliomas after three-dimensional conformal radiotherapy. J Clin Oncol 2002;20:1635–42.

[54] Hochberg FH, Pruitt A. Assumptions in the radiotherapy of glioblastoma. Neurology 1980;30:907–11.

[55] deGuzman AF, Kearns WT, Shaw E, et al. Radiation safety issues with high activities of liquid I-125: techniques and experience. J Appl Clin Med Phys 2003;4:143–8.

[56] Tatter SB, Shaw EG, Rosenblum ML, et al. An inflatable balloon catheter and liquid 125I radiation source (GliaSite Radiation Therapy System) for treatment of recurrent malignant glioma: multicenter safety and feasibility trial. J Neurosurg 2003;99: 297–303.

[57] Stieber V, Tatter S, Mikkelsen T, et al. A phase I dose-escalation trial of GliaSite brachytherapy with conventional radiation therapy for newly diagnosed glioblastoma multiforme. Presented at the ASCO Meeting Abstracts. Orlando (FL), May 13–17, 2005

[58] Chakravarti A, Erkkinen MG, Nestler U, et al. Temozolomide-mediated radiation enhancement in glioblastoma: a report on underlying mechanisms. Clin Cancer Res 2006;12:4738–46.

[59] Cairncross G, Berkey B, Shaw E, et al. Phase III trial of chemotherapy plus radiotherapy compared with radiotherapy alone for pure and mixed anaplastic oligodendroglioma: Intergroup Radiation Therapy Oncology Group Trial 9402. J Clin Oncol 2006;24:2707–14.

[60] Prados MD, Seiferheld W, Sandler HM, et al. Phase III randomized study of radiotherapy plus procarbazine, lomustine, and vincristine with or without BUdR for treatment of anaplastic astrocytoma: final report of RTOG 9404. Int J Radiat Oncol Biol Phys 2004;58: 1147–52.

[61] Medical Research Council Brain Tumor Working Party. Randomized trial of procarbazine, lomustine, and vincristine in the adjuvant treatment of high-grade astrocytoma: a Medical Research Council trial. J Clin Oncol 2001;19:509–18.

[62] Karim AB, Afra D, Cornu P, et al. Randomized trial on the efficacy of radiotherapy for cerebral low-grade glioma in the adult: European Organization for Research and Treatment of Cancer Study 22845 with the Medical Research Council study BRO4: an interim analysis. Int J Radiat Oncol Biol Phys 2002;52:316–24.

[63] Karim AB, Maat B, Hatlevoll R, et al. A randomized trial on dose-response in radiation therapy of low-grade cerebral glioma: European Organization for Research and Treatment of Cancer (EORTC) Study 22844. Int J Radiat Oncol Biol Phys 1996;36: 549–56.

[64] Shaw E, Arusell R, Scheithauer B, et al. Prospective randomized trial of low- versus high-dose radiation therapy in adults with supratentorial low-grade glioma: initial report of a North Central Cancer Treatment Group/Radiation Therapy Oncology Group/Eastern Cooperative Oncology Group study. J Clin Oncol 2002;20:2267–76.

[65] Pignatti F, van den BM, Curran D, et al. Prognostic factors for survival in adult patients with cerebral low-grade glioma. J Clin Oncol 2002;20:2076–84.

[66] Shaw EG, Berkey B, Coons SW, et al. Initial report of Radiation Therapy Oncology Group (RTOG) 9802: prospective studies in adult low-grade glioma (LGG). J Clin Oncol (Meeting Abstracts) 2006;24:1500.

[67] Klein M, Heimans JJ, Aaronson NK, et al. Effect of radiotherapy and other treatment-related factors on mid-term to long-term cognitive sequelae in low-grade gliomas: a comparative study. Lancet 2002;360:1361–8.

[68] Brown PD, Buckner JC, O'Fallon JR, et al. Effects of radiotherapy on cognitive function in patients with low-grade glioma measured by the Folstein mini-mental state examination. J Clin Oncol 2003;21:2519–24.

[69] Kiebert GM, Curran D, Aaronson NK, et al. Quality of life after radiation therapy of cerebral low-grade gliomas of the adult: results of a randomised phase III trial on dose response (EORTC trial 22844). EORTC Radiotherapy Co-operative Group. Eur J Cancer 1998;34:1902–9.

[70] Laack NN, Brown PD, Ivnik RJ, et al. Cognitive function after radiotherapy for supratentorial low-grade glioma: a North Central Cancer Treatment Group prospective study. Int J Radiat Oncol Biol Phys 2005;63(4):1175–83.

[71] Klein LE, Roca RP, McArthur J, et al. Diagnosing dementia. Univariate and multivariate analyses of the mental status examination. J Am Geriatr Soc 1985;33:483–8.

[72] Weiss L, Sagerman RH, King GA, et al. Controversy in the management of optic nerve glioma. Cancer 1987;59:1000–4.

[73] Alshail E, Rutka JT, Becker LE, et al. Optic chiasmatic-hypothalamic glioma. Brain Pathol 1997;7:799–806.

[74] Dutton JJ. Gliomas of the anterior visual pathway. Surv Ophthalmol 1994;38:427–52.

[75] Jakobiec FA, Depot MJ, Kennerdell JS, et al. Combined clinical and computed tomographic diagnosis of orbital glioma and meningioma. Ophthalmology 1984;91:137–55.

[76] Housepian FM, Chi TL. Neurofibromatosis and optic pathways gliomas. J Neurooncol 1993;15:51–5.

[77] Lewis RA, Gerson LP, Axelson KA, et al. von Recklinghausen neurofibromatosis. II. Incidence of optic gliomata. Ophthalmology 1984;91:929–35.

[78] Listernick R, Charrow J, Greenwald M, et al. Natural history of optic pathway tumors in children with neurofibromatosis type 1: a longitudinal study. J Pediatr 1994;125:63–6.

[79] Alvord EC Jr, Lofton S. Gliomas of the optic nerve or chiasm. Outcome by patients' age, tumor site, and treatment. J Neurosurg 1988;68:85–98.

[80] Erkal HS, Serin M, Cakmak A. Management of optic pathway and chiasmatic-hypothalamic gliomas in children with radiation therapy. Radiother Oncol 1997;45:11–5.

[81] Grabenbauer GG, Schuchardt U, Buchfelder M, et al. Radiation therapy of optico-hypothalamic gliomas (OHG)–radiographic response, vision and late toxicity. Radiother Oncol 2000;54:239–45.

[82] Zebrack BJ, Gurney JG, Oeffinger K, et al. Psychological outcomes in long-term survivors of childhood brain cancer: a report from the Childhood Cancer Survivor Study. J Clin Oncol 2004;22:999–1006.

[83] Robison LL, Green DM, Hudson M, et al. Long-term outcomes of adult survivors of childhood cancer. Cancer 2005;104:2557–64.

[84] Robison LL. The Childhood Cancer Survivor Study: a resource for research of long-term outcomes among adult survivors of childhood cancer. Minn Med 2005;88:45–9.

[85] Jenkin D, Angyalfi S, Becker L, et al. Optic glioma in children: surveillance, resection, or irradiation? Int J Radiat Oncol Biol Phys 1993;25:215–25.

[86] Kovalic JJ, Grigsby PW, Shepard MJ, et al. Radiation therapy for gliomas of the optic nerve and chiasm. Int J Radiat Oncol Biol Phys 1990;18:927–32.

[87] Pierce SM, Barnes PD, Loeffler JS, et al. Definitive radiation therapy in the management of symptomatic patients with optic glioma. Survival and long-term effects. Cancer 1990;65: 45–52.

[88] Demaerel P, de Ruyter N, Casteels I, et al. Visual pathway glioma in children treated with chemotherapy. Eur J Paediatr Neurol 2002;6:207–12.

[89] Stafford SL, Perry A, Leavitt JA, et al. Anterior visual pathway meningiomas primarily resected between 1978 and 1988: the Mayo Clinic Rochester experience. J Neuroophthalmol 1998;18:206–10.

[90] Stafford SL, Perry A, Suman VJ, et al. Primarily resected meningiomas: outcome and prognostic factors in 581 Mayo Clinic patients, 1978 through 1988. Mayo Clin Proc 1998;73: 936–42.

[91] Perry A, Stafford SL, Scheithauer BW, et al. Meningioma grading: an analysis of histologic parameters. Am J Surg Pathol 1997;21:1455–65.

[92] Kondziolka D, Flickinger JC, Perez B. Judicious resection and/or radiosurgery for parasagittal meningiomas: outcomes from a multicenter review. Gamma knife Meningioma Study Group. Neurosurgery 1998;43:405–13.

[93] Roberti F, Sekhar LN, Kalavakonda C, et al. Posterior fossa meningiomas: surgical experience in 161 cases. Surg Neurol 2001;56:8–20.

[94] Margalit NS, Lesser JB, Moche J, et al. Meningiomas involving the optic nerve: technical aspects and outcomes for a series of 50 patients. Neurosurgery 2003;53:523–32.

[95] Pitz S, Becker G, Schiefer U, et al. Stereotactic fractionated irradiation of optic nerve sheath meningioma: a new treatment alternative. Br J Ophthalmol 2002;86:1265–8.

[96] Turbin RE, Thompson CR, Kennerdell JS, et al. A long-term visual outcome comparison in patients with optic nerve sheath meningioma managed with observation, surgery, radiotherapy, or surgery and radiotherapy. Ophthalmology 2002;109:890–9.

[97] Debus J, Wuendrich M, Pirzkall A, et al. High efficacy of fractionated stereotactic radiotherapy of large base-of-skull meningiomas: long-term results. J Clin Oncol 2001;19:3547–53.

[98] Mendenhall WM, Morris CG, Amdur RJ, et al. Radiotherapy alone or after subtotal resection for benign skull base meningiomas. Cancer 2003;98:1473–82.

[99] Glaholm J, Bloom HJ, Crow JH. The role of radiotherapy in the management of intracranial meningiomas: the Royal Marsden Hospital experience with 186 patients. Int J Radiat Oncol Biol Phys 1990;18:755–61.

[100] Baumert BG, Villa S, Studer G, et al. Early improvements in vision after fractionated stereotactic radiotherapy for primary optic nerve sheath meningioma. Radiother Oncol 2004; 72:169–74.

[101] Condra KS, Buatti JM, Mendenhall WM, et al. Benign meningiomas: primary treatment selection affects survival. Int J Radiat Oncol Biol Phys 1997;39:427–36.

[102] Goldsmith BJ. Meningioma. In: Leibel SJ, Phillips TI, editors. Textbook of radiation oncology: principles. 1st edition. New York: Elsevier; 1998. p. 324–40.

[103] Goldsmith BJ, Wara WM, Wilson CB, et al. Postoperative irradiation for subtotally resected meningiomas. A retrospective analysis of 140 patients treated from 1967 to 1990. J Neurosurg 1994;80:195–201.

[104] Milosevic MF, Frost PJ, Laperriere NJ, et al. Radiotherapy for atypical or malignant intracranial meningioma. Int J Radiat Oncol Biol Phys 1996;34:817–22.

[105] Chamberlain MC. Adjuvant combined modality therapy for malignant meningiomas. J Neurosurg 1996;84:733–6.

[106] Narayan S, Cornblath WT, Sandler HM, et al. Preliminary visual outcomes after three-dimensional conformal radiation therapy for optic nerve sheath meningioma. Int J Radiat Oncol Biol Phys 2003;56:537–43.

[107] Becker G, Jeremic B, Pitz S, et al. Stereotactic fractionated radiotherapy in patients with optic nerve sheath meningioma. Int J Radiat Oncol Biol Phys 2002;54:1422–9.

[108] Flickinger JC, Kondziolka D, Maitz AH, et al. Gamma knife radiosurgery of imaging-diagnosed intracranial meningioma. Int J Radiat Oncol Biol Phys 2003;56:801–6.

[109] Stafford SL, Pollock BE, Foote RL, et al. Meningioma radiosurgery: tumor control, outcomes, and complications among 190 consecutive patients. Neurosurgery 2001;49:1029–37.

[110] Pollock BE, Stafford SL, Utter A, et al. Stereotactic radiosurgery provides equivalent tumor control to Simpson grade 1 resection for patients with small- to medium-size meningiomas. Int J Radiat Oncol Biol Phys 2003;55:1000–5.

[111] Eustacchio S, Trummer M, Fuchs I, et al. Preservation of cranial nerve function following Gamma knife radiosurgery for benign skull base meningiomas: experience in 121 patients with follow-up of 5 to 9.8 years. Acta Neurochir Suppl 2002;84:71–6.

[112] Shin M, Kurita H, Sasaki T, et al. Analysis of treatment outcome after stereotactic radiosurgery for cavernous sinus meningiomas. J Neurosurg 2001;95:435–9.

[113] Iwai Y, Yamanaka K, Ishiguro T. Gamma knife radiosurgery for the treatment of cavernous sinus meningiomas. Neurosurgery 2003;52:517–24.

[114] Lee JY, Niranjan A, McInerney J, et al. Stereotactic radiosurgery providing long-term tumor control of cavernous sinus meningiomas. J Neurosurg 2002;97:65–72.

[115] Stieber VW, deGuzman AF. Pituitary. In: Perez C, Brady L, Schmidt-Ullrich R, et al, editors. Principles and practice of radiation oncology. New York: Lippincott Williams and Wilkins; 2003.

[116] Turner HE, Stratton IM, Byrne JV, et al. Audit of selected patients with nonfunctioning pituitary adenomas treated without irradiation–a follow-up study. Clin Endocrinol (Oxf) 1999;51:281–4.

[117] Kovalic JJ, Grigsby PW, Fineberg BB. Recurrent pituitary adenomas after surgical resection: the role of radiation therapy. Radiology 1990;177:273–5.

[118] Zhang N, Pan L, Wang EM, et al. Radiosurgery for growth hormone-producing pituitary adenomas. J Neurosurg 2000;93(Suppl 3):6–9.

[119] Izawa M, Hayashi M, Nakaya K, et al. Gamma knife radiosurgery for pituitary adenomas. J Neurosurg 2000;93(Suppl 3):19–22.

[120] Mitsumori M, Shrieve DC, Alexander E III, et al. Initial clinical results of LINAC-based stereotactic radiosurgery and stereotactic radiotherapy for pituitary adenomas. Int J Radiat Oncol Biol Phys 1998;42:573–80.

[121] Shin M, Kurita H, Sasaki T, et al. Stereotactic radiosurgery for pituitary adenoma invading the cavernous sinus. J Neurosurg 2000;93(Suppl 3):2–5.

[122] Landolt AM, Haller D, Lomax N, et al. Stereotactic radiosurgery for recurrent surgically treated acromegaly: comparison with fractionated radiotherapy. J Neurosurg 1998;88:1002–8.

[123] Landolt AM, Lomax N. Gamma knife radiosurgery for prolactinomas. J Neurosurg 2000;93(Suppl 3):14–8.

[124] Witt TC. Stereotactic radiosurgery for pituitary tumors. Neurosurg Focus 2003;14:e10.

[125] Pan L, Zhang N, Wang EM, et al. Gamma knife radiosurgery as a primary treatment for prolactinomas. J Neurosurg 2000;93(Suppl 3):10–3.

[126] Sheehan JM, Vance ML, Sheehan JP, et al. Radiosurgery for Cushing's disease after failed transsphenoidal surgery. J Neurosurg 2000;93:738–42.

[127] Rahn T, Thoren M, Hall K, et al. Stereotactic radiosurgery in Cushing's syndrome: acute radiation effects. Surg Neurol 1980;14:85–92.

[128] Brada M, Rajan B, Traish D, et al. The long-term efficacy of conservative surgery and radiotherapy in the control of pituitary adenomas. Clin Endocrinol (Oxf) 1993;38:571–8.

[129] Halberg FE, Sheline GE. Radiation therapy of pituitary tumors. Endocrinol Metab Clin 1997;16:667–84.

[130] Zierhut D, Flentje M, Adolph J, et al. External radiotherapy of pituitary adenomas. Int J Radiat Oncol Biol Phys 1995;33:307–14.

[131] Urdaneta N, Chessin H, Fischer JJ. Pituitary adenomas and craniopharyngiomas: analysis of 99 cases treated with radiation therapy. Int J Radiat Oncol Biol Phys 1976;1:895–902.

[132] Gittoes NJ, Bates AS, Tse W, et al. Radiotherapy for non-function pituitary tumours. Clin Endocrinol (Oxf) 1998;48:331–7.

[133] Milker-Zabel S, Debus J, Thilmann C, et al. Fractionated stereotactically guided radiotherapy and radiosurgery in the treatment of functional and nonfunctional adenomas of the pituitary gland. Int J Radiat Oncol Biol Phys 2001;50:1279–86.

[134] Tsang RW, Brierley JD, Panzarella T, et al. Role of radiation therapy in clinical hormonally-active pituitary adenomas. Radiother Oncol 1996;41:45–53.

[135] Grigsby PW, Simpson JR, Stokes S, et al. Results of surgery and irradiation or irradiation alone for pituitary adenomas. J Neurooncol 1988;6:129–34.

[136] Orth DN, Liddle GW. Results of treatment in 108 patients with Cushing's syndrome. N Engl J Med 1971;285:243–7.

[137] Tsagarakis S, Grossman A, Plowman PN, et al. Megavoltage pituitary irradiation in the management of prolactinomas: long-term follow-up. Clin Endocrinol (Oxf) 1991;34: 399–406.

[138] Merchant TE, Kiehna EN, Sanford RA, et al. Craniopharyngioma: the St. Jude Children's Research Hospital experience 1984-2001. Int J Radiat Oncol Biol Phys 2002;53:533–42.

[139] Sanford RA. Craniopharyngioma: results of survey of the American Society of Pediatric Neurosurgery. Pediatr Neurosurg 1994;21(Suppl 1):39–43.

[140] Schulz-Ertner D, Frank C, Herfarth KK, et al. Fractionated stereotactic radiotherapy for craniopharyngiomas. Int J Radiat Oncol Biol Phys 2002;54:1114–20.

[141] Stripp DC, Maity A, Janss AJ, et al. Surgery with or without radiation therapy in the management of craniopharyngiomas in children and young adults. Int J Radiat Oncol Biol Phys 2004;58:714–20.

[142] Kobayashi T, Kida Y, Mori Y, et al. Long-term results of gamma knife surgery for the treatment of craniopharyngioma in 98 consecutive cases. J Neurosurg 2005;103:482–8.

[143] Stafford SL, Kozelsky TF, Garrity JA, et al. Orbital lymphoma: radiotherapy outcome and complications. Radiother Oncol 2001;59:139–44.

[144] Uy NW, Woo SY, Teh BS, et al. Intensity-modulated radiation therapy (IMRT) for meningioma. Int J Radiat Oncol Biol Phys 2002;53:1265–70.

[145] Monje ML, Mizumatsu S, Fike JR, et al. Irradiation induces neural precursor-cell dysfunction. Nat Med 2002;8:955–62.

[146] Silber JH, Radcliffe J, Peckham V, et al. Whole-brain irradiation and decline in intelligence: the influence of dose and age on IQ score. J Clin Oncol 1992;10:1390–6.

[147] Jankovic M, Brouwers P, Valsecchi MG, et al. Association of 1800 cGy cranial irradiation with intellectual function in children with acute lymphoblastic leukaemia. ISPACC. International Study Group on Psychosocial Aspects of Childhood Cancer. Lancet 1994;344: 224–7.

[148] Leber KA, Bergloff J, Pendl G. Dose-response tolerance of the visual pathways and cranial nerves of the cavernous sinus to stereotactic radiosurgery. J Neurosurg 1998;88:43–50.

[149] Stafford SL, Pollock BE, Leavitt JA, et al. A study on the radiation tolerance of the optic nerves and chiasm after stereotactic radiosurgery. Int J Radiat Oncol Biol Phys 2003;55: 1177–81.

[150] Kleinberg L, Grossman SA, Piantadosi S, et al. Phase I trial to determine the safety, pharmacodynamics, and pharmacokinetics of RSR13, a novel radioenhancer, in newly diagnosed glioblastoma multiforme. J Clin Oncol 1999;17:2593–603.

[151] Tishler RB, Loeffler JS, Lunsford LD, et al. Tolerance of cranial nerves of the cavernous sinus to radiosurgery. Int J Radiat Oncol Biol Phys 1993;27:215–21.

[152] Al Mefty O, Topsakal C, Pravdenkova S, et al. Radiation-induced meningiomas: clinical, pathological, cytokinetic, and cytogenetic characteristics. J Neurosurg 2004;100: 1002–13.

[153] Jones A. Radiation oncogenesis in relation to the treatment of pituitary tumours. Clin Endocrinol (Oxf) 1991;35:379–97.

[154] Brada M, Ford D, Ashley S, et al. Risk of second brain tumour after conservative surgery and radiotherapy for pituitary adenoma. BMJ 1992;304:1343–6.

[155] Danoff BF, Cowchock FS, Marquette C, et al. Assessment of the long-term effects of primary radiation therapy for brain tumors in children. Cancer 1982;49:1580–6.

[156] Pirzkall A, Li X, Oh J, et al. 3D MRSI for resected high-grade gliomas before RT: tumor extent according to metabolic activity in relation to MRI. Int J Radiat Oncol Biol Phys 2004;59:126–37.

[157] Pirzkall A, McKnight TR, Graves EE, et al. MR-spectroscopy guided target delineation for high-grade gliomas. Int J Radiat Oncol Biol Phys 2001;50:915–28.

[158] McKnight TR, Noworolski SM, Vigneron DB, et al. An automated technique for the quantitative assessment of 3D-MRSI data from patients with glioma. J Magn Reson Imaging 2001;13:167–77.

[159] Pirzkall A, Nelson SJ, McKnight TR, et al. Metabolic imaging of low-grade gliomas with three-dimensional magnetic resonance spectroscopy. Int J Radiat Oncol Biol Phys 2002;53: 1254–64.

[160] Graves EE, Nelson SJ, Vigneron DB, et al. A preliminary study of the prognostic value of proton magnetic resonance spectroscopic imaging in gamma knife radiosurgery of recurrent malignant gliomas. Neurosurgery 2000;46:319–26.

[161] Graves EE, Pirzkall A, Nelson SJ, et al. Registration of magnetic resonance spectroscopic imaging to computed tomography for radiotherapy treatment planning. Med Phys 2001;28: 2489–96.

[162] Nelson SJ, Graves E, Pirzkall A, et al. In vivo molecular imaging for planning radiation therapy of gliomas: an application of 1H MRSI. J Magn Reson Imaging 2002;16:464–76.

[163] Barker FG, Davis RL, Chang SM, et al. Necrosis as a prognostic factor in glioblastoma multiforme. Cancer 1996;77:1161–6.

[164] Kamada K, Houkin K, Abe H, et al. Differentiation of cerebral radiation necrosis from tumor recurrence by proton magnetic resonance spectroscopy. Neurol Med Chir (Tokyo) 1997;37:250–6.

[165] Nelson SJ, Huhn S, Vigneron DB, et al. Volume MRI and MRSI techniques for the quantitation of treatment response in brain tumors: presentation of a detailed case study. J Magn Reson Imaging 1997;7:1146–52.

[166] Nelson SJ, Vigneron DB, Dillon WP. Serial evaluation of patients with brain tumors using volume MRI and 3D 1H MRSI. NMR Biomed 1999;12:123–38.

[167] Taylor JS, Langston JW, Reddick WE, et al. Clinical value of proton magnetic resonance spectroscopy for differentiating recurrent or residual brain tumor from delayed cerebral necrosis. Int J Radiat Oncol Biol Phys 1996;36:1251–61.

[168] Schlemmer HP, Bachert P, Henze M, et al. Differentiation of radiation necrosis from tumor progression using proton magnetic resonance spectroscopy. Neuroradiology 2002;44: 216–22.

[169] Dowling C, Bollen AW, Noworolski SM, et al. Preoperative proton MR spectroscopic imaging of brain tumors: correlation with histopathologic analysis of resection specimens. AJNR Am J Neuroradiol 2001;22:604–12.

ELSEVIER
SAUNDERS

NEUROLOGIC
CLINICS

Neurol Clin 25 (2007) 1035–1071

# Medical Management of Brain Tumor Patients

Jan Drappatz, MD[a,b,*], David Schiff, MD[c],
Santosh Kesari, MD, PhD[a,b],
Andrew D. Norden, MD[a,b], Patrick Y. Wen, MD[a,b]

[a]Division of Neuro-Oncology, Department of Neurology,
Brigham and Women's Hospital, 75 Francis Street, Boston, MA 02115, USA
[b]Center for Neuro-Oncology, Dana-Farber/Brigham and Women's Cancer Center,
SW430D, 44 Binney Street, Boston, MA 02115, USA
[c]Neuro-Oncology Center, University of Virginia Health Sciences Center,
Box 800432, Charlottesville, VA 22908-0432, USA

Neurologists play an important role in providing effective, compassionate supportive care for patients who have brain tumors. The most common management problems include the treatment of seizures, peritumoral edema, venous thromboembolism (VTE), medication side effects, fatigue, cognitive dysfunction, and depression. Despite their importance, there are few definitive studies addressing these issues. This review summarizes the current medical management of patients who have brain tumor [1].

## Seizures

### Epidemiology and pathophysiology

The incidence of seizures among patients who have brain tumor is related to tumor type and ranges from 30% to 70% [2,3]. Low-grade gliomas present more frequently with seizures (60% to 85%) than high-grade primary brain tumors (20% to 40%) or metastases (15% to 20%) [4–7]. Cortical tumors more likely cause seizures than infratentorial, deep gray, or white matter lesions [5]. Several mechanisms are implicated in seizure development. These include an imbalance between inhibitory and abnormal excitatory, mainly glutamatergic, mechanisms [8,9]; changes in peritumoral

* Corresponding author. Center for Neuro-Oncology, Dana-Farber Brigham and Women's Cancer Center, SW430D, 44 Binney Street, Boston, MA 02115.
E-mail address: jdrappatz@partners.org (J. Drappatz).

0733-8619/07/$ - see front matter © 2007 Elsevier Inc. All rights reserved.
doi:10.1016/j.ncl.2007.07.015 neurologic.theclinics.com

brain tissue; and the relative deafferentation of cortical areas, known to induce epileptogenic foci, often distant from the tumor site (secondary epileptogenesis) [7,9]. Seizures are a major cause of morbidity associated with brain tumors. Status epilepticus is uncommon, typically occurring at the time of diagnosis or progression. It is associated with a high mortality, similar to status epilepticus from other causes, and is influenced by age and tumor histology [10].

## Prophylactic treatment

The use of prophylactic antiepileptic drugs (AEDs) in patients who have brain tumor often is based on individual preference of treating physicians rather than clinical evidence. A meta-analysis of five randomized trials, including a total of 403 patients diagnosed with glial tumors, meningiomas, and brain metastases [11–15], found no benefit supporting anticonvulsant prophylaxis with phenobarbital, phenytoin, or valproic acid in patients who had no history of seizures, regardless of the type of tumor [16]. A meta-analysis of randomized, controlled trials exploring the potential value of anticonvulsant prophylaxis after supratentorial surgery favored the use of phenytoin to prevent early seizures, including patients who have brain tumor and are undergoing surgery. There was no evidence, however, that long-term treatment with phenytoin or carbamazepine reduced the incidence of late seizures compared with placebo or no treatment [17]. Similar findings also were obtained in patients undergoing craniotomy for a variety of other conditions, including vascular malformations and abscesses.

Known adverse effects with anticonvulsant therapy encompass rash (including Stevens-Johnson syndrome), myelosuppression, ataxia, hepato-toxicity, osteomalacia, tremor, cognitive dysfunction, and drug-drug inter-actions. The incidence and severity of these side effects is higher in patients who have brain tumor than in other patients receiving anticonvul-sants [18,19]. Overall, 23.8% of patients who have brain tumor and are taking AEDs experience side effects severe enough to warrant a change in or discontinuation of AED therapy [18].

Considering the lack of evidence supporting the use of prophylactic anti-convulsants, the American Academy of Neurology issued a practice param-eter stating that prophylactic AEDs should not be administered routinely to patients who have newly diagnosed brain tumors (standard) and should be tapered and discontinued in the first postoperative week in patients who have not experienced a seizure (guideline) [18]. Despite these recommenda-tions, 89% of patients in a recent study that looked at practice patterns in patients who had adult glioma received AEDs, although only 32% presented with seizures [20].

Long-term treatment with AEDs is indicated once patients who have brain tumor suffer a seizure resulting from the high risk for recurrence. Even if complete seizure control cannot be achieved, AED therapy may decrease severity and frequency. The selection of a particular AED requires consideration of the treatment patients are receiving. Several of the anticonvulsants used commonly (phenytoin, carbamazepine, oxcarbamazepine, and phenobarbital) induce cytochrome P450 (CYP450) enzymes, leading to a clinically significant reduction in the plasma levels of many antineoplastic drugs. Valproic acid is a CYP450 inhibitor and may decrease clearance of other drugs metabolized by this pathway. Most of the newer agents (levetiracetam, gabapentin, pregabilin, lamotrigine, topiramate, tiagabine, and zonisamide) do not induce the CYP450 system and increasingly are used in patients who have brain tumor. Enzyme-inducing AEDs (EIAEDs) also interact with dexamethasone, which frequently is used to treat peritumoral edema. Dexamethasone induces CYP450 enzymes, potentially lowering levels of AEDs metabolized by the CYP450 system. Conversely, the use of EIAEDs may result in the need to increase the dose of dexamethasone to produce the same therapeutic effect [21–23].

The general principles for management of epilepsy apply to patients who have brain tumor. Patients should be treated with a single agent at the lowest dose that controls seizures effectively. Table 1 lists commonly used AEDs with their doses, side effects, and the Food and Drug Administration (FDA)-approved indication. If the initial drug does not work at highest tolerated dose, then patients should be switched to monotherapy with a second drug. The use of multiple AEDs should be reserved for refractory cases as side effects increase with the number of AEDs used. Although the FDA has approved the marketing of some AEDs for adjunctive use only, many of the non-EIAEDs frequently are used as monotherapy [24]. Few studies exist comparing efficacy of different anticonvulsants. The selection of the AED for individual patients usually is made based on considerations of side-effect profile, pharmacokinetic properties, administration, and mode of action.

Some AEDs have useful concomitant effects. Topiramate and zonisamide can cause weight loss, whereas topiramate may alleviate chronic headaches in some patients. Lamotrigine and valproic acid are mood stabilizers.

*Antiepileptic drugs interactions with antineoplastic agents*

Many chemotherapy agents used commonly in patients who have brain tumor, such as cisplatin, carboplatin, carmustine, and methotrexate, interact with AEDs, such as phenytoin, reducing their bioavailability [25–27]. The mechanisms implied include impaired AED absorption, CYP450 enzyme induction, and altered protein binding. EIAEDs in return accelerate the metabolism of many chemotherapeutic agents, including thiotepa, taxanes, and irinotecan [28–30], and many of the newer targeted molecular agents, such as imatinib, gefitinib, temsirolimus, erlotinib, and tipifarnib [31–34]. Glucocorticoids, such as dexamethasone, also induce the CYP450 system [35]. If given with dexamethasone or prednisone, phenytoin concentrations should be monitored closely, and the dose should be adjusted if necessary.

Table 1
Antiepileptic drugs used for patients who have brain tumor

| Enzyme-inducing antiepileptics | Dose | Adverse effects | Approved for monotherapy in the United States |
|---|---|---|---|
| Carbamazapine (Tegretol, Tegretol XR, Carbatrol) | 400–2400 mg/d (twice a day–4 times a day) (TPC: 8–12 µg/mL) | Drowsiness, dizziness, diplopia, bone marrow suppression (especially leucopenia), rash, hyponatremia, hepatotoxicity, arrhythmia | Yes |
| Oxcarbazepine (Trileptal) | 1200–2400 mg/day (twice a day–4 times a day) (TPC: 12–30 µg/mL) | Drowsiness, dizziness, diplopia, rash, nausea, hyponatremia, lymphadenopathy, hepatotoxicity | Yes |
| Phenytoin (Dilantin, Phenytek) | 15–20mg/kg load and then 3–5 mg/kg/day (every day–twice a day) (TPC: 10–20 µg/mL) | Drowsiness, dizziness, rash, gingival hyperplasia, hirsutism, bone marrow suppression, hepatotoxicity, neuropathy, cerebellar degeneration, folate deficiency, osteomalacia, lupus, lymphadenopathy | Yes |
| Phenobarbital | 10–20 mg/kg load and then 1–3 mg/kg/day (every day) (TPC: 15–40 µg/mL) | Sedation, dizziness, impaired cognitive function, hyperactivity, rash, bone marrow suppression (rare), hepatotoxicity (rare), frozen shoulder, Dupuytren's contracture, reduced libido | Yes |
| Primidone (Mysoline) | 750–2000 mg (3 times a day) (TPC: primidone 5–12 µg/mL; phenobarbital 15–40 µg/mL) | Similar to phenobarbital | Yes |

| Drug | Dose | Side effects | |
|---|---|---|---|
| Clonazepam (Klonopin) | 2–20 mg/day (every day–4 times a day) | Drowsiness, ataxia, behavior problems, hyperactivity, hypersalivation, seizure exacerbation, hepatotoxicity, blood dyscrasia | No |
| Felbamate (Felbatol) | 1200–3600 mg/day (3 times a day–4 times a day) | Substantial risk for aplastic anemia or liver failure; drowsiness, headache, nausea, constipation | Yes (rarely used) |
| Gabapentin (Neurontin) | 900–4800 mg/day (3 times a day–4 times a day)[a] | Drowsiness, dizziness, fatigue, ataxia | No |
| Lamotrigine (Lamictal) | 300–500 mg/day; 100–150 mg/day if taking valproic acid (every day–twice a day) (TPC: 3–14 µg/mL) | Drowsiness, dizziness, fatigue, ataxia, rash, hepatotoxicity | Conversion to monotherapy |
| Levetiracetam (Keppra) | 1000–3000 mg/day (twice a day)[a] | Drowsiness, fatigue, nervousness, headaches | No |
| Pregabalin (Lyrica) | 150–600 mg/day (twice a day–4 times a day) | Drowsiness, dizziness, edema, impaired concentration, blurred vision, weight gain, ataxia, possible dependency | No |
| Tiagabine (Gabitril) | 32–56 mg/day (twice a day–4 times a day)[a] | Drowsiness, dizziness, fatigue, nervousness, tremor, decreased concentration | No |
| Topiramate (Topamax) | 200–400 mg/day (twice a day)[a] | Drowsiness, fatigue, decreased concentration, parasthesias, weight loss, kidney stones | Yes |

(continued on next page)

Table 1 (*continued*)

| Non-enzyme-inducing antiepileptics | Dose | Side effects | Approved for monotherapy for partial or secondary generalized seizures in the United States |
|---|---|---|---|
| Valproic acid (Depakote, Depakene) | 15–60 mg/kg/day (2–4 times a day) (TPC: 50–100 μg/mL) | Drowsiness, nausea, tremor, thrombocytopenia, hepatotoxicity, weight gain, hair loss, pancreatitis | Yes |
| Zonisamide (Zonegran) | 200–600 mg/day (every day–twice a day) (TPC: 10–30 μg/mL) | Drowsiness, dizziness, anorexia, nausea, headache, difficulty concentrating, weight loss, renal stones | No |

*Abbreviation:* TPC, target plasma concentration.

[a] Therapeutic plasma concentration not established.

*Modified from* Wen PY, Schiff D, Kesari S, et al. Medical management of patients with brain tumors. J Neurooncol 2006;80:313; with permission.

Temozolomide is not known to interact with anticonvulsants. Valproic acid inhibits the glucuronidation of 7-ethyl-10-hydroxycamptothecin (SN-38), the active metabolite of irinotecan, leading to a 270% increase in the area under the concentration-time curve of SN-38 in rats [36]. Additionally, it inhibits histone deacetylase, a target of several therapeutic agents in development, such as vorinostat; its use in patients receiving these drugs, therefore, should be avoided [37].

## Surgical management of seizures

Seizures in patients who have brain tumor occasionally may be refractory to medical management. Surgical treatment of brain tumor–related epilepsy generally is indicated only in patients who have slow-growing tumors with a good prognosis. The best results are obtained when the pathologic lesion and adjacent epileptogenic cortex are resected [38].

# Cerebral edema

## Pathophysiology

Cerebral edema may be defined broadly as a pathologic increase in the amount of total brain water content leading to an increase in brain volume [39]. It occurs when plasma-like fluid enters the brain extracellular space through impaired capillary endothelial tight junctions in tumors (vasogenic edema) [40] and is a significant cause of morbidity and mortality. The molecular constituents of brain endothelial tight junctions consist of transmembrane proteins occludin, claudin 1 and 5, and junctional adhesion molecules that bind their counterparts on neighboring cells, "gluing" the cells together and creating the blood-brain barrier (BBB) [40]. Intracellularly, the occludins and claudins bind to zonula occluden (ZO) 1, ZO2, and ZO3, which in turn are attached to the actin cytoskeleton [40]. Normal astrocytes help to maintain a normal BBB [41], which is illustrated in Fig. 1. In high-grade tumors, the deficiency of normal astrocytes leads to defective endothelial tight junctions, resulting in BBB disruption, allowing passage of fluid into the extracellular space [40]. In addition, tumor cells produce factors, such as vascular endothelial growth factor (VEGF) [42,43] and scatter factor/hepatocyte growth factor [44,45], which increase the permeability of tumor vessels by downregulation of occludin and ZO1 [40,44,46,47]. In addition, the membrane water channel protein, aquaporin-4 (AQP4), is upregulated around malignant brain tumors [40]. AQP4-mediated transcellular water movement is important for fluid clearance in vasogenic brain edema, suggesting AQP4 activation or upregulation as a novel therapeutic target in vasogenic brain edema [40,48]. High VEGF expression is reported in human anaplastic astrocytoma and glioblastoma (GBM) [49,50], meningiomas [44], and brain metastases [51]. VEGF is important especially when tumors

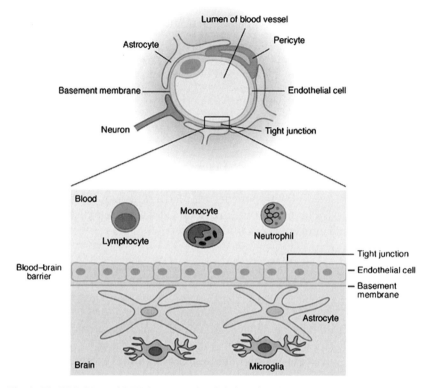

Fig. 1. The BBB. Normal BBB demonstrating tight junctions between endothelial cells forming a barrier between the circulation and the brain parenchyma. Peritumoral edema formation occurs through defective endothelial junctions of an abnormal BBB. (*From* Francis K, van Beek J, Canova C, et al. Innate immunity and brain inflammation: the key role of complement. Expert Rev Mol Med 2003;5:1–19; © Copyright 2003, Cambridge University Press; available at: http://www-ermm.cbcu.cam.ac.uk/03006264h.htm; with permission.)

outgrow their blood supply. Hypoxia is the driving force for VEGF production in glioblastomas and the most important trigger for angiogenesis and cerebral edema formation in glioblastoma [52].

*Diagnosis and treatment of cerebral edema*

Cerebral edema tends to extend along white matter tracts. CT and MRI are helpful in the diagnosis of edema (Fig. 2). Therapy includes tumor-directed measures, such as debulking surgery, radiotherapy (RT), chemotherapy, and the use of corticosteroids. Ingraham and coworkers pioneered the use of cortisone to treat postoperative cerebral edema in neurosurgical patients in 1952. He first used steroids in an attempt to ameliorate postoperative adrenal insufficiency in patients undergoing craniotomy for craniopharyngioma resection and noted the favorable effect on postoperative

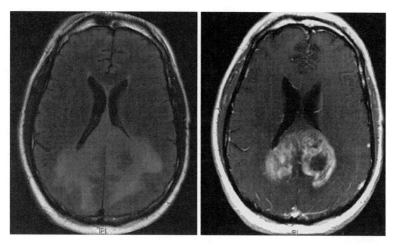

Fig. 2. Fluid-attenuated inversion recovery (FLAIR) (*left*) axial MRI sequences from a patient who had a glioblastoma involving the corpus callosum. There is hyperintense signal abnormality involving the splenium of the corpus callosum, tracking into the cerebral white matter, in a pattern consistent with vasogenic brain edema. T1-weighted, gadolinium-enhanced, axial image (*right*) demonstrates heterogeneous contrast enhancement within the tumor and surrounding hypointense signal.

cerebral edema [53]. Galicich and colleagues [54] and French and Galicich [55] introduced dexamethasone therapy as the standard treatment for tumor-associated edema. Despite their well-known side effects (Table 2), better alternatives do not exist and corticosteroids have remained the mainstay of treatment ever since.

The mechanism of action of corticosteroids is not well understood. It has been argued that their antiedema effect is the result of reduction of the permeability of tumor capillaries by causing dephosphorylation of the tight junction component proteins occludin and ZO1 [40,56]. Corticosteroids usually are indicated in any patients who have brain tumor who have symptomatic peritumoral edema. Dexamethasone is used most commonly as it has little mineralocorticoid activity and, possibly, a lower risk for infection and cognitive impairment compared with other corticosteroids [57]. The choice of starting dose of a corticosteroid largely is arbitrary and depends on the clinical context. The usual starting dose is a 10-mg load, followed by 16 mg per day in patients who have significant symptomatic edema. Lower doses may be as effective, especially for less severe edema [58]. The dose may be increased up to 100 mg per day if necessary [59]. Dexamethasone can be given twice daily, although many clinicians prescribe it 4 times daily. As a general rule, patients should be treated with the smallest effective dose for the shortest time possible to avoid the harmful effects of steroids. For asymptomatic patients who have peritumoral edema on imaging studies, corticosteroids are unnecessary. Dexamethasone usually produces

Table 2
Complications of corticosteroids

| Systemic complications of corticosteroids | Neurologic complications of corticosteroids |
|---|---|
| General | Common |
| • Increased appetite | • Myopathy |
| • Weight gain | • Behavioral changes |
| • Cushingoid features (moon face, centripetal obesity, buffalo hump) | • Visual blurring |
| | • Tremor |
| • Increased susceptibility to infections | • Insomnia |
| • Candidiasis | • Reduced taste and olfaction |
| Bone | • Cerebral atrophy |
| • Osteoporosis | Uncommon |
| • Avascular necrosis | • Psychosis |
| Cardiac/vascular | • Hallucinations |
| • Hypertension | • Hiccups |
| • Increased cardiovascular and cerebrovascular disease | • Dementia |
| | • Seizures |
| Eye | • Dependence |
| • Cataracts | • Epidural lipomatosis |
| • Glaucoma | |
| • Central serous chorioretinopathy | |
| Gastrointestinal | |
| • Peptic ulceration | |
| • GI bleeding | |
| Genitourinary and reproductive | |
| • Menstrual irregularities | |
| • Infertility | |
| Hematologic | |
| • Neutrophilia | |
| • Lymphopenia | |
| Metabolic | |
| • Hyperglycemia | |
| • Hypokalemia | |
| • Hyperlipidemia | |
| • Fluid retention | |
| Skin | |
| • Hirsutism | |
| • Fragile skin | |
| • Purpura | |
| • Acne | |
| • Striae | |

*Adapted from* Wen PY, Schiff D, Kesari S, et al. Medical management of patients with brain tumors. J Neurooncol 2006;80:313; with permission.

symptomatic improvement within 24 to 72 hours. Generalized symptoms, such as headache and lethargy, tend to respond better than focal ones. Improvement on CT and MRI studies often lags behind clinical improvement. Contrast enhancement of tumors typically decreases, suggesting partial restoration of the BBB [60], whereas tumor perfusion can increase because of reduced peritumoral water content and local tissue pressure [61]. Using diffusion tensor MRI, administration of corticosteroids decreases peritumoral extracellular water content in edematous brain without affecting the water content of contralateral normal brain [62].

Occasionally, when there is significant mass effect and impending herniation, other measures may be required until corticosteroids have had a chance to take effect or until patients undergo debulking surgery. These include elevation of the head of the bed, fluid restriction, mannitol, hypertonic saline, diuretics, and hyperventilation [63,64].

After more surgical debulking, steroids should be tapered. The taper can start within a week after surgery but should be delayed in symptomatic patients undergoing RT. In general, patients who have brain tumors exerting significant mass effect should receive steroids for 24 hours before starting RT to reduce intracranial pressure and minimize neurologic symptoms.

## Adverse effects of corticosteroids

Steroids can cause deleterious side effects and drug-drug interactions. A common and clinically important interaction exists with EIAEDs, which may decrease steroid effectiveness [21,65]. Dexamethasone also may induce specific CYP450 isozymes, potentially interacting with other agents metabolized by this system.

The characteristic features of long-term steroid use include truncal obesity, moon facies, buffalo hump, acne, purpura, and striae distensae and, although undesirable, rarely produce significant morbidity. Potentially serious and debilitating adverse effects include proximal myopathy [66], osteoporosis and avascular bone necrosis [67,68], diabetes mellitus [69], cognitive dysfunction [70], gastrointestinal (GI) hemorrhage [71], bowel perforation [72], and opportunistic infections, such as oropharyngeal candidiasis [73] and *Pneumocystis jirovecii* pneumonia (PJP) [74]. Corticosteroids rarely mask life-threatening emergencies, such as sepsis or meningitis. Longer duration of treatment (more than 3 weeks), higher doses, and hypoalbuminemia are associated with greater toxicity [75].

## Gastrointestinal complications

Many patients who have brain tumor and are receiving corticosteroids are treated with histamine ($H_2$) blockers or proton pump inhibitors to prevent GI bleeding or peptic ulcer disease. A relationship between corticosteroids and these complications remains, however, somewhat controversial [76,77]. Studies evaluating GI complications in patients receiving steroids have found a low incidence of peptic ulceration and GI bleeding when corticosteroids are used alone [78]. The risk is increased when patients also are taking nonsteroidal anti-inflammatories (NSAIDs). The use of proton-pump inhibitors and $H_2$ blockers in patients who have brain tumor, therefore, should be restricted to high-risk patients (ie, in the perioperative setting, patients who have a previous history of GI bleed or peptic ulceration or patients receiving anticoagulation or NSAIDs).

Occasionally, corticosteroids also can cause pancreatitis and fatty liver disease Bowel perforation is uncommon but, because corticosteroids mask many of the inflammatory signs of perforation, this diagnosis should be considered in any patients who have abdominal pain, fever, or unexplained leukocytosis.

## Musculoskeletal complications

Steroid myopathy is a common and often disabling complication of steroid therapy in patients who have brain tumor [79,80], with an incidence of 7% to 60% [79]. Although individual susceptibility varies, it is more common in the geriatric population and after prolonged periods of high doses of corticosteroids. The largest published series reported symptomatic steroid myopathy in 10.6% of patients [80]. Symptoms include muscle atrophy and weakness, especially in the proximal lower extremities. Two types of steroid myopathy exist, acute and chronic. The chronic form is more common and presents with insidious onset of muscle weakness, whereas the acute form presents with abrupt symptoms and rhabdomyolysis while patients are receiving high dose steroids [81]. Patients typically report difficulties arising from the seated position. Assessment of hip flexor strength is the most sensitive clinical test for steroid myopathy, but upper extremity muscles, neck muscles, and even respiratory muscles can be involved [82]. Muscle enzymes, electromyography, and muscle biopsy often are normal. Occasionally, electromyography demonstrates myopathic changes or biopsy reveals atrophy of type IIb muscle fibers, variation of the fiber size, and centralization of the nuclei without evidence of inflammation [79]. Glucocorticosteroids inhibit protein synthesis, primarily in type II muscle fibers [83], the fibers characterized by high glycolytic and low oxidative capacity. The main inhibitory mechanism includes downregulation of factors involved in peptide initiation, increased protein catabolism, and induction of glutamine synthetase activity [83,84], leading to alterations in amino acid and carbohydrate metabolism. Steroids also inhibit antiapoptotic effects of insulin-like growth factor (IGF)-I [85], thereby contributing to protein catabolism and muscle apoptosis observed in acute myopathy [86]. Steroid myopathy is less common in patients treated with phenytoin, perhaps as a result of induction of hepatic metabolism of dexamethasone by phenytoin, reducing the effective exposure of muscle cells to the glucocorticoid [80,87].

The development of steroid myopathy can be avoided or minimized by using the lowest possible dose of corticosteroids. Once patients become symptomatic, treatment generally is limited to physical therapy. If possible, corticosteroids should be discontinued or tapered to the lowest possible dose. Gradual recovery of strength can take up to several months.

Use of nonfluorinated steroids, such as prednisone and methylpredniso-lone instead of dexamethasone, may lower the risk for steroid myopathy. Regular exercise can attenuate the symptoms.

Patients receiving chronic corticosteroids (equivalent to 2.5- to 5-mg prednisone or more) are at risk for developing osteoporosis and fractures [88,89]. Age and estrogen deficiency increase the risk for fracture. The mechanism of bone loss is multifactorial, but the most important effects include reduction in osteoblasts and increased osteocyte and osteoblast apoptosis leading to decreased bone formation and turnover [90]. Molecular mechanisms, such as downregulation of IGF-1 and prostaglandin E2, both of which stimulate bone growth, also are implicated.

The diagnosis of osteoporosis is made with a bone mineral density (BMD) test. Calcium and vitamin D supplementation have been evaluated in randomized trials. A 2000 Cochrane systematic review, based on five trials, including 274 patients, showed improvement in vertebral BMD only but no improvement in femoral BMD or fractures [91]. Nevertheless, the American College of Rheumatology recommends calcium and vitamin D supplementation for all patients taking chronic glucocorticoids [92]. Patients receiving chronic corticosteroid therapy should be given calcium supplements (1500 mg per day) with vitamin D (800 IU daily) or an activated form of vitamin D (eg, alfacalcidiol at 1 μg per day or calcitriol at 0.5 μg per day) [92]. Bisphosphonates, such as etidronate, alendronate, ibandronate, risedronate, and zoledonate, have been studied extensively for the treatment of glucocorticoid-induced fractures since the mid-1990s [93]. A Cochrane systematic review demonstrated a positive effect on BMD; however, results regarding fractures were inconclusive [91]. A recent systematic review demonstrated a risk reduction of vertebral fractures from 1.4% to 11% with bisphosphonates [93]. Other therapies include calcitonin, which is less effective than bisphosphonates [94], and teriparatide, a human recombinant 1-34 parathyroid hormone [95]. Although there is no definitive evidence, high-risk patients (65 years and older or who have history of fractures) might benefit from preventive use of bisphosphonates. For patients who develop severe pain from compression fractures, kyphoplasty [96] may play a role. Another complication of steroid use is avascular necrosis of the hip or other bones.

*Psychiatric complications*

Two large meta-analyses found that mild psychiatric symptoms may develop in as many as 28% of patients and severe reactions in 6% of patients receiving steroids [97,98]. The corticosteroid-induced psychiatric symptoms reported most commonly are affective, including mania and depression. Frequently, patients receiving short-term corticosteroid therapy present with euphoria or hypomania, whereas chronic therapy tends to create depressive symptoms [98,99]. Severe episodes of depression can include suicidal ideation. Cognitive deficits with increased distractability and memory impairment also are described [100] and believed related to hippocampal dysfunction [101]. The corticosteroid dosage is the most important risk factor for the development of psychiatric symptoms. The incidence of psychiatric disturbance was 1.3% in patients receiving 40 mg per day or less of prednisone and 18.4% in patients receiving more than 80 mg per day of prednisone [102]. A history of prior psychiatric illness, however, seems not to predict occurrence of steroid-induced psychiatric symptoms [103]. Discontinuation of corticosteroid therapy usually leads to a full recovery. Psychosis, aggression, or agitation should be treated with atypical antipsychotics, such as olanzapine or quetiapine. Patients who have persistent affective symptoms who are receiving chronic corticosteroid therapy should be maintained at the lowest effective corticosteroid dose and treated with antidepressants for depression and a mood stabilizer for manic symptoms. Patients who have affective symptoms must be evaluated for suicidal ideation [98].

## Immunosuppressive effects and infectious complications of corticosteroids

Corticosteroids are immunosuppressive drugs. The use of moderate to high doses of glucocorticoids can result in clinically significant suppression of the immune system and susceptibility to opportunistic infections. *Pneumocystis jirovecii* is an archiascomycetous fungus capable of causing life-threatening pneumonitis in immunocompromised patients [104,105]. It formerly was known as *Pneumocystis carinii* but the species infecting humans was renamed *Pneumocystis jirovecii* with *Pneumocystis carinii* being reserved for one of two species infecting rats. PJP is most common in patients who have AIDS and in other immunosuppressed patients, such as organ transplant recipients and patients who have hematologic malignancies [106]. Patients who have a CD4 count below 200 cells per cubic millimeter are particularly at risk. Although PJP is rare in patients who have brain tumor, patients receiving corticosteroids or prolonged courses of daily temozolomide are at increased risk for developing PJP [107–111]. Small cohort studies estimate the incidence in patients who have brain tumor at between 1.7% [107] and 6.2% [109]. Patients are susceptible particularly when steroids are tapered.

The clinical presentation of PJP is that of an acute pneumonia, but the diagnosis should be considered in any patients at risk for developing new respiratory symptoms. Diagnostic work-up and treatment of PJP are reviewed elsewhere [106]. All patients who have brain tumor and are receiving chronic steroids or prolonged daily courses of temozolomide should receive prophylactic therapy against PJP. Trimethoprim-sulfamethoxazole (TMP-SMZ) is highly effective in preventing PJP when administered as a single double-strength tablet (160 mg of TMP plus 800 mg of SMZ) twice a day for

3 consecutive days each week or once daily 3 times a week during steroid administration and for 1 additional month afterward [105,106]. Aerosolized pentamidine, dapsone or atovaquone are alternatives that should be considered in patients allergic to TMP-SMZ (Table 3).

Candidiasis is the most common opportunistic infection secondary to immunosuppression from steroids. Most candidal infections are mucocutaneous or oropharyngeal and easily treated with nystatin, clotrimazole, or topical antifungal agents. Occasionally, esophageal or systemic candidiasis may occur and require systemic therapy with agents, such as fluconazole or itraconazole.

### Other steroid side effects

Epidural lipomatosis is a rare disorder seen in patients receiving chronic steroid treatment in which excess adipose tissue is deposited within the epidural space and occasionally is described in patients who have brain tumor [112]. It can present as back pain, radiculopathy, or frank spinal cord compression. Treatment is directed at decreasing the steroid dose and in severe cases, multilevel decompressive laminectomy might become necessary to alleviate the neurologic symptoms caused by spinal cord compression [113]. Longer-term corticosteroid use may result in occurrence of glaucoma [114] and cataract formation [115], the severity of which corresponds to the dose and duration of therapy [116,117]. Corticosteroids also can cause hiccups [75,118]. These occasionally can be troublesome and require treatment metoclopramide, chlorpromazine, or baclofen [119]. Glucocorticoid use also is associated with hyperglycemia. Mild blood sugar elevations often can be managed with oral agents. Marked hyperglycemia,

Table 3
Prophylaxis of *Pneumocystis jirovecii* pneumonia

| Regimen | Dose |
|---|---|
| TMP-SMZ | Double strength (800-mg SMZ and 160-mg TMP) 3 times weekly or single strength (400-mg SMZ and 80-mg TMP) daily |
| Aerosolized pentamidine | 300 mg monthly |
| Dapsone | 50 mg twice daily or 100 mg daily |
| Dapsone + pyrimethamine + leucovorin | 50 mg daily Dapsone 50 mg or 100 mg once daily Pyrimethamine 50 mg every week Leucovorin 25 mg every week |
| Dapsone + pyrimethamine + leucovorin | Dapsone 200 mg every week Pyrimethamine 75 mg every week Leucovorin 25 mg every week |
| Atovaquone | 1500 mg daily |

*From* Wen PY, Schiff D, Kesari S, et al. Medical management of patients with brain tumors. J Neurooncol 2006;80:313; with permission.

especially in diabetic patients, usually requires insulin [120]. Steroid pseudo-rheumatism [121] is caused by withdrawal from corticosteroids. It is manifested by diffuse arthralgias. Reintroduction of steroids followed by a slower taper or treatment with NSAIDs may lead to improvement.

*Novel therapies for cerebral edema*

The deleterious effects associated with corticosteroids are the driving force in the quest for alternative therapies for cerebral edema. Corticotropin-releasing factor (CRF) reduces peritumoral edema by a direct effect on blood vessels through CRF 1 and 2 receptors. Phase I/II trials of this agent suggest that it is relatively well tolerated [122,123]. Several phase III trials are in progress examining the efficacy of this drug in the treatment of acute and chronic peritumoral edema.

Preliminary studies suggest that cyclooxygenase-2 (COX-2) inhibitors may be effective in treating cerebral edema [124–126]. Further clinical studies using COX-2 inhibitors for peritumoral edema have been delayed because of the cardiovascular complications of this class of drugs. VEGF increases vascular permeability and, therefore, plays an important role in the pathogenesis of peritumoral edema [127]. Inhibitors of VEGF, such as VEGF antibodies (eg, bevacizumab [Avastin]) [128] or inhibitors of VEGF receptors (eg, AZD2171 [Recentin]) [129], reduce tumor-related edema. These classes of drugs eventually may prove more effective and less toxic alternatives to corticosteroids.

## Thromboembolic complications

*Epidemiology and pathophysiology*

VTE is the second leading cause of death in patients who have cancer [130]. The association between brain tumors and thromboembolic disease is a well-known phenomenon and contributes significantly to morbidity and mortality. The incidence of deep vein thrombosis (DVT) or pulmonary emboli (PE) in patients who have brain tumor varies significantly in different studies (3% to 60%) [131–134]. In patients who have high-grade gliomas outside the perioperative period, the incidence is approximately 20% to 30% [134–138]. This risk generally is greater in the postoperative period and in patients who have hemiplegia, patients older than 60 years, glioblastoma histology, large tumor size, use of chemotherapy, hormonal therapy, operation length greater than 4 hours, and A or AB blood group types [139]. In contrast to adults, children who have brain tumors have a low incidence of VTE [140]. Timely diagnosis and initiation of therapy of VTE is essential. Left untreated, nearly 50% of all patients who have symptomatic, proximal DVTs develop PE [141], with mortality rates of 10% to 34% [142–144]. The VTE risk persists throughout the clinical course of these patients. A prospective study of 77 patients who had high-grade glioma reported a 21% risk for DVT at 12 months, which increased to 32% at 24 months [135].

The pathogenesis of VTE in patients who have brain tumor is not understood completely [145,146]. Normal brain tissue is a rich source of tissue factor (TF), the cell surface receptor of factor VII/VIIa that plays a central role in the initiation of the coagulation cascade [147]. Higher-grade tumors express higher levels of TF, leading to greater activation of the coagulation cascade [148]. The release of brain-derived TF and other procoagulants and fibrinolytic inhibitors from tumor and surrounding cerebral tissue into the systemic circulation is believed to activate the coagulation cascade and result in chronic disseminated intravascular coagulation [148–150]. Elevated levels of D-dimer, homocysteine, lipoprotein a, VEGF, tissue-type plasminogen activator, and plasminogen activator inhibitor are found in patients who have malignant gliomas and contribute to the hypercoaguable state [139].

## Diagnosis

Duplex ultrasonography in combination with clinical evaluation generally provides an adequately precise and noninvasive approach to diagnosing DVT [151]. For proximal DVT, ultrasonography has sensitivities of 89% to 96% and specificities of 94% to 99% [152]. For symptomatic calf DVT, however, the sensitivity drops to 73% to 93% [152,153] and for asymptomatic patients, ultrasonography has a sensitivity of only 50% [152]. Repeat ultrasound or venography may be required for patients who have suspected calf vein DVT and a negative or technically inadequate ultrasound. Contrast venography still is considered the gold standard to rule out the diagnosis of DVT but is performed rarely [154]. For patients who have a low clinical suspicion of DVT, a normal D-dimer is sufficient in excluding DVT and an ultrasound can be omitted safely in these cases [155].

The diagnosis of PE involves a combination of clinical assessment and imaging studies. For patients who have an at least intermediate pretest probability of PE, imaging is necessary. Standard tests include ventilation-perfusion scan, helical CT, and pulmonary angiography. Helical CT, although highly specific, has variably reported sensitivities ranging from 66% to 93% and, therefore, may not be sufficiently sensitive to exclude PE in patients who have a high pretest probability [156–159]. Current-generation CT angiography may offer higher sensitivity [160]. Nevertheless, further imaging studies, such as lower-extremity ultrasonography and pulmonary angiography, are needed in patients who have a high pretest likelihood of PE and a negative CT scan. It is likely that accuracy of CT will improve as the technology evolves.

## Prophylactic treatment

Because of the high risk for developing VTE, patients who have brain tumor and are undergoing craniotomy require adequate prophylaxis. The methods used for VTE prophylaxis are mechanical, pharmacologic (ie, unfractioned heparin or low-molecular-weight heparin [LMWH]), or a combination of both. The optimal prophylactic regimen is not established. Mechanical methods include early ambulation, compression stockings, electrical calf muscle stimulation [161], and intermittent external pneumatic compression devices. Each of these helps limit venous stasis and enhance systemic fibrinolysis. Studies of mechanical prophylaxis in neurosurgery patients demonstrate up to a 50% reduction in VTE compared with controls [162–164], with the greatest effect derived from the use of pneumatic compression, although failure rates in some studies are as high as 9.5% [165]. Studies in patients who have undergone craniotomy comparing pneumatic compression devices with heparin suggest that heparin reduces the frequency of DVT and PE by 40% to 50% [166,167]. The rate of major postoperative intracranial hemorrhage may increase from its baseline of 1% to 3.9% to as high as 10.9% when heparin is introduced [131,168,169]. A meta-analysis of four trials of thromboprophylaxis predominantly in patients who have brain tumor found that LMWH and unfractionated heparins (UFH) reduced the risk for VTE from 12.5% to 6.2% and carried only a 2% risk for major bleeding [170]. Nonetheless, many neurosurgeons continue to associate LMWH with bleeding complications and use mechanical methods only [171,172].

The high incidence of VTE in patients who have malignant gliomas beyond the perioperative period potentially could be reduced with prophylactic anticoagulation, although whether or not this reduction would outweigh the potential risks is unclear. A recent trial (PRODIGE study) attempted to randomize patients who have malignant gliomas to treatment with dalteparin or placebo to determine the benefits of primary prophylaxis [173]. However, the study had to be terminated prematurely, and, although patients receiving dalteparin had a lower rate of VTE, the difference did not reach statistical significance.

*Symptomatic treatment*

The main objectives in the treatment of VTE are to prevent PE, improve lower limb circulation, and resolve leg edema and associated pain. UFH and LMWH in particular are used widely for the treatment of VTE and reducing the frequency of recurrent thromboembolic complications. Meta-analyses comparing UFH and LMWH for the treatment of DVT show better outcomes, with a reduction of major bleeding complications, in patients treated with LMWH [174,175].

Only patients who have strict contraindications for therapeutic anticoagulation should be treated with inferior vena cava (IVC) filters. IVC filters have a higher complication rate and are less effective in preventing PE compared with anticoagulation. A retrospective study of patients who have brain tumors identified complications in up to 62% of patients after IVC filter placement, including procedure-associated morbidity (ie, pneumothorax, infection, bleeding, and IVC wall damage), and thrombotic events, including a 12% risk for recurrent PE, 26% incidence of IVC thrombosis, and 10% postphlebitic syndrome [176]. Four out of 10 patients who have brain metastases who received IVC filters in a case series reported by Schiff and DeAngelis had recurrent VTE [177]. The use of IVC filters, therefore, should be reserved for patients who have recent craniotomy, intracranial hemorrhage, frequent falls, poor compliance, or prolonged thrombocytopenia from chemotherapy. In patients who have temporary contraindications, an IVC filter followed by delayed anticoagulation may limit future thromboembolic complications.

Many studies have demonstrated the relative safety of properly monitored anticoagulation in patients who have primary and metastatic brain tumors [177–181]; this topic is reviewed extensively in the neurosurgical and neuro-oncologic literature [145,146,178,182–185]. The incidence of cerebral hemorrhage in these studies generally was not increased significantly in anticoagulated patients [178,180], whereas systemic bleeding generally was minor and infrequent [177,186]. When hemorrhagic complications occur, they are seen most commonly in the context of supratherapeutic anticoagulation [187,188]. Table 4 lists the anticoagulants that are used most commonly in the treatment of VTE and Fig. 3 shows their mechanisms of action.

Warfarin remains the standard long-term anticoagulant used in patients who have brain tumor. Until recently, the majority of patients receiving anticoagulation for VTE were treated initially with heparin or LMWHs and then converted to warfarin. As patients who have brain tumor frequently receive concurrent therapy with medications that interact with warfarin, close monitoring of the international normalized ratio (INR) is necessary. The use of LMWHs in lieu of warfarin avoids the difficulties of fluctuating INRs because of the many drug-drug interactions with warfarin. The role of LMWH in patients who have brain tumor is evolving. Although there is no evidence indicating that LMWHs are more effective or safer than oral anticoagulant therapy in patients who have brain tumors, there is accumulating evidence that LMWHs are more effective and safer in cancer patients in general. In a randomized trial of secondary prevention of VTE in patients who have systemic cancer, warfarin, when compared with enoxaparin (1.5 mg/kg daily), was associated with a higher frequency of bleeding; there were six deaths resulting from hemorrhage in the warfarin group compared with none in the enoxaparin group [189]. In the Randomized Comparison of Low-Molecular-Weight Heparin versus Oral Anticoagulant Therapy for the Prevention of Recurrent Venous Thromboemoblism in Patients with Cancer (CLOT) trial, dalteparin was more effective than warfarin in the prevention of VTE in patients who had cancer and bleeding complications were similar in each group [190]. The study included 27 patients who had brain tumor. Dalteparin, compared with warfarin, also was associated with improved survival among patients who had solid tumor and who had VTE, although there was no difference between groups when metastatic disease was present [191]. Moreover, dalteparin did not increase the risk for bleeding complications in

Table 4
Agents used in the treatment of venous throembolism

| Agent | Dose | Monitoring | Reversal | Half-life | Comments |
|---|---|---|---|---|---|
| Unfractionated heparin | Treatment: bolus 40–80 U/kg IV then 18 U/kg/h IV infusion[a]; prophylaxis: 5000 U SC every 12 h | Goal aPTT 1.5–2.5 × ULN; check 4 × day, then every 24 h when aPTT stable | Protamine 1 mg/100 U slow IV infusion (>10 min) | 1 h | HIT is more common (>1% of patients) |
| Dalteparin | Treatment: 200 U/kg SC daily or 100 U/kg SC every 12 h; prophylaxis: 2500–5000 U SC every 24 h | Anti-Xa levels (rarely used) | Protamine 1 mg/100 U slow IV infusion (reverses 74% of anti-Xa activity); rhFVIIa (90 μg/kg IV) | 3–5 h | HIT less common (<1%); use caution in obese patients and with CrCl<30 mL/min |
| Enoxaparin | Treatment: 1 mg/kg SC (maximum 100 mg every 12 h); prophylaxis: 40 mg SC daily | Anti-Xa levels (rarely used) | Protamine 1 mg/100 U slow IV infusion (reverses 54% of anti-Xa activity); rhFVIIa (90 μg/kg IV) | 4.5 h | HIT less common (<1%); avoid daily dosing (1.5 mg/kg) for initial treatment; use caution in obese patients and with CrCl<30 mL/min |
| Tinzaparin | Treatment: 175 U SC daily | Anti-Xa levels (rarely used) | Protamine 1 mg/100 U slow IV infusion (reverses 85% of anti-Xa activity); rhFVIIa (90 μg/kg IV) | 3–5 h | HIT less common (<1%); use caution use caution in obese patients and with CrCl<30 mL/min |
| Fondaparinux | Treatment: 5–10 mg SC daily, 5 mg (<50 kg), 7.5 mg (50–100 kg), 10 mg (>100 kg); prophylaxis: 2.5 mg SC daily | Anti Xa levels (rarely used) | rhFVIIa (90 μg/kg IV) | 17–21 h | No reported cases of HIT with its use |

| | Treatment | Monitoring | Reversal | Half-life | Comments |
|---|---|---|---|---|---|
| Warfarin | Treatment: start 5 mg by mouth daily and adjust dose to PT/INR | Goal INR 2–3 | Vitamin K: 1–5 mg by mouth for INR correction; 10-mg slow IV infusion for life-threatening bleeding; FFP (10–15 mL/kg IV) or rhFVIIa (30–90 µg/kg) for life-threatening bleeding | 20–60 h | Multiple drug interactions |
| Lepirudin | Treatment: bolus 0.4 mg/kg (up to 44 mg) IV then 0.15 mg/kg/h (up to 16.5 mg/h) IV infusion; reduce dose with renal insufficiency: avoid if CrCl <15 mL/min | Goal aPTT 1.5–2.5 ULN; check aPTT ratio 4 h after initiation and after dose changes then at least daily | rhFVIIa (90 µg/kg IV) | 0.8–2 h | Indication: HIT treatment; anaphylaxis risk with repeat exposure within 3–4 mo |
| Argatroban | Treatment: 2 µg/kg/min IV if normal hepatic function; with compromised hepatic function, 0.5 µg/kg/min IV | Goal aPTT ratio 1.5–3 × ULN; check aPTT ratio 2–4 hrs after initiation and after dose changes then at least daily | rhFVIIa (90 µg/kg IV) | 30–50 min | Indication: HIT treatment |

*Abbreviations:* aPTT, activated partial thromboplastin time; CrCl, creatine clearance; IV, intravenously; PT, prothrombin time; rhFVIIa, recombinant factor VIIa; SC, subcutaneously; ULN, upper limit of normal.

<sup>a</sup> An UFH bolus should be used only in patients at serious risk for deterioration from PE. A minibolus of 40 U/kg is safer than a full bolus.

*Modified from* Gerber DE, Grossman SA, Streiff MB. Management of venous thromboembolism in patients with primary and metastatic brain tumors. J Clin Oncol 2006;24:1310; with permission.

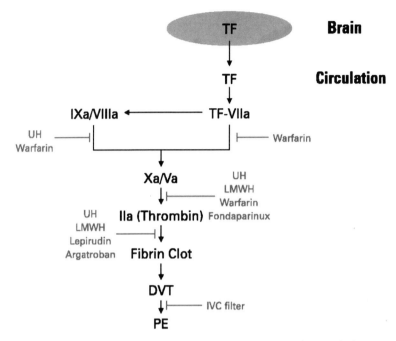

Fig. 3. Mechanism of VTE in patients who have brain tumors. Pharmacologic treatment modalities are indicated at their sites of action. Clotting factors are listed by roman numerals. UH, unfractionated heparin. (*From* Gerber DE, Grossman SA, Streiff MB. Management of venous thromboembolism in patients with primary and metastatic brain tumors. J Clin Oncol 2006;24:1310; with permission.)

patients who had brain metastases in one study of patients who had VTE and disseminated cancer [192]. At the authors' institution, LMWH is favored over warfarin for secondary prevention of VTE, although more evidence is desirable before applying this approach routinely in this patient population. Before initiation of therapeutic anticoagulation, a screening head CT or MRI should be performed to rule out recent intracranial bleeding (Fig. 4 illustrates treatment algorithm). Evidence of recent spontaneous bleeding generally is considered a contraindication to anticoagulation. Anticoagulation probably should be avoided in patients who have brain metastases from melanoma, choriocarcinoma, or renal or thyroid cancer, as these tumors are associated with an increased rate of hemorrhage.

Currently FDA-approved LMWHs for treatment of VTE include enoxaparin, dalteparin, tinzaparin, and nadroparin [153]. The advantages of LMWH compared with UFH are better bioavailability and longer half-life, more predictable dose response, reduced requirements for laboratory monitoring, lower frequency of heparin-induced thrombocytopenia (HIT), and perhaps less heparin-associated osteopenia [188,193]. Because of their improved safety and ease of use, stable patients who have DVT usually are treated with LMWH in an outpatient setting while transitioning to

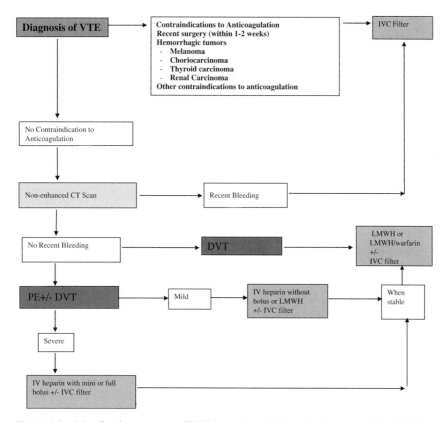

Fig. 4. Algorithm for the treatment of VTE in patients who have brain tumor. (*Modified from* Wen PY, Schiff D, Kesari S, et al. Medical management of patients with brain tumors. J Neuro-oncol 2006;80:313; with permission.)

oral anticoagulation with warfarin to reach therapeutic INR levels [194–196]. There also is evidence that LMWHs are modestly superior to UFH for initial treatment of DVT and at least as effective as UFH for treatment of PE [152]. Outpatient therapy probably is safe and effective [152,197]. Treatment with UFH usually is reserved for patients who have serious PEs and high-risk patients where the longer half-life and less complete protamine reversibility of LMWHs make them less attractive as early treatment in patients. When administering UFH, a bolus of UFH should be reserved for high-risk patients who have symptomatic PE where the risk for progressive thrombosis outweighs the potential bleeding risk associated with more aggressive initial anticoagulation. The duration of anticoagulation depends on the persistence of the underlying hypercoaguable state. As most primary brain tumors and metastatic cancers are incurable, anticoagulation is continued indefinitely in the majority of these patients. When the underlying cause of the hypercoaguable state no longer exists, anticoagulation can be discontinued after approximately 6 months.

Patients who have HIT must not receive heparin products. In lieu of heparin, direct thrombin inhibitors, such as lepirudin, argatroban, or bivalirudin, and the heparinoid danaparoid (not approved in the United States) could be considered, although little data exist to guide their use in patients who have brain tumors. Fondaparinux is a synthetic pentasaccharide, which binds to antithrombin, thereby indirectly selectively inhibiting factor Xa. Fondaparinux demonstrates efficacy compared with LMWH in randomized clinical trials and is FDA approved for the prevention and treatment of VTE. Because it does not bind to platelets or platelet factor 4, it should not produce HIT, and although not FDA approved for this indication, its use might be considered in patients who have brain tumor who have developed HIT.

*Intracranial hemorrhage*

The most feared complication of anticoagulation in patients who have brain tumor is intracranial hemorrhage. Any change in neurologic symptoms or onset of headaches should prompt immediate brain imaging. If hemorrhage is confirmed, anticoagulation needs to be reversed and a neurosurgical consultation obtained. Protamine reverses UFH completely. It reverses LMWH incompletely, however, and has an even less effect on fondaparinux and the direct thrombin inhibitors [145,198]. Vitamin K reverses the effect of warfarin but requires hours to days to take effect [199]. Therefore, blood products, such as fresh frozen plasma, recombinant human factor VIIa, or prothrombin complex concentrates, should be used as part of initial therapy [200–202]. Recombinant factor VIIa also may reverse the anticoagulant effects of LMWHs, direct thrombin inhibitors, and fondaparinux [203,204].

**Neurocognitive symptoms**

The majority of patients who have brain tumor experience distressing neurocognitive symptoms. These symptoms include fatigue, depression, and cognitive impairment and contribute to a marked reduction of quality of life [205]. Appropriate assessment of these symptoms, with particular consideration of their multidimensional nature, is critical in all patients who have brain tumor to allow for timely identification and development of a rational therapeutic strategy. Potential etiologic factors and comorbidities need to be examined with specific attention to factors that may be correctable (ie, anemia, nutritional status, endocrine dysfunction, depression, and anxiety).

*Fatigue*

Fatigue affects the quality of life adversely in the majority of patients who have brain tumor [206,207]. In one survey of patients who had primary brain tumors, 42% reported "quite a bit low" or "very low" energy levels on the Functional Assessment of Cancer Therapy-Brain scale [205] and increased levels of fatigue correlated strongly with decreased quality of life. Several studies assessing the quality of life in patients who had malignant gliomas found that fatigue was the symptom reported most frequently and as most troublesome [207,208]. Fatigue tends to be more common in patients who have high-grade gliomas than for those who have lower-grade tumors [209] and is troublesome especially after treatment with RT [210,211]. Fatigue tends to increase with the number of radiation fractions, reaching a maximum at the end of RT. Fatigue in patients who have brain tumor during RT often is perceived as inevitable and something that needs to be endured. This fatigue provides an opportunity, however, for intervention to improve the quality of life of these patients. Fatigue also is associated with an adverse prognosis [212,213].

AED use, chemotherapy, anemia, metabolic disturbances, depression, endocrine dysfunction, and weight gain from chronic steroid use all contribute to fatigue. It is important to exclude hypothyroidism and hypocortisolism, reduce or eliminate AEDs, and treat anemia and depression. Psychostimulants may play a role in the treatment of brain-tumor related fatigue. The psychostimulants available include methylphenidate, pemoline, dextroamphetamine, and modafinil. These drugs generally are well tolerated in patients who have brain tumor, although potentially they lower the seizure threshold. Modafinil does not have proconvulsant effects. It benefits patients who have fatigue from various causes [214–222] and acts as an augmenter of antidepressants, especially in patients who have residual tiredness or fatigue [223–226]. A pilot study of modafinil for treatment of neurobehavioral dysfunction and fatigue in adult patients who had brain tumors showed improvement across cognitive, mood, and fatigue outcome measures, and the drug was well tolerated [227]. This drug potentially has a role in the treatment of fatigue during RT.

## Cognitive impairment

Cognitive deficits are common in patients who have brain tumors and include problems, such as poor short-term memory, distractibility, personality change, emotional lability, loss of executive function, and decreased psychomotor speed. These complaints can be tumor related and exacerbated by chemotherapy and RT and antiepileptics and corticosteroids [228]. Whole-brain RT alone or in combination with high-dose chemotherapy results in greater cognitive decline than partial RT or high-dose chemotherapy alone [229]. The MRI scan in these patients often demonstrates periventricular white matter changes (Fig. 5). Patients undergoing treatment should have a baseline cognitive assessment so that changes can be identified and patient reports quantified [228]. The cognitive impairment may be associated with behavioral disturbances and require psychiatric intervention and

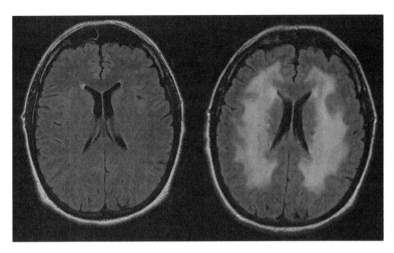

Fig. 5. Fluid-attenuated inversion recovery (FLAIR) axial MRI sequences from a 52-year-old man who had primary central nervous system lymphoma. The left image demonstrates normal white matter. The right image 3 months later after 6 doses of high-dose methotrexate demonstrates development of confluent abnormal T2 hyperintensity in the subcortical and periventricular white matter extending into the internal capsules bilaterally with preservation of the corpus callosum. The patient was symptomatic with memory loss, inattention, and word-finding difficulties.

social service support. Medications, such as methylphenidate, may be helpful in improving motivation, attention, and neurologic functioning [230]. Donepezil, an acetylcholinesterase inhibitor approved for Alzheimer's disease, improves cognitive functioning, including memory, mood, and quality of life in patients who have brain tumor after RT [231]. Other acetylcholinesterase inhibitors and glutamate inhibitors, such as memantine, also may be helpful with memory loss. Atypical antipsychotics, such as quetiapine, risperdone, and olanzapine, often are used to treat psychotic symptoms, anger, agitation, and poor impulse control [232]. Patients who have cognitive impairment, frontal gait disorder, and urinary incontinence, should be evaluated for the presence of communicating hydrocephalus and may benefit from ventriculoperitoneal shunting [233].

*Depression*

Depression is a common symptom in patients who have brain tumor. Depression may be related to frontal lobe tumor location or medications (dexamethasone and levetiracetam, in particular), or it may be part of the psychologic response to the tumor diagnosis. Estimates of the rates of depression vary between studies and depend on the assessment method. In the Glioma Outcomes Project there was significant discrepancy between the rates of depression reported by patients and physicians [234]. Among the 598 patients who had malignant glioma, physicians diagnosed depression using the *Diagnostic and Statistical Manual of Mental Disorders, Fourth Edition* criteria in 15% of the study subjects in the early postoperative period. A total of 93% of these patients, however, reported symptoms of depression during this period [234]. As survival was shorter among depressed patients [234], the importance of diagnosis and treatment cannot be underestimated. Depressed patients require adequate psychosocial support and should be considered for antidepressant pharmacotherapy. Commonly used antidepressants include selective serotonin reuptake inhibitors (fluoxetine, fluvoxamine, paroxetine, sertraline, citalopram, and escitalopram), serotonin/norepinephrine reuptake inhibitors (duloxetine, milnacipran, and venlafaxine), and noradrenergic and specific serotonergic antidepressants (mirtazepine) and generally are well tolerated. The norepinephrine-dopamine reuptake inhibitor, buproprion, is associated with lowering of the seizure threshold and should be avoided in patients who have brain tumor.

## Summary

Seizures, cerebral edema, thromboembolic complications, neurocognitive dysfunction, and depression are common challenges in patients who have brain tumor and account for significant morbidity and mortality. Effective medical management of these complications can improve quality of life significantly. Current evidence suggests that anticoagulation for VTE in patients who have brain tumor does not increase the risk for intracranial hemorrhage significantly, unless there is a clear contraindication. Further studies are required, however, to define the optimal prophylaxis and treatment of VTE. AEDs should be given only to patients who have had a seizure. There is no evidence that prophylactic AEDs are beneficial in patients who have brain tumor who have not had seizures. To minimize interactions with other drugs, non-EIAEDs should be considered. Corticosteroids treat brain tumor–related edema effectively but have unfavorable side effects and should be used in the smallest effective dose and for the shortest duration possible. Fatigue and depression often are not recognized or treated in patients who have primary brain tumor, but effective therapy can have a major impact on patient quality of life.

## References

[1] Wen PY, Schiff D, Kesari S, et al. Medical management of patients with brain tumors. J Neurooncol 2006;80(3):313–32.
[2] Hauser WA, Annegers JF, Kurland LT. Incidence of epilepsy and unprovoked seizures in Rochester, Minnesota: 1935–1984. Epilepsia 1993;34(3):453–68.
[3] Morris HH, Estes ML, Gilmore R, et al. Chronic intractable epilepsy as the only symptom of primary brain tumor. Epilepsia 1993;34(6):1038–43.
[4] Cascino GD. Epilepsy and brain tumors: implications for treatment. Epilepsia 1990; 31(Suppl 3):S37–44.

[5] Herman ST. Epilepsy after brain insult: targeting epileptogenesis. Neurology 2002; 59(9 Suppl. 5):S21–6.

[6] Moots PL, Maciunas RJ, Eisert DR, et al. The course of seizure disorders in patients with malignant gliomas. Arch Neurol 1995;52(7):717–24.

[7] Vecht CJ, van Breemen M. Optimizing therapy of seizures in patients with brain tumors. Neurology 2006;67(12 Suppl 4):S10–3.

[8] Bateman DE, Hardy JA, McDermott JR, et al. Amino acid neurotransmitter levels in gliomas and their relationship to the incidence of epilepsy. Neurol Res 1988;10(2): 112–4.

[9] Wolf HK, Roos D, Blumcke I, et al. Perilesional neurochemical changes in focal epilepsies. Acta Neuropathol (Berl) 1996;91(4):376–84.

[10] Cavaliere R, Farace E, Schiff D. Clinical implications of status epilepticus in patients with neoplasms. Arch Neurol 2006;63(12):1746–9.

[11] Forsyth PA, Weaver S, Fulton D, et al. Prophylactic anticonvulsants in patients with brain tumour. Can J Neurol Sci 2003;30(2):106–12.

[12] Franceschetti S, Binelli S, Casazza M, et al. Influence of surgery and antiepileptic drugs on seizures symptomatic of cerebral tumours. Acta Neurochir (Wien) 1990;103(1–2): 47–51.

[13] Glantz MJ, Cole BF, Friedberg MH, et al. A randomized, blinded, placebo-controlled trial of divalproex sodium prophylaxis in adults with newly diagnosed brain tumors. Neurology 1996;46(4):985–91.

[14] Lee ST, Lui TN, Chang CN, et al. Prophylactic anticonvulsants for prevention of immediate and early postcraniotomy seizures. Surg Neurol 1989;31(5):361–4.

[15] North JB, Penhall RK, Hanieh A, et al. Phenytoin and postoperative epilepsy. A double-blind study. J Neurosurg 1983;58(5):672–7.

[16] Sirven JI, Wingerchuk DM, Drazkowski JF, et al. Seizure prophylaxis in patients with brain tumors: a meta-analysis. Mayo Clin Proc 2004;79(12):1489–94.

[17] Temkin NR. Antiepileptogenesis and seizure prevention trials with antiepileptic drugs: meta-analysis of controlled trials. Epilepsia 2001;42(4):515–24.

[18] Glantz MJ, Cole BF, Forsyth PA, et al. Practice parameter: anticonvulsant prophylaxis in patients with newly diagnosed brain tumors. Report of the Quality Standards Subcommittee of the American Academy of Neurology. Neurology 2000;54(10):1886–93.

[19] Batchelor TT, Byrne TN. Supportive care of brain tumor patients. Hematol Oncol Clin North Am 2006;20(6):1337–61.

[20] Chang SM, Parney IF, Huang W, et al. Patterns of care for adults with newly diagnosed malignant glioma. Jama 2005;293(5):557–64.

[21] Chalk JB, Ridgeway K, Brophy T, et al. Phenytoin impairs the bioavailability of dexamethasone in neurological and neurosurgical patients. J Neurol Neurosurg Psychiatr 1984; 47(10):1087–90.

[22] Lawson LA, Blouin RA, Smith RB, et al. Phenytoin-dexamethasone interaction: a previously unreported observation. Surg Neurol 1981;16(1):23–4.

[23] Werk EE Jr, Choi Y, Sholiton L, et al. Interference in the effect of dexamethasone by diphenylhydantoin. N Engl J Med 1969;281(1):32–4.

[24] Sperling MR, Ko J. Seizures and brain tumors. Semin Oncol 2006;33(3):333–41.

[25] Dofferhoff AS, Berendsen HH, vd Naalt J, et al. Decreased phenytoin level after carboplatin treatment. Am J Med 1990;89(2):247–8.

[26] Fincham RW, Schottelius DD. Decreased phenytoin levels in antineoplastic therapy. Ther Drug Monit 1979;1(2):277–83.

[27] Grossman SA, Sheidler VR, Gilbert MR. Decreased phenytoin levels in patients receiving chemotherapy. Am J Med 1989;87(5):505–10.

[28] Chang TK, Chen G, Waxman DJ. Modulation of thiotepa antitumor activity in vivo by alteration of liver cytochrome P450-catalyzed drug metabolism. J Pharmacol Exp Ther 1995;274(1):270–5.

[29] Prados MD, Yung WK, Jaeckle KA, et al. Phase 1 trial of irinotecan (CPT-11) in patients with recurrent malignant glioma: a North American Brain Tumor Consortium study. Neuro-oncol 2004;6(1):44–54.

[30] Vecht CJ, Wagner GL, Wilms EB. Interactions between antiepileptic and chemotherapeutic drugs. Lancet Neurol 2003;2(7):404–9.

[31] Cloughesy TF, Wen PY, Robins HI, et al. Phase II trial of tipifarnib in patients with recurrent malignant glioma either receiving or not receiving enzyme-inducing antiepileptic drugs: a North American Brain Tumor Consortium Study. J Clin Oncol 2006;24(22): 3651–6.

[32] Prados MD, Lamborn K, Yung WK, et al. A phase 2 trial of irinotecan (CPT-11) in patients with recurrent malignant glioma: a North American Brain Tumor Consortium study. Neuro-oncol 2006;8(2):189–93.

[33] Prados MD, Lamborn KR, Chang S, et al. Phase 1 study of erlotinib HCl alone and combined with temozolomide in patients with stable or recurrent malignant glioma. Neuro-oncol 2006;8(1):67–78.

[34] Wen PY, Yung WK, Lamborn KR, et al. Phase I/II study of imatinib mesylate for recurrent malignant gliomas: North American Brain Tumor Consortium Study 99-08. Clin Cancer Res 2006;12(16):4899–907.

[35] McCune JS, Hawke RL, LeCluyse EL, et al. In vivo and in vitro induction of human cytochrome P4503A4 by dexamethasone. Clin Pharmacol Ther 2000;68(4):356–66.

[36] Gupta E, Wang X, Ramirez J, et al. Modulation of glucuronidation of SN-38, the active metabolite of irinotecan, by valproic acid and phenobarbital. Cancer Chemother Pharmacol 1997;39(5):440–4.

[37] Camphausen K, Cerna D, Scott T, et al. Enhancement of in vitro and in vivo tumor cell radiosensitivity by valproic acid. Int J Cancer 2005;114(3):380–6.

[38] Cascino GD. Surgical treatment for epilepsy. Epilepsy Res 2004;60(2–3):179–86.

[39] Fishman RA. Brain edema. N Engl J Med 1975;293(14):706–11.

[40] Papadopoulos MC, Saadoun S, Binder DK, et al. Molecular mechanisms of brain tumor edema. Neuroscience 2004;129(4):1011–20.

[41] Janzer RC, Raff MC. Astrocytes induce blood-brain barrier properties in endothelial cells. Nature 1987;325(6101):253–7.

[42] Bates DO, Lodwick D, Williams B. Vascular endothelial growth factor and microvascular permeability. Microcirculation 1999;6(2):83–96.

[43] Machein MR, Plate KH. VEGF in brain tumors. J Neurooncol 2000;50(1–2):109–20.

[44] Lamszus K, Lengler U, Schmidt NO, et al. Vascular endothelial growth factor, hepatocyte growth factor/scatter factor, basic fibroblast growth factor, and placenta growth factor in human meningiomas and their relation to angiogenesis and malignancy. Neurosurgery 2000;46(4):938–47 [discussion: 938–47].

[45] Arrieta O, Garcia E, Guevara P, et al. Hepatocyte growth factor is associated with poor prognosis of malignant gliomas and is a predictor for recurrence of meningioma. Cancer 2002;94(12):3210–8.

[46] Behzadian MA, Windsor LJ, Ghaly N, et al. VEGF-induced paracellular permeability in cultured endothelial cells involves urokinase and its receptor. Faseb J 2003;17(6): 752–4.

[47] Wang W, Dentler WL, Borchardt RT. VEGF increases BMEC monolayer permeability by affecting occludin expression and tight junction assembly. Am J Physiol Heart Circ Physiol 2001;280(1):H434–40.

[48] Wang F, Feng XC, Li YM, et al. Aquaporins as potential drug targets. Acta Pharmacol Sin 2006;27(4):395–401.

[49] Ludwig HC, Feiz-Erfan I, Bockermann V, et al. Expression of nitric oxide synthase isozymes (NOS I-III) by immunohistochemistry and DNA in situ hybridization. Correlation with macrophage presence, vascular endothelial growth factor (VEGF) and oedema volumetric data in 220 glioblastomas. Anticancer Res 2000;20(1A):299–304.

[50] Lafuente JV, Adan B, Alkiza K, et al. Expression of vascular endothelial growth factor (VEGF) and platelet-derived growth factor receptor-beta (PDGFR-beta) in human gliomas. J Mol Neurosci 1999;13(1–2):177–85.

[51] Ludwig HC, Ahkavan-Shigari R, Rausch S, et al. Oedema extension in cerebral metastasis and correlation with the expression of nitric oxide synthase isozymes (NOS I-III). Anticancer Res 2000;20(1A):305–10.

[52] Plate KH, Breier G, Risau W. Molecular mechanisms of developmental and tumor angiogenesis. Brain Pathol 1994;4(3):207–18.

[53] Ingraham FD, Matson DD, Mc LR. Cortisone and ACTH as an adjunct to the surgery of craniopharyngiomas. N Engl J Med 1952;246(15):568–71.

[54] Galicich JH, French LA, Melby JC. Use of dexamethasone in treatment of cerebral edema associated with brain tumors. J Lancet 1961;81:46–53.

[55] French LA, Galicich JH. The use of steroids for control of cerebral edema. Clin Neurosurg 1964;10:212–23.

[56] Romero IA, Radewicz K, Jubin E, et al. Changes in cytoskeletal and tight junctional proteins correlate with decreased permeability induced by dexamethasone in cultured rat brain endothelial cells. Neurosci Lett 2003;344(2):112–6.

[57] Batchelor T, DeAngelis LM. Medical management of cerebral metastases. Neurosurg Clin N Am 1996;7(3):435–46.

[58] Vecht CJ, Hovestadt A, Verbiest HB, et al. Dose-effect relationship of dexamethasone on Karnofsky performance in metastatic brain tumors: a randomized study of doses of 4, 8, and 16 mg per day. Neurology 1994;44(4):675–80.

[59] Vick NA, Wilson CB. Total care of the patient with a brain tumor with consideration of some ethical issues. Neurol Clin 1985;3(4):705–10.

[60] Zaki HS, Jenkinson MD, Du Plessis DG, et al. Vanishing contrast enhancement in malignant glioma after corticosteroid treatment. Acta Neurochir (Wien) 2004;146(8):841–5.

[61] Bastin ME, Carpenter TK, Armitage PA, et al. Effects of dexamethasone on cerebral perfusion and water diffusion in patients with high-grade glioma. AJNR Am J Neuroradiol 2006;27(2):402–8.

[62] Lu S, Ahn D, Johnson G, et al. Peritumoral diffusion tensor imaging of high-grade gliomas and metastatic brain tumors. AJNR Am J Neuroradiol 2003;24(5):937–41.

[63] Rabinstein AA. Treatment of cerebral edema. Neurologist 2006;12(2):59–73.

[64] Gomes JA, Stevens RD, Lewin JJ 3rd, et al. Glucocorticoid therapy in neurologic critical care. Crit Care Med 2005;33(6):1214–24.

[65] Gattis WA, May DB. Possible interaction involving phenytoin, dexamethasone, and antineoplastic agents: a case report and review. Ann Pharmacother 1996;30(5):520–6.

[66] Afifi AK, Bergman RA, Harvey JC. Steroid myopathy. Clinical, histologic and cytologic observations. Johns Hopkins Med J 1968;123(4):158–73.

[67] Adachi JD, Bensen WG, Cividino A. Corticosteroid-induced osteoporosis. J Am Med Womens Assoc 1998;53(1):25–30, 40.

[68] Gebhard KL, Maibach HI. Relationship between systemic corticosteroids and osteonecrosis. Am J Clin Dermatol 2001;2(6):377–88.

[69] Rizza RA, Mandarino LJ, Gerich JE. Cortisol-induced insulin resistance in man: impaired suppression of glucose production and stimulation of glucose utilization due to a postreceptor detect of insulin action. J Clin Endocrinol Metab 1982;54(1):131–8.

[70] Brunner R, Schaefer D, Hess K, et al. Effect of high-dose cortisol on memory functions. Ann N Y Acad Sci 2006;1071:434–7.

[71] Piper JM, Ray WA, Daugherty JR, et al. Corticosteroid use and peptic ulcer disease: role of nonsteroidal anti-inflammatory drugs. Ann Intern Med 1991;114(9):735–40.

[72] Warshaw AL, Welch JP, Ottinger LW. Acute perforation of the colon associated with chronic corticosteroid therapy. Am J Surg 1976;131(4):442–6.

[73] Davies AN, Brailsford S, Beighton D. Corticosteroids and oral candidosis. Palliat Med 2001;15(6):521.

[74] Stuck AE, Minder CE, Frey FJ. Risk of infectious complications in patients taking gluco-corticosteroids. Rev Infect Dis 1989;11(6):954–63.

[75] Weissman DE, Dufer D, Vogel V, et al. Corticosteroid toxicity in neuro-oncology patients. J Neurooncol 1987;5(2):125–8.

[76] Marcus P, McCauley DL. Steroid therapy and H2-receptor antagonists: pharmacoeconomic implications. Clin Pharmacol Ther 1997;61(5):503–8.

[77] Spiro HM. Is the steroid ulcer a myth? N Engl J Med 1983;309(1):45–7.

[78] Carson JL, Strom BL, Schinnar R, et al. The low risk of upper gastrointestinal bleeding in patients dispensed corticosteroids. Am J Med 1991;91(3):223–8.

[79] Batchelor TT, Taylor LP, Thaler HT, et al. Steroid myopathy in cancer patients. Neurology 1997;48(5):1234–8.

[80] Dropcho EJ, Soong SJ. Steroid-induced weakness in patients with primary brain tumors. Neurology 1991;41(8):1235–9.

[81] Hanson P, Dive A, Brucher JM, et al. Acute corticosteroid myopathy in intensive care patients. Muscle Nerve 1997;20(11):1371–80.

[82] van Balkom RH, van der Heijden HF, van Herwaarden CL, et al. Corticosteroid-induced myopathy of the respiratory muscles. Neth J Med 1994;45(3):114–22.

[83] Owczarek J, Jasinska M, Orszulak-Michalak D. Drug-induced myopathies. An overview of the possible mechanisms. Pharmacol Rep 2005;57(1):23–34.

[84] Hickson RC, Czerwinski SM, Wegrzyn LE. Glutamine prevents downregulation of myosin heavy chain synthesis and muscle atrophy from glucocorticoids. Am J Physiol 1995; 268(4 Pt 1):E730–4.

[85] Gayan-Ramirez G, Vanderhoydonc F, Verhoeven G, et al. Acute treatment with corticosteroids decreases IGF-1 and IGF-2 expression in the rat diaphragm and gastrocnemius. Am J Respir Crit Care Med 1999;159(1):283–9.

[86] Singleton JR, Baker BL, Thorburn A. Dexamethasone inhibits insulin-like growth factor signaling and potentiates myoblast apoptosis. Endocrinology 2000;141(8):2945–50.

[87] Stern LZ, Gruener R, Amundsen P. Diphenylhydantoin for steroid-induced muscle weakness. Jama 1973;223(11):1287–8.

[88] van Staa TP, Leufkens HG, Cooper C. The epidemiology of corticosteroid-induced osteoporosis: a meta-analysis. Osteoporos Int 2002;13(10):777–87.

[89] Van Staa TP, Leufkens HG, Abenhaim L, et al. Use of oral corticosteroids and risk of fractures. J Bone Miner Res 2000,15(6):993–1000.

[90] Weinstein RS, Jilka RL, Parfitt AM, et al. Inhibition of osteoblastogenesis and promotion of apoptosis of osteoblasts and osteocytes by glucocorticoids. Potential mechanisms of their deleterious effects on bone. J Clin Invest 1998;102(2):274–82.

[91] Homik J, Cranney A, Shea B, et al. Bisphosphonates for steroid induced osteoporosis. Cochrane Database Syst Rev 2000;(2):CD001347.

[92] Recommendations for the prevention and treatment of glucocorticoid-induced osteoporosis: 2001 update. American College of Rheumatology Ad Hoc Committee on Glucocorticoid-Induced Osteoporosis. Arthritis Rheum 2001;44(7):1496–503.

[93] Gourlay M, Franceschini N, Sheyn Y. Prevention and treatment strategies for glucocorticoid-induced osteoporotic fractures. Clin Rheumatol 2007;26(2):144–53.

[94] Tascioglu F, Colak O, Armagan O, et al. The treatment of osteoporosis in patients with rheumatoid arthritis receiving glucocorticoids: a comparison of alendronate and intranasal salmon calcitonin. Rheumatol Int 2005;26(1):21–9.

[95] Lane NE, Sanchez S, Modin GW, et al. Bone mass continues to increase at the hip after parathyroid hormone treatment is discontinued in glucocorticoid-induced osteoporosis: results of a randomized controlled clinical trial. J Bone Miner Res 2000;15(5):944–51.

[96] Lavelle W, Carl A, Lavelle ED, et al. Vertebroplasty and kyphoplasty. Med Clin North Am 2007;91(2):299–314.

[97] Lewis DA, Smith RE. Steroid-induced psychiatric syndromes. A report of 14 cases and a review of the literature. J Affect Disord 1983;5(4):319–32.

[98] Warrington TP, Bostwick JM. Psychiatric adverse effects of corticosteroids. Mayo Clin Proc 2006;81(10):1361–7.

[99] Wada K, Yamada N, Sato T, et al. Corticosteroid-induced psychotic and mood disorders: diagnosis defined by DSM-IV and clinical pictures. Psychosomatics 2001;42(6):461–6.

[100] Hall RC, Popkin MK, Stickney SK, et al. Presentation of the steroid psychoses. J Nerv Ment Dis 1979;167(4):229–36.

[101] Lupien SJ, McEwen BS. The acute effects of corticosteroids on cognition: integration of animal and human model studies. Brain Res Brain Res Rev 1997;24(1):1–27.

[102] Drug-induced convulsions. Report from Boston Collaborative Drug Surveillance Program. Lancet 1972;2(7779):677–9.

[103] Stiefel FC, Breitbart WS, Holland JC. Corticosteroids in cancer: neuropsychiatric complications. Cancer Invest 1989;7(5):479–91.

[104] Edman JC, Kovacs JA, Masur H, et al. Ribosomal RNA sequence shows Pneumocystis carinii to be a member of the fungi. Nature 1988;334(6182):519–22.

[105] Thomas CF Jr, Limper AH. Pneumocystis pneumonia. N Engl J Med 2004;350(24): 2487–98.

[106] Kovacs JA, Gill VJ, Meshnick S, et al. New insights into transmission, diagnosis, and drug treatment of Pneumocystis carinii pneumonia. Jama 2001;286(19):2450–60.

[107] Henson JW, Jalaj JK, Walker RW, et al. Pneumocystis carinii pneumonia in patients with primary brain tumors. Arch Neurol 1991;48(4):406–9.

[108] Schiff D. Pneumocystis pneumonia in brain tumor patients: risk factors and clinical features. J Neurooncol 1996;27(3):235–40.

[109] Slivka A, Wen PY, Shea WM, et al. Pneumocystis carinii pneumonia during steroid taper in patients with primary brain tumors. Am J Med 1993;94(2):216–9.

[110] Stupp R, Dietrich PY, Ostermann Kraljevic S, et al. Promising survival for patients with newly diagnosed glioblastoma multiforme treated with concomitant radiation plus temozolomide followed by adjuvant temozolomide. J Clin Oncol 2002;20(5):1375–82.

[111] Cohen MH, Johnson JR, Pazdur R. Food and Drug Administration Drug approval summary: temozolomide plus radiation therapy for the treatment of newly diagnosed glioblastoma multiforme. Clin Cancer Res 2005;11(19 Pt 1):6767–71.

[112] Clancey JK. Spinal epidural lipomatosis: a case study. J Neurosci Nurs 2004;36(4):208–9, 213.

[113] Zampella EJ, Duvall ER, Sekar BC, et al. Symptomatic spinal epidural lipomatosis as a complication of steroid immunosuppression in cardiac transplant patients. Report of two cases. J Neurosurg 1987;67(5):760–4.

[114] Smith CL. "Corticosteroid glaucoma" a summary and review of the literaure. Am J Med Sci 1966;252(2):239–44.

[115] Sundmark E. The occurrence of posterior subcapsular cataracts in patients on long-term systemic corticosteroid therapy. Acta Ophthalmol (Copenh) 1963;41:515–23.

[116] Black RL, Oglesby RB, Von Sallmann L, et al. Posterior subcapsular cataracts induced by corticosteroids in patients with rheumatoid arthritis. Jama 1960;174:166–71.

[117] Hadjikoutis S, Morgan JE, Wild JM, et al. Ocular complications of neurological therapy. Eur J Neurol 2005;12(7):499–507.

[118] Cersosimo RJ, Brophy MT. Hiccups with high dose dexamethasone administration: a case report. Cancer 1998;82(2):412–4.

[119] Lewis JH. Hiccups: causes and cures. J Clin Gastroenterol 1985;7(6):539–52.

[120] Braithwaite SS, Barr WG, Rahman A, et al. How to avoid metabolic emergencies. Postgrad Med 1998;104(5):163–6, 171, 166–75.

[121] Rotstein J, Good RA. Steroid pseudorheumatism. AMA Arch Intern Med 1957;99(4): 545–55.

[122] Villalona-Calero MA, Eckardt J, Burris H, et al. A phase I trial of human corticotropin-releasing factor (hCRF) in patients with peritumoral brain edema. Ann Oncol 1998;9(1): 71–7.

[123] Tjuvajev J, Uehara H, Desai R, et al. Corticotropin-releasing factor decreases vasogenic brain edema. Cancer Res 1996;56(6):1352–60.

[124] Badie B, Schartner JM, Hagar AR, et al. Microglia cyclooxygenase-2 activity in experimental gliomas: possible role in cerebral edema formation. Clin Cancer Res 2003;9(2):872–7.

[125] Khan RB, Krasin MJ, Kasow K, et al. Cyclooxygenase-2 inhibition to treat radiation-induced brain necrosis and edema. J Pediatr Hematol Oncol 2004;26(4):253–5.

[126] Portnow J, Suleman S, Grossman SA, et al. A cyclooxygenase-2 (COX-2) inhibitor compared with dexamethasone in a survival study of rats with intracerebral 9L gliosarcomas. Neuro-oncol 2002;4(1):22–5.

[127] Josko J, Knefel K. The role of vascular endothelial growth factor in cerebral oedema formation. Folia Neuropathol 2003;41(3):161–6.

[128] Gonzalez J, Kumar AJ, Conrad CA, et al. Effect of bevacizumab on radiation necrosis of the brain. Int J Radiat Oncol Biol Phys 2007;67(2):323–6.

[129] Batchelor TT, Sorensen AG, di Tomaso E, et al. AZD2171, a pan-VEGF receptor tyrosine kinase inhibitor, normalizes tumor vasculature and alleviates edema in glioblastoma patients. Cancer Cells 2007;11(1):83–95.

[130] Pruemer J. Prevalence, causes, and impact of cancer-associated thrombosis. Am J Health Syst Pharm 2005;62(22 Suppl 5):S4–6.

[131] Constantini S, Kornowski R, Pomeranz S, et al. Thromboembolic phenomena in neurosurgical patients operated upon for primary and metastatic brain tumors. Acta Neurochir (Wien) 1991;109(3–4):93–7.

[132] Ruff RL, Posner JB. Incidence and treatment of peripheral venous thrombosis in patients with glioma. Ann Neurol 1983;13(3):334–6.

[133] Sawaya R, Zuccarello M, Elkalliny M, et al. Postoperative venous thromboembolism guganand brain tumors: Part I. Clinical profile. J Neurooncol 1992;14(2):119–25.

[134] Simanek R, Vormittag R, Hassler M, et al. Venous thromboembolism and survival in patients with high-grade glioma. Neuro-oncol 2007;9(2):89–95.

[135] Brandes AA, Scelzi E, Salmistraro G, et al. Incidence of risk of thromboembolism during treatment high-grade gliomas: a prospective study. Eur J Cancer 1997;33(10):1592–6.

[136] Cheruku R, Tapazoglou E, Ensley J, et al. The incidence and significance of thromboembolic complications in patients with high-grade gliomas. Cancer 1991;68(12):2621–4.

[137] Levitan N, Dowlati A, Remick SC, et al. Rates of initial and recurrent thromboembolic disease among patients with malignancy versus those without malignancy. Risk analysis using Medicare claims data. Medicine (Baltimore) 1999;78(5):285–91.

[138] Marras LC, Geerts WH, Perry JR. The risk of venous thromboembolism is increased throughout the course of malignant glioma: an evidence-based review. Cancer 2000; 89(3):640–6.

[139] Sciacca FL, Ciusani E, Silvani A, et al. Genetic and plasma markers of venous thromboembolism in patients with high grade glioma. Clin Cancer Res 2004;10(4):1312–7.

[140] Tabori U, Beni-Adani L, Dvir R, et al. Risk of venous thromboembolism in pediatric patients with brain tumors. Pediatr Blood Cancer 2004;43(6):633–6.

[141] Alpert JS, Dalen JE. Epidemiology and natural history of venous thromboembolism. Prog Cardiovasc Dis 1994;36(6):417–22.

[142] Horlander KT, Mannino DM, Leeper KV. Pulmonary embolism mortality in the United States, 1979–1998: an analysis using multiple-cause mortality data. Arch Intern Med Jul 28 2003;163(14):1711–7.

[143] Goldhaber SZ, Visani L, De Rosa M. Acute pulmonary embolism: clinical outcomes in the International Cooperative Pulmonary Embolism Registry (ICOPER). Lancet 1999; 353(9162):1386–9.

[144] Naess IA, Christiansen SC, Romundstad P, et al. Incidence and mortality of venous thrombosis: a population-based study. J Thromb Haemost 2007;5(4):692–9.

[145] Gerber DE, Grossman SA, Streiff MB. Management of venous thromboembolism in patients with primary and metastatic brain tumors. J Clin Oncol 2006;24(8):1310–8.

[146] Walsh DC, Kakkar AK. Thromboembolism in brain tumors. Curr Opin Pulm Med 2001; 7(5):326–31.

[147] Thoron L, Arbit E. Hemostatic changes in patients with brain tumors. J Neurooncol 1994; 22(2):87–100.

[148] Hamada K, Kuratsu J, Saitoh Y, et al. Expression of tissue factor correlates with grade of malignancy in human glioma. Cancer 1996;77(9):1877–83.

[149] Iberti TJ, Miller M, Abalos A, et al. Abnormal coagulation profile in brain tumor patients during surgery. Neurosurgery 1994;34(3):389–94 [discussion: 385–94].

[150] Sawaya R, Highsmith RF. Postoperative venous thromboembolism and brain tumors: Part III. Biochemical profile. J Neurooncol 1992;14(2):113–8.

[151] McRae SJ, Ginsberg JS. Update in the diagnosis of deep-vein thrombosis and pulmonary embolism. Curr Opin Anaesthesiol 2006;19(1):44–51.

[152] Segal JB, Eng J, Tamariz LJ, et al. Review of the evidence on diagnosis of deep venous thrombosis and pulmonary embolism. Ann Fam Med 2007;5(1):63–73.

[153] Bates SM, Ginsberg JS. Clinical practice. Treatment of deep-vein thrombosis. N Engl J Med 2004;351(3):268–77.

[154] Palareti G, Cosmi B, Legnani C. Diagnosis of deep vein thrombosis. Semin Thromb Hemost 2006;32(7):659–72.

[155] Wells PS, Anderson DR, Rodger M, et al. Evaluation of D-dimer in the diagnosis of suspected deep-vein thrombosis. N Engl J Med 2003;349(13):1227–35.

[156] Qaseem A, Snow V, Barry P, et al. Current diagnosis of venous thromboembolism in primary care: a clinical practice guideline from the American Academy of Family Physicians and the American College of Physicians. Ann Fam Med 2007;5(1):57–62.

[157] Rathbun SW, Raskob GE, Whitsett TL. Sensitivity and specificity of helical computed tomography in the diagnosis of pulmonary embolism: a systematic review. Ann Intern Med 2000;132(3):227–32.

[158] Quiroz R, Kucher N, Zou KH, et al. Clinical validity of a negative computed tomography scan in patients with suspected pulmonary embolism: a systematic review. Jama 2005; 293(16):2012–7.

[159] Roy PM, Colombet I, Durieux P, et al. Systematic review and meta-analysis of strategies for the diagnosis of suspected pulmonary embolism. Bmj 2005;331(7511):259.

[160] Stein PD, Fowler SE, Goodman LR, et al. Multidetector computed tomography for acute pulmonary embolism. N Engl J Med 2006;354(22):2317–27.

[161] Bostrom S, Holmgren E, Jonsson O, et al. Post-operative thromboembolism in neurosurgery. A study on the prophylactic effect of calf muscle stimulation plus dextran compared to low-dose heparin. Acta Neurochir (Wien) 1986;80(3–4):83–9.

[162] Bucci MN, Papadopoulos SM, Chen JC, et al. Mechanical prophylaxis of venous thrombosis in patients undergoing craniotomy: a randomized trial. Surg Neurol 1989;32(4):285–8.

[163] Skillman JJ, Collins RE, Coe NP, et al. Prevention of deep vein thrombosis in neurosurgical patients: a controlled, randomized trial of external pneumatic compression boots. Surgery 1978;83(3):354–8.

[164] Turpie AG, Hirsh J, Gent M, et al. Prevention of deep vein thrombosis in potential neurosurgical patients. A randomized trial comparing graduated compression stockings alone or graduated compression stockings plus intermittent pneumatic compression with control. Arch Intern Med 1989;149(3):679–81.

[165] Chan AT, Atiemo A, Diran LK, et al. Venous thromboembolism occurs frequently in patients undergoing brain tumor surgery despite prophylaxis. J Thromb Thrombolysis 1999;8(2):139–42.

[166] Flinn WR, Sandager GP, Silva MB Jr, et al. Prospective surveillance for perioperative venous thrombosis. Experience in 2643 patients. Arch Surg May 1996;131(5):472–80.

[167] Agnelli G, Piovella F, Buoncristiani P, et al. Enoxaparin plus compression stockings compared with compression stockings alone in the prevention of venous thromboembolism after elective neurosurgery. N Engl J Med 1998;339(2):80–5.

[168] Cerrato D, Ariano C, Fiacchino F. Deep vein thrombosis and low-dose heparin prophylaxis in neurosurgical patients. J Neurosurg 1978;49(3):378–81.

[169] Comerota AJ, Chouhan V, Harada RN, et al. The fibrinolytic effects of intermittent pneumatic compression: mechanism of enhanced fibrinolysis. Ann Surg 1997;226(3):306–13 [discussion: 304–313].

[170] Iorio A, Agnelli G. Low-molecular-weight and unfractionated heparin for prevention of venous thromboembolism in neurosurgery: a meta-analysis. Arch Intern Med 2000;160(15): 2327–32.

[171] Carman TL, Kanner AA, Barnett GH, et al. Prevention of thromboembolism after neurosurgery for brain and spinal tumors. South Med J 2003;96(1):17–22.

[172] Stephens PH, Healy MT, Smith M, et al. Prophylaxis against thromboembolism in neurosurgical patients: a survey of current practice in the United Kingdom. Br J Neurosurg 1995; 9(2):159–63.

[173] Perry JR, Rogers L, Laperriere N, et al. PRODIGE: a phase III randomized placebo-controlled trial of thromboprophylaxis using dalteparin low molecular weight heparin (LMWH) in patients with newly diagnosed malignant glioma. J Clin Oncol 2007;25(18S):2011.

[174] Rocha E, Martinez-Gonzalez MA, Montes R, et al. Do the low molecular weight heparins improve efficacy and safety of the treatment of deep venous thrombosis? A meta-analysis. Haematologica 2000;85(9):935–42.

[175] Mismetti P, Laporte S, Darmon JY, et al. Meta-analysis of low molecular weight heparin in the prevention of venous thromboembolism in general surgery. Br J Surg 2001;88(7):913–30.

[176] Levin JM, Schiff D, Loeffler JS, et al. Complications of therapy for venous thromboembolic disease in patients with brain tumors. Neurology 1993;43(6):1111–4.

[177] Schiff D, DeAngelis LM. Therapy of venous thromboembolism in patients with brain metastases. Cancer 1994;73(2):493–8.

[178] Olin JW, Young JR, Graor RA, et al. Treatment of deep vein thrombosis and pulmonary emboli in patients with primary and metastatic brain tumors. Anticoagulants or inferior vena cava filter? Arch Intern Med 1987;147(12):2177–9.

[179] Choucair AK, Silver P, Levin VA. Risk of intracranial hemorrhage in glioma patients receiving anticoagulant therapy for venous thromboembolism. J Neurosurg 1987;66(3):357–8.

[180] Quevedo JF, Buckner JC, Schmidt JL, et al. Thromboembolism in patients with high-grade glioma. Mayo Clin Proc 1994;69(4):329–32.

[181] Ruff RL, Posner JB. The incidence of systemic venous thrombosis and the risk of anticoagulation in patients with malignant gliomas. Trans Am Neurol Assoc 1981;106:223–6.

[182] Pruitt AA. Treatment of medical complications in patients with brain tumors. Curr Treat Options Neurol 2005;7(4):323–36.

[183] Knovich MA, Lesser GJ. The management of thromboembolic disease in patients with central nervous system malignancies. Curr Treat Options Oncol 2004;5(6):511–7.

[184] Norris LK, Grossman SA. Treatment of thromboembolic complications in patients with brain tumors. J Neurooncol 1994;22(2):127–37.

[185] Wen PY, Marks PW. Medical management of patients with brain tumors. Curr Opin Oncol 2002;14(3):299–307.

[186] Coon WW, Willis PW 3rd. Hemorrhagic complications of anticoagulant therapy. Arch Intern Med 1974;133(3):386–92.

[187] Levine MN, Raskob G, Beyth RJ, et al. Hemorrhagic complications of anticoagulant treatment: the Seventh ACCP Conference on Antithrombotic and Thrombolytic Therapy. Chest 2004;126(3 Suppl):287S–310S.

[188] Hirsh J, Warkentin TE, Shaughnessy SG, et al. Heparin and low-molecular-weight heparin: mechanisms of action, pharmacokinetics, dosing, monitoring, efficacy, and safety. Chest 2001;119(1 Suppl):64S–94S.

[189] Meyer G, Marjanovic Z, Valcke J, et al. Comparison of low-molecular-weight heparin and warfarin for the secondary prevention of venous thromboembolism in patients with cancer: a randomized controlled study. Arch Intern Med 2002;162(15):1729–35.

[190] Lee AY, Levine MN, Baker RI, et al. Low-molecular-weight heparin versus a coumarin for the prevention of recurrent venous thromboembolism in patients with cancer. N Engl J Med 2003;349(2):146–53.

[191] Wakelee HA, Sikic BI. Activity of novel cytotoxic agents in lung cancer: epothilones and topoisomerase I inhibitors. Clin Lung Cancer 2005;7(Suppl 1):S6–12.

[192] Monreal M, Zacharski L, Jimenez JA, et al. Fixed-dose low-molecular-weight heparin for secondary prevention of venous thromboembolism in patients with disseminated cancer: a prospective cohort study. J Thromb Haemost 2004;2(8):1311–5.

[193] Linenberger ML, Wittkowsky AK. Thromboembolic complications of malignancy. Part 2: management. Oncology (Williston Park) 2005;19(8):1077–84 [discussion: 1084, 1078–87].

[194] Dunn AS, Coller B. Outpatient treatment of deep vein thrombosis: translating clinical trials into practice. Am J Med 1999;106(6):660–9.

[195] Koopman MM, Prandoni P, Piovella F, et al. Treatment of venous thrombosis with intravenous unfractionated heparin administered in the hospital as compared with subcutaneous low-molecular-weight heparin administered at home. The Tasman Study Group. N Engl J Med 1996;334(11):682–7.

[196] Levine M, Gent M, Hirsh J, et al. A comparison of low-molecular-weight heparin administered primarily at home with unfractionated heparin administered in the hospital for proximal deep-vein thrombosis. N Engl J Med 1996;334(11):677–81.

[197] Kovacs MJ, Anderson D, Morrow B, et al. Outpatient treatment of pulmonary embolism with dalteparin. Thromb Haemost 2000;83(2):209–11.

[198] Crowther MA, Berry LR, Monagle PT, et al. Mechanisms responsible for the failure of protamine to inactivate low-molecular-weight heparin. Br J Haematol 2002;116(1):178–86.

[199] Warkentin TE, Crowther MA. Reversing anticoagulants both old and new. Can J Anaesth 2002;49(6):S11–25.

[200] Aguilar MI, Hart RG, Kase CS, et al. Treatment of warfarin-associated intracerebral hemorrhage: literature review and expert opinion. Mayo Clin Proc 2007;82(1):82–92.

[201] Dickneite G. Prothrombin complex concentrate versus recombinant factor VIIa for reversal of coumarin anticoagulation. Thromb Res 2007;119(5):643–51.

[202] Ingerslev J, Vanek T, Culic S. Use of recombinant factor VIIa for emergency reversal of anticoagulation. J Postgrad Med 2007;53(1):17–22.

[203] Firozvi K, Deveras RA, Kessler CM. Reversal of low-molecular-weight heparin-induced bleeding in patients with pre-existing hypercoagulable states with human recombinant activated factor VII concentrate. Am J Hematol 2006;81(8):582–9.

[204] Gerotziafas GT, Depasse F, Chakroun T, et al. Recombinant factor VIIa partially reverses the inhibitory effect of fondaparinux on thrombin generation after tissue factor activation in platelet rich plasma and whole blood. Thromb Haemost 2004;91(3):531–7.

[205] Heimans JJ, Taphoorn MJ. Impact of brain tumour treatment on quality of life. J Neurol 2002;249(8):955–60.

[206] Pelletier G, Verhoef MJ, Khatri N, et al. Quality of life in brain tumor patients: the relative contributions of depression, fatigue, emotional distress, and existential issues. J Neurooncol 2002;57(1):41–9.

[207] Osoba D, Aaronson NK, Muller M, et al. Effect of neurological dysfunction on health-related quality of life in patients with high-grade glioma. J Neurooncol 1997;34(3):263–78.

[208] Osoba D, Brada M, Prados MD, et al. Effect of disease burden on health-related quality of life in patients with malignant gliomas. Neuro-oncol 2000;2(4):221–8.

[209] Salo J, Niemela A, Joukamaa M, et al. Effect of brain tumour laterality on patients' perceived quality of life. J Neurol Neurosurg Psychiatry 2002;72(3):373–7.

[210] Hickok JT, Roscoe JA, Morrow GR, et al. Frequency, severity, clinical course, and correlates of fatigue in 372 patients during 5 weeks of radiotherapy for cancer. Cancer 2005; 104(8):1772–8.

[211] Lovely MP, Miaskowski C, Dodd M. Relationship between fatigue and quality of life in patients with glioblastoma multiformae. Oncol Nurs Forum 1999;26(5):921–5.

[212] Rogers MP, Orav J, Black PM. The use of a simple Likert scale to measure quality of life in brain tumor patients. J Neurooncol 2001;55(2):121–31.

[213] Brown PD, Ballman KV, Rummans TA, et al. Prospective study of quality of life in adults with newly diagnosed high-grade gliomas. J Neurooncol 2006;76(3):283–91.

[214] Carter GT, Weiss MD, Lou JS, et al. Modafinil to treat fatigue in amyotrophic lateral sclerosis: an open label pilot study. Am J Hosp Palliat Care 2005;22(1):55–9.

[215] Fishbain DA, Cutler RB, Lewis J, et al. Modafinil for the treatment of pain-associated fatigue: review and case report. J Pain Palliat Care Pharmacother 2004;18(2):39–47.

[216] Kraft GH, Bowen J. Modafinil for fatigue in MS: a randomized placebo-controlled double-blind study. Neurology 2005;65(12):1995–7 [author reply: 1995–7].

[217] Rabkin JG, McElhiney MC, Rabkin R, et al. Modafinil treatment for fatigue in HIV+ patients: a pilot study. J Clin Psychiatry 2004;65(12):1688–95.

[218] Rammohan KW, Lynn DJ. Modafinil for fatigue in MS: a randomized placebo-controlled double-blind study. Neurology 2005;65(12):1995–7 [author reply: 1995–7].

[219] Schwartz TL, Azhar N, Cole K, et al. An open-label study of adjunctive modafinil in patients with sedation related to serotonergic antidepressant therapy. J Clin Psychiatry 2004;65(9):1223–7.

[220] Sevy S, Rosenthal MH, Alvir J, et al. Double-blind, placebo-controlled study of modafinil for fatigue and cognition in schizophrenia patients treated with psychotropic medications. J Clin Psychiatry 2005;66(7):839–43.

[221] Stankoff B, Waubant E, Confavreux C, et al. Modafinil for fatigue in MS: a randomized placebo-controlled double-blind study. Neurology 2005;64(7):1139–43.

[222] Zifko UA, Rupp M, Schwarz S, et al. Modafinil in treatment of fatigue in multiple sclerosis. Results of an open-label study. J Neurol 2002;249(8):983–7.

[223] Ashton AK. Modafinil augmentation of phenelzine for residual fatigue in dysthymia. Am J Psychiatry 2004;161(9):1716–7.

[224] DeBattista C, Lembke A, Solvason HB, et al. A prospective trial of modafinil as an adjunctive treatment of major depression. J Clin Psychopharmacol 2004;24(1):87–90.

[225] Lundt L. Modafinil treatment in patients with seasonal affective disorder/winter depression: an open-label pilot study. J Affect Disord 2004;81(2):173–8.

[226] Price CS, Taylor FB. A retrospective chart review of the effects of modafinil on depression as monotherapy and as adjunctive therapy. Depress Anxiety 2005;21(4):149–53.

[227] Kaleita TA, Wellisch DK, Graham CA, et al. Pilot study of modafinil for treatment of neurobehavioral dysfunction and fatigue in adult patients with brain tumors. J Clin Oncol 2006;24(18S):1503 [abstract].

[228] Wefel JS, Kayl AE, Meyers CA. Neuropsychological dysfunction associated with cancer and cancer therapies: a conceptual review of an emerging target. Br J Cancer 2004;90(9): 1691–6.

[229] Correa DD. Cognitive functions in brain tumor patients. Hematol Oncol Clin North Am 2006;20(6):1363–76.

[230] Meyers CA, Weitzner MA, Valentine AD, et al. Methylphenidate therapy improves cognition, mood, and function of brain tumor patients. J Clin Oncol 1998;16(7):2522–7.

[231] Shaw EG, Rosdhal R, D'Agostino RB Jr, et al. Phase II study of donepezil in irradiated brain tumor patients: effect on cognitive function, mood, and quality of life. J Clin Oncol 2006;24(9):1415–20.

[232] Lee MA, Leng ME, Tiernan EJ. Risperidone: a useful adjunct for behavioural disturbance in primary cerebral tumours. Palliat Med 2001;15(3):255–6.

[233] Thiessen B, DeAngelis LM. Hydrocephalus in radiation leukoencephalopathy: results of ventriculoperitoneal shunting. Arch Neurol 1998;55(5):705–10.

[234] Litofsky NS, Farace E, Anderson F Jr, et al. Depression in patients with high-grade glioma: results of the Glioma Outcomes Project. Neurosurgery 2004;54(2):358–66 [discussion: 357–66].

ELSEVIER
SAUNDERS

NEUROLOGIC
CLINICS

Neurol Clin 25 (2007) 1073–1088

# Management of Patients with Low-Grade Gliomas

Mark R. Gilbert, MD[a],*, Frederick F. Lang, MD[b]

[a]Department of Neuro-Oncology, University of Texas MD Anderson Cancer Center,
1515 Holcombe Boulevard, Houston, Texas 77030, USA
[b]Department of Neurosurgery, University of Texas MD Anderson Cancer Center,
1515 Holcombe Boulevard, Houston, Texas 77030, USA

The accurate diagnosis and management of patients who have infiltrating low-grade gliomas (LGGs) is increasing in importance. Recent advances in molecular characterization, imaging, and treatment of these tumors underscore this current focus of investigations. LGGs are primary brain tumors arising within the brain parenchyma and rarely disseminate outside the central nervous system. Pathologically, they include astrocytomas, oligodendrogliomas, and mixed oligoastrocytomas, all classified as grade 2 by the World Health Organization (WHO) grading system [1]. Although considered low grade with a low proliferate rate and homogeneous cellular morphology by histologic evaluation, these tumors often undergo malignant transformation to a higher-grade glial tumor; therefore, they no longer are considered benign neoplasms [2,3].

Typically, LGGs are well demonstrated on routine MRI as a nonenhancing mass that is hypointense on T1 sequences and hyperintense on T2 or fluid-attenuated inversion-recovery (FLAIR) imaging (as shown in Fig. 1) [4]. These lesions are not as well defined on CT of the brain, likely accounting for the increase in early diagnosis of these lesions over the past 2 decades commensurate with the improved availability of MRI. The new era of earlier diagnosis has led some physicians to advocate early intervention with surgical resection, radiation, or chemotherapy. The hope of this early approach is that with limited disease, cure may be possible. Conversely, others advocate observation, given the slow growth of the tumor and the potential morbidities associated with radical surgical resection and radiotherapy. Early diagnosis has not been shown clearly to alter prognosis but does

---

* Corresponding author.
*E-mail address:* mrgilbert@mdanderson.org (M.R. Gilbert).

0733-8619/07/$ - see front matter © 2007 Elsevier Inc. All rights reserved.
doi:10.1016/j.ncl.2007.07.007      *neurologic.theclinics.com*

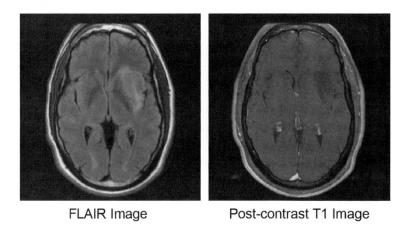

FLAIR Image                    Post-contrast T1 Image

Fig. 1. MRI of a LGG.

complicate interpretation of treatment results because of lead-time bias; those patients diagnosed early may seem to live longer even if the natural history of the tumor is not altered by the therapeutic interventions. Furthermore, there are recent data suggesting that a subset of patients may benefit from chemotherapy, a treatment previously considered ineffective.

Although controversy exists regarding the optimal management of patients who have LGGs, recent randomized trials and large cooperative group efforts are beginning to provide some guidelines. Additionally, recent advances in molecular profiling of these tumors are helping to define prognosis and likelihood of response to therapy better. These important discoveries, paralleling the findings in WHO grade 3 gliomas, are changing individual patient treatment and having an impact on clinical trial designs by changing tumor classification and stratification [5,6]. This article reviews the recent results and discusses some of the controversies in management.

### Histologic and molecular classification

Primary brain tumors rarely spread outside the central nervous system. Therefore, use of the conventional T (*t*umor size), N (*n*odal involvement), M (*m*etastases) system commonly used for solid tumors is of little benefit for staging primary brain tumors, such as glial malignancies. Instead, grading systems traditionally have used histologic features to stratify patients for prognostic and treatment purposes. Although several systems exist, the one developed by the WHO is used most commonly [1]. Glial tumors are graded from I to IV with grade I restricted to noninfiltrative tumors, such as pilocytic astrocytoma, often curable by surgical resection. Grade II tumors, in which LGGs are classified, are significantly different from grade I in that they are infiltrative, rarely curable by surgical resection, and have the potential to undergo malignant transformation to a higher-grade neoplasm.

Within the grade II group, the most common tumors are glial in origin. This includes astrocytomas, oligodendrogliomas, and the mixed oligoastrocytomas. This subclassification is based on the morphologic appearance of the tumor cells and has prognostic and therapeutic importance. Most series demonstrate a median survival of 6 to 8 years for astrocytomas and 9 to 12 years for oligodendrogliomas [7]. Patients who have mixed oligoastrocytomas have a reported outcome that falls between the astrocytomas and pure oligodendrogliomas. In all three histologic subtypes, malignant transformation to a higher-grade tumor occurs in the majority of cases and accounts for the subsequent short survival [2,3].

Recently, molecular changes have been uncovered in LGGs that have allowed more accurate subclassification. The most prominent has been the association between the loss of heterozygosity of the 1p and 19q chromosomes (1p19q LOH) and prognosis in oligodendrogliomas. A recent study demonstrated that the 1p19q LOH is mediated by a translocation t(1;19)(q10;p10) [8] Patients harboring tumors with this codeletion have a far better prognosis than those who have oligodendrogliomas without these changes (reviewed by Aldape and colleagues [9]). 1p 19q LOH has been associated with a marked increase in treatment response in anaplastic (grade III) oligodendrogliomas; however, this has not been studied extensively for grade II tumors. Mutation of the p53 tumor suppressor gene is seen in more than 60% of astrocytomas and is related inversely to the presence of 1p19q LOH [10]. Loss of heterozygosity at 6q, 13q and 22q also is reported.

## Clinical prognostic factors

Several studies have attempted to determine prognostic factors, recognizing that grade II gliomas have a wide prognostic range with survival as short as 1 year to greater than 10 to 12 years. Pignatti and colleagues determined five factors, including age, histology, presence of neurologic deficits before surgery, tumor diameter, and tumor crossing the midline as significant determinants of outcome. There was a direct correlation of the number of poor factors with survival [11]. As shown in Table 1, patients who had no poor prognostic factors had a median survival of 9 years, whereas patients who had all 5 poor prognostic factors had a median survival of less than 1 year. The study by Bauman and colleagues [12] performed a recursive partitioning analysis of potential prognostic factors on data from 401 patients who had LGG. Four groups were identified with distinct survival differences (shown in Table 2).

As described previously, molecular factors also have a great impact on prognosis, as illustrated by 1p19q LOH. Other analyses have found a correlation between measures of tumor proliferation, such as Ki-67 and

Table 1
Clinical prognostic factors for low-grade glioma

| Negative prognostic factors | |
| --- | --- |
| Age >40 years | |
| Largest diameter of tumor >6 cm | |
| Tumor crosses midline | |
| Histology is astrocytoma | |
| Neurologic deficits are present | |
| **Median survival by score (sum of negative prognostic factors)** | **Median survival in years** |
| 0 | 9.2 |
| 1 | 8.8 |
| 2 | 5.8 |
| 3 | 3.5 |
| 4 | 1.9 |
| 5 | 0.7 |

*Data from* Pignatti F, van den Bent M, Curran D, et al. Prognostic factors for survival in adult patients with cerebral low-grade glioma. J Clin Oncol 2002;20:2076–84.

proliferative cell nuclear antigen levels and survival [13]. Those tumors with a higher proliferative rate were associated with a worse prognosis.

## Signs and symptoms

Patients who have brain tumors usually present with generalized or focal signs or symptoms, although occasionally the diagnosis is made coincidentally. Generalized symptoms, such as headaches, nausea, vomiting, and altered level of consciousness, arise as a consequence of increased intracranial pressure or seizures. Focal signs often are the consequence of tumor infiltration or dysfunction arising from displacement of brain parenchyma by the tumor mass. Although 30% of patients who have primary brain tumors (all types) present with seizures, 50% to 90% of patients who have LGGs present with seizures. This high rate of seizures may be the result

Table 2
Results of a recursive partitioning analysis demonstrating the impact of clinical factors on survival

| Group | KPS | Patient age | Tumor enhancement | Median survival |
| --- | --- | --- | --- | --- |
| 1 | <70 | >40 years | NS | 12 months |
| 2 | ≥70 | >40 years | Yes | 46 months |
| 3 | <70 | 18–40 years | NS | 87 months |
| | ≥70 | >40 years | No | |
| 4 | ≥70 | 18–40 years | NS | 128 months |

*Abbreviations:* KPS, Karnofsky Performance Status score; NS, presence or absence of enhancement was not a significant factor.

*Data from* Bauman G, Lote K, Larson D, et al. Pretreatment factors predict overall survival for patients with low-grade glioma: a recursive partitioning analysis. Int J Radiat Oncol Biol Phys 1999;45:923–9.

of the frequent involvement of the cerebral cortex by these low-grade tumors. Headaches or focal neurologic deficits are present in approximately one third of patients. Cognitive or behavioral changes and papilledema are reported at presentation in approximately 10% of patients.

The differential diagnosis of a nonenhancing abnormality noted on MRI is extensive. These include multiple sclerosis, stroke, infectious diseases (including viral encephalitis, toxoplasmosis, and cysticercosis), and other idiopathic conditions, such as sarcoidosis and Behçet's disease. As recently reviewed by Omuro and coworkers [14], imaging, including advanced technology (such as magnetic resonance spectroscopy, diffusion-weighted imaging, apparent diffusion coefficient maps, and positron emission tomography) often cannot distinguish reliably many of these diseases from gliomas. Investigations looking for systemic processes or other manifestations of the disease may be critical in excluding these illnesses.

Additionally, since the advent of MRI, there is a cohort of patients found to have incidental nonenhancing abnormalities that frequently are unrelated to the primary reason for the imaging study. For example, some patients who have head trauma or a new-onset headache syndrome undergo a brain MRI that reveals a small, nonenhancing lesion that is unlikely related to the trauma or causing symptoms, such as headache. In these patients, the decision regarding the timing of proceeding with an extensive diagnostic evaluation, including a surgical procedure, is difficult. Often, serial imaging evaluations are performed and the decision to proceed with tissue sampling procedure, biopsy, or tumor resection is based on growth of the lesion or a change in the imaging appearance, such as the development of contrast enhancement.

## Patient management

Patients who have clinical or imaging-based evidence of increased intracranial pressure often benefit from the administration of corticosteroids. Dexamethasone is used most commonly because of the low level of mineralicorticoid effects combined with potent glucocorticoid effects. Patients presenting with seizures require treatment with anticonvulsants. The choice of anticonvulsant may have an important impact on the treatment of the tumor. Several anticonvulsants used commonly, such as phenytoin, carbamazepine, and phenobarbital, are well known to increase activity within the hepatic cytochrome P450 system (CYP-450) [15]. This augmentation of the CYP-450 system markedly may alter the pharmacokinetics of certain cancer chemotherapy agents, such as paclitaxel, irinotecan, and the newer tyrosine kinase signal transduction modulators, such as imatinib, gefitinib, and tipifarnib. Valproic acid has been found to inhibit CYP-450 enzymes, although the decrease in chemotherapy clearance often is not clinically significant. Anticonvulsants may have an additional impact on cancer treatment. Carbamazepine and valproic acid are associated with myelotoxicity manifest primarily as leukopenia with carbamazepine and thrombocytopenia with valproic acid. The newer generation of anticonvulsants, such as leviteractam, lamotigen, and topiramate, do not alter CYP-450 activity and rarely are associated with myelotoxicity. Recent studies are demonstrating efficacy of these newer agents in the treatment of tumor-associated seizures [16].

Prophylactic use of anticonvulsants in patients who have brain tumors remains controversial. A consensus statement from the American Academy of Neurology was based on a metaanalysis of four randomized studies comparing prophylactic use of anticonvulsants with no treatment [17]. Prophylactic administration of anticonvulsants did not reduce the incidence of seizures. The conclusions of this meta-analysis may not be directly applicable to patients who have LGGs, however, because (1) the studies used for the analysis included patients who had brain metastases and who had a much lower likelihood of developing seizures; (2) early generation anticonvulsants were used without documentation of adequate blood concentrations; and (3) each study included a relatively small number of patients. The impact of the newer generation of anticonvulsants on seizure prevention has not been studied adequately in patients who have brain tumor, particularly those who have LGGs where the incidence of seizures is high.

## Treatment

### Surgery

Surgery is critical to the management of LGGS, as it is necessary for establishing a diagnosis. There remains debate, however, about the extent of surgery on the outcome of patients who have LGGs. The choice of aggressively removing diffuse LGGs to achieve a gross total or subtotal resection, rather than performing a stereotactic biopsy, has been one of the most controversial debates among neurosurgical oncologists.

The decision to proceed with resection versus a biopsy often is dependent on location and growth characteristics of the lesion. Biopsies often are undertaken for deep-seated lesions (eg, tumors within the brainstem or thalamus), those confined to eloquent cortex (eg, a lesion located directly in the motor cortex), or widespread infiltrative lesions, particularly if they extend across the midline. Even for patients who have tumors in surgically accessible locations, the debate of biopsy versus tumor resection continues, however. This debate is heated, particularly for lesions in regions of the brain where surgical resection is feasible but may be associated with significant morbidity, such as the insula cortex [18]. No level I evidence exists that supports either approach. The invasive nature of diffuse LGGs and the frequent juxtaposition to or within critically "eloquent" brain regions often precludes complete tumor removal and certainly prevents resection of a margin. Because even aggressive resections may leave tumor cells behind, many neurosurgeons opt against any intervention more than a biopsy; however, other neurosurgeons advocate radical removal, or at least subtotal removal, to minimize tumor burden and reduce symptoms, in particular seizures.

Over the past decade, there has been an increasing trend to more extensive tumor resection. This may be related partly to advances in imaging technologies, including functional imaging that provide preoperative localization of motor, sensory, visual, and language function. Additionally, advances in intraoperative navigational systems improve the ability to define tumor margins and the advent of intraoperative imaging, such as MRI, may result in more extensive tumor resection by identifying residual tumor that is not apparent on visual inspection. Recent studies suggest that these technologic advances have permitted increased tumor resection while reducing surgical morbidity and mortality [19].

Although improved survival has not been proved by more extensive tumor resection, there is evidence that radical resection improves the accuracy of diagnosis. A study of 81 patients who underwent a biopsy for diagnosis and then underwent an extensive resection revealed that in 38% of cases the grade of tumor was changed after a larger tissue sample was obtained at surgery [20]. The new diagnosis changed prognosis in all 31 patients and altered the treatment regimen in 21 of the patients studied. In situations where extensive resection is not safe or feasible and where biopsy is indicated, use of multivoxel spectroscopy may increase the likelihood of sampling the most malignant region of the tumor by targeting the voxel with the highest choline to creatine ratio [21].

There also is evidence that extensive tumor resection may have a positive impact on patients' quality of life. Although only a few studies have addressed this area, there are data supporting a decrease in seizure frequency [22]. Additionally, anecdotal experience suggests that patients who have a complete or near complete resection have better palliation of symptoms and less postoperative edema than patients who undergo biopsy or only a partial resection.

The impact of surgical removal of LGGs on patient survival remains unclear. For high-grade gliomas, two recent phase III studies have indicated that radical resection improves patient survival compared with biopsy or subtotal resection [23,24]. Whether or not these results translate to low-grade tumors is not known and there is no randomized trial in LGGs that addresses this question specifically. There are, however, many reports that used retrospective analyses to examine this issue [3,25–30]. These studies have been summarized in several reviews, the most comprehensive of which was by Keles and colleagues [31]. They identified 30 English-language articles on LGGs published between 1970 and 2000 that incorporated statistical analyses and addressed the issue of extent of resection. The investigators found that there was a general trend for more of the recently published articles to support extensive resections, whereas many of the older articles showed no difference between gross total resection and biopsy. To reduce known biases, the investigators then eliminated studies that included pediatric patients, that contained WHO grade I astrocytomas, or that evaluated small numbers of patients ( <75). They were left with only five articles they deemed valid studies, all of which demonstrated that extent of resection was a statistically significant variable in univariate analyses, and in four of the five studies it was a significant variable in multivariate analyses. Even in these studies, however, the extent of tumor resection often was not determined precisely. Extent of resection is measured best by comparing preoperative and postoperative MRI, ideally using volumetric computational analyses. Few studies have used postoperative images to document the extent of resection [3,26,28–30]. In one of the better studies in the literature, Berger and colleagues [28], used a computerized image analysis technique to determine the preoperative and postoperative radiographic tumor volumes in a series of 53 patients who had diffuse LGGs. The investigators found that the extent of resection influenced significantly the incidence of recurrence and the time to tumor progression. Specifically, none of the patients who had undergone a total resection (N = 13) recurred during a mean follow-up of 54 months. In contrast, 14.8% of patients who had residual tumor whose volume was less than 10 cm$^3$ (N = 27) recurred and 46% of patients who had residual tumor whose volume was greater than 10 cm$^3$ recurred.

Current data suggest that biopsy and radical resection are appropriate options for treating patients who have diffuse LGGs. Because of the potential advantages of maximal removal in terms of diagnosis, symptom control, and cytoreduction, however, there is an increasing trend to recommend maximal tumor removal, especially in patients who have large tumors that cause neurologic deficits, as long as neurologic function is preserved. Effective surgery requires maximal use of surgical adjuncts for defining the spatial limits of the tumor (ie, computer-assisted surgery or intraoperative ultrasound) and for assessing functional brain (ie, cortical and subcortical mapping techniques usually with awake craniotomy).

*Radiation therapy*

Radiation therapy has been the standard treatment of LGGs for several decades. Despite widespread acknowledgment that this modality may result in tumor stabilization or reduction, however, controversy exists about optimal dosing and timing of treatment. The recent publications of results from three large international cooperative group trials and the recent completion of a fourth large randomized trial provide guidance for developing treatment algorithms.

*Radiotherapy dosing*

The European Organization for Research and Treatment of Cancer (EORTC) in their trial, EORTC 22,844, compared low-dose radiation with high-dose radiation [32]. This study accrued 379 patients who were randomized to receive 45 Gy over 5 weeks or 59.4 Gy over 6.6 weeks of conventional, limited-field, external beam radiotherapy. The two arms were well matched by age, gender, and percent of patients who had oligodendrogliomas or mixed oligoastrocytomas. No difference in overall survival or 5-year progression-free survival (PFS) was detected between the two treatment arms. Similarly, an intergroup study with involvement of the North Central Cancer Treatment Group, the Radiation Therapy Oncology Group (RTOG), and the Eastern Cooperative Oncology Group (ECOG) randomized 211 patients to 50.5 Gy in 28 fractions or 64.8 Gy in 36 fractions using conventional, limited-field, external beam radiotherapy [33]. The two treatment arms were well matched for histology, age, gender, and performance status. Similar to the EORTC trial, no differences in survival or PFS were noted. More radiation-induced neurotoxicity was noted with the higher-dose regimen. As a consequence of these studies, patients who have LGG typically are treated with a radiotherapy regimen that has a total dose of 50 to 54 Gy.

*Timing of radiotherapy*

The typical slow growth of LGGs has led to a controversy regarding the timing of radiotherapy. Expectation of progressive tumor enlargement, albeit potentially over a long period of time, supports the view that early treatment should be undertaken. Conversely, given the variable growth rate of these tumors, others advocate serial observation, reserving initiation of treatment until there is clear evidence of tumor growth. A randomized clinical trial, EORTC 22,845, a collaboration between the EORTC and the Brain Tumor Working Group of the Medical Research Council of the United Kingdom, was launched in 1986 to assess the impact of early versus late initiation of radiotherapy [34,35]. The study accrued 311 patients who were randomized to undergo serial observation, reserving treatment for clear evidence of tumor progression, or receive immediate (within 8 weeks of surgery) treatment with radiation using a dosing schedule of 54 Gy over 6 weeks. The groups were well matched by extent of tumor resection. The results demonstrated a statistically significant difference in PFS with a 5-year PFS of 55% in the treated group versus 34.6% in the observation arm. There was no difference in overall survival, however, between the two groups. Unfortunately, this study did not include formal measures of quality of life using established quality of life instruments, measures of neurocognitive function, or assessment of symptom burden, including the impact of these symptoms on daily activities (interference items) [36–38]. An improvement in seizure control was noted for the group treated with radiotherapy and although no differences in performance status outcome were noted, concern remains that the patients treated early with radiotherapy are more likely to develop neurocognitive decline as a consequence of radiation toxicity and the development of leukoencephalopathy.

More recently, an intergroup study led by the RTOG (RTOG 98-02) specifically identified patients believed to have a good prognosis to undergo only serial observation [39]. This group only included patients who were 40 years of age or younger who had undergone complete tumor resection, as estimated by a treating neurosurgeon. The initial analysis of this study arm (accrual = 111 patients) recently has been presented and submitted for publication. The overall survival rate at 5 years is 93% with 5-year PFS rate of 48%. Three factors were identified, however, that predicted outcome. Preoperative tumor diameter greater than 4 cm, astrocytic histology (versus mixed or oligodendroglial), and postoperative residual (on central review) greater than or equal to 1 cm was associated with a significantly higher risk for early progression. The group with all three poor prognostic factors had a 5-year PFS rate of 13% compared with the group with all favorable factors demonstrating a 5-year PFS rate of 70%. These results support an observation strategy for selected patients who have LGG but contemplation of additional clinical and tumor factors needs to be considered in making the decision.

*Chemotherapy*

The role of chemotherapy in the management of LGGs is evolving. Historically, this group of tumors was considered poorly responsive to traditional cytotoxic chemotherapy. This lack of response is believed a consequence of a low rate of cell proliferation, similar to the low-grade, indolent lymphomas. Few studies have been performed to evaluate chemotherapy for newly diagnosed LGGs systematically. The Southwest Oncology Group performed the only published randomized trial [40]. Sixty-six patients who had LGGs and measurable tumor were randomized to external beam radiation or radiation plus lomustine (CCNU). There was no difference in survival between the two arms, and the radiation-only arm had a higher objective response rate (79% versus 54%). This study did not complete accrual, however, and there was a trend toward improved survival in the combined radiation and chemotherapy group.

More recently, a series of phase II studies have been published demonstrating objective responses in patients who had recurrent LGGs. A summary of published studies is shown in Table 3 [41–46]. Objective response rates as high as 80% have been reported with the use of the combination of procarbazine, CCNU, and vincristine (PCV); complete responses, however, are rare. Similar results, presented in Table 3, also have been reported with the use of temozolomide, an oral alkylating agent that has a favorable toxicity profile. Careful review reveals that many of the tumors treated in these published studies were found to have contrast enhancement, an atypical feature for a LGG, raising the concern that the presumed recurrence was the consequence of malignant transformation or radiation-induced necrosis. Several of these studies, however, demonstrate clearly that oligodendroglial tumors and those with mixed oligoastrocytic histology are far more likely to respond to chemotherapy. Furthermore, similar to

Table 3
Trials of chemotherapy for low-grade glioma

| Study | No. of patients | Pathology | Enhancement (%) | Prior radiation therapy or chemotherapy | Chemotherapy Regimen | Response rate (%) | 1 year PFS |
|---|---|---|---|---|---|---|---|
| Buckner et al [41] | 28 | O, OA | 46 | No | PCV | 52 | 91 |
| Soffietti et al [42] | 26 | O, OA | 73 | Yes | PCV | 62 | 80 |
| Quinn et al [43] | 46 | A, O, AA | 70 | Yes | TMZ | 61 | 76 |
| Pace et al [44] | 43 | A, O, AA | 60 | Yes | TMZ | 47 | 39 |
| Brada et al [48] | 30 | A, O, AA | 0 | No | TMZ | 10 | >90 |
| Hoang-Xuan et al [47] | 60 | O, OA | 11 | No | TMZ | 31 | 73 |
| Van den Bent et al [45] | 32 | O, OA | 100 | Yes[a] | TMZ | 22 | 11 |

*Abbreviations:* A, astrocytoma; O, oligodendroglioma; OA, oligoastrocytoma; TMZ, temozolomide.
[a] All patients received prior PCV.
*Data from* Lang FF, Gilbert MR. Diffusely infiltrative low-grade gliomas in adults. J Clin Oncol 2006;24(8):1236–45.

grade III oligodendrogliomas, tumors demonstrating allelic loss of the 1p and 19q arms are more likely to respond to a chemotherapy regimen [47].

Temozolomide has been used as the primary therapy in patients who have newly diagnosed LGG [48]. Twenty-nine patients who had incompletely resected LGG were enrolled on the study. Nineteen patients had tumors with an astrocytic or mixed histology; the remaining 10 patients had an oligodendroglioma. The overall objective response rate was 58%, combining partial and minor responses. Although progression during treatment was rare, the 3-year PFS rate was only 66%, suggesting that chemotherapy alone was not a sufficient treatment for patients who had residual LGG after partial resection. No data regarding the 1p 19q chromosomal status were provided for these patients.

There are ongoing efforts to define further the subgroup of patients who have LGG who are likely to benefit from chemotherapy. Methylguanine-methyltransferase (MGMT) is a DNA repair enzyme, and high expression of this enzyme has been correlated with resistance to chemotherapy, including temozolomide. A recent study demonstrated a significant correlation of hypermethylation of the promoter region of the MGMT gene with improved outcome in patients who had glioblastoma who were treated with a combination of radiation therapy and temozolomide [49]. Methylation of the promoter region prevents gene transcription and tumor cells with methylated promoter have low levels of MGMT activity. A recent study correlated response to temozolomide in patients who had newly diagnosed LGG with the methylation status of the promoter region of the MGMT gene [50]. A total of 68 patients were enrolled with 62% having an oligodendroglioma and the remainder an astrocytoma (12%) or a mixed histology tumor (26%). There was combined allelic loss of 1p and 19q in 36% and intact chromosome in the remaining 64%. MGMT was hypermethylated in 63 of the 68 patients (92%). Despite the large numeric imbalance, there was a statistically significant difference in progression-free survival between the methylated and unmethylated MGMT groups (29.5 months versus 6 months, respectively; $P < .0001$). Allelic status of 1p and 19q also demonstrated a statistical difference in PFS. Those with allelic loss had a PFS of 35 months compared with 23 months for those without loss ($P = .04$). There was no statistical difference in PFS when comparing outcome based on histology.

Several prospective randomized clinical trials currently are underway to address the role of chemotherapy for patients who have LGG. RTOG 98-02 is a three-arm trial that completed accrual in 2002. In addition to the observation arm for good risk patients (described previously), patients who have residual tumor or those over 40 years of age were randomized to receive radiation therapy (54 Gy) plus 6 cycles of adjuvant PCV or radiation alone. More than 250 patients were accrued to the randomized component and the results of the trial are maturing. Tumor tissue was collected on the majority of patients and it is anticipated that 1p 19q LOH status and MGMT promoter methylation data will be determined and used in the analysis of outcome.

The RTOG is completing a phase II study of concurrent radiation plus daily temozolomide followed by 6 months of adjuvant temozolomide for patients who have poor-risk LGG. Using the prognostic factors defined by Pignatti and colleagues [11] (described previously), patients who have three or more poor prognostic factors are eligible. The EORTC recently opened an important study, protocol 22,041, a randomized trial comparing upfront radiation therapy (50.4 Gy) with upfront chemotherapy using temozolomide. Patients will be stratified on the basis of 1p allelic loss with the primary outcome measure of PFS with treatment-related changes in quality of life measures and neurocognitive function as the secondary objectives.

The role of chemotherapy in the management of patients who have LGG remains to be defined. Although some clinical trials demonstrate a high response rate, this has not yet been shown to have an impact on patient outcome as symptomatic improvement or prolongation of survival. Much of the impetus to develop an effective chemotherapy regimen results from the concern regarding the late toxicities associated with radiotherapy to the brain. Furthermore, caution should be exercised in proceeding with more intensive treatments, such as the concurrent chemotherapy and radiotherapy regimen. Although this treatment has proved superior to radiation alone for patients who have glioblastoma, early reports suggest that the incidence of treatment-related brain injury may be higher than with radiation therapy alone [51,52]. This increased risk for late toxicity may be an important consideration, particularly in patients who have favorable prognosis LGG. The additional studies (described previously) and continued improvements in molecular classification should assist in optimizing treatment of patients who have LGG.

## References

[1] Kleihues P, Cavenee WK, editors. Pathology and genetics of tumours of the nervous system. Lyon (France): IARC Press; 2000.

[2] Vertosick FT Jr, Selker RG, Arena VC. Survival of patients with well-differentiated astrocytomas diagnosed in the era of computed tomography. Neurosurgery 1991;28(4): 496–501.

[3] McCormack BM, Miller DC, Budzilovich GN, et al. Treatment and survival of low-grade astrocytoma in adults–1977–1988. Neurosurgery 1992;31(4):636–42 [discussion: 642].

[4] Henson JW, Gonzalez RG. Neuroimaging in glioma therapy. Expert Rev Neurother 2004; 4(4):665–71.

[5] Cairncross G, Berkey B, Shaw E, et al. A phase III trial of chemotherapy plus radiotherapy (RT) versus RT alone for pure and mixed anaplastic oligodendroglioma (RTOG 9402): an intergroup trial by the RTOG, NCCTG, SWOG, NCIC CTG and ECOG. J Clin Oncol 2006;80:27–35.

[6] van den Bent MJ, Carpentier AF, Brandes AA, et al. Adjuvant PCV improves progression free survival but not overall survival in newly diagnosed anaplastic oligodendrogliomas and oligoastrocytomas: a randomized EORTC phase III trial. J Clin Oncol 2006.

[7] Ohgaki H, Kleihues P. Population-based studies on incidence, survival rates, and genetic alterations in astrocytic and oligodendroglial gliomas. J Neuropathol Exp Neurol 2005; 64(6):479–89.

[8] Jenkins RB, Blair H, Ballman KV, et al. A t(1;19)(q10;p10) mediates the combined deletions of 1p and 19q and predicts a better prognosis of patients with oligodendroglioma. Cancer Res 2006;66(20):9852–61.

[9] Aldape K, Burger PC, Perry A. Clinicopathologic aspects of 1p/19q loss and the diagnosis of oligodendroglioma. Arch Pathol Lab Med 2007;131(2):242–51.

[10] Okamoto Y, Di Patre PL, Burkhard C, et al. Population-based study on incidence, survival rates, and genetic alterations of low-grade diffuse astrocytomas and oligodendrogliomas. Acta Neuropathol (Berl) 2004;108(1):49–56.

[11] Pignatti F, van den Bent M, Curran D, et al. Prognostic factors for survival in adult patients with cerebral low-grade glioma. J Clin Oncol 2002;20(8):2076–84.

[12] Bauman G, Lote K, Larson D, et al. Pretreatment factors predict overall survival for patients with low-grade glioma: a recursive partitioning analysis. Int J Radiat Oncol Biol Phys 1999; 45(4):923–9.

[13] Maiuri F, Del Basso De Caro ML, Iaconetta G, et al. Prognostic and survival-related factors in patients with well-differentiated oligodendrogliomas. Zentralbl Neurochir 2006;67(4): 204–9.

[14] Omuro AM, Leite CC, Mokhtari K, et al. Pitfalls in the diagnosis of brain tumours. Lancet Neurol 2006;5(11):937–48.

[15] Gilbert MR, Supko JG, Batchelor T, et al. Phase I clinical and pharmacokinetic study of irinotecan in adults with recurrent malignant glioma. Clin Cancer Res 2003;9(8): 2940–9.

[16] Newton HB, Goldlust SA, Pearl D. Retrospective analysis of the efficacy and tolerability of levetiracetam in brain tumor patients. J Neurooncol 2006;78(1):99–102.

[17] Glantz MJ, Cole BF, Forsyth PA, et al. Practice parameter: anticonvulsant prophylaxis in patients with newly diagnosed brain tumors. Report of the Quality Standards Subcommittee of the American Academy of Neurology. Neurology 2000;54(10):1886–93.

[18] Lang FF, Olansen NE, DeMonte F, et al. Surgical resection of intrinsic insular tumors: complication avoidance. J Neurosurg 2001;95(4):638–50.

[19] Sawaya R, Hammoud M, Schoppa D, et al. Neurosurgical outcomes in a modern series of 400 craniotomies for treatment of parenchymal tumors. Neurosurgery 1998;42(5):1044–55 [discussion: 1055–6].

[20] Jackson RJ, Fuller GN, Abi-Said D, et al. Limitations of stereotactic biopsy in the initial management of gliomas. Neuro oncol 2001;3(3):193–200.

[21] Hall W, Truwit C. 1.5 T Spectroscopy-supported brain biopsy. Neurosurg Clin N Am 2005; 16:165–72.

[22] Ammirati M, Vick N, Liao YL, et al. Effect of the extent of surgical resection on survival and quality of life in patients with supratentorial glioblastomas and anaplastic astrocytomas. Neurosurgery 1987;21(2):201–6.

[23] Stummer W, Novotny A, Stepp H, et al. Fluorescence-guided resection of glioblastoma multiforme by using 5-aminolevulinic acid-induced porphyrins: a prospective study in 52 consecutive patients. J Neurosurg 2000;93(6):1003–13.

[24] Vuorinen V, Hinkka S, Farkkila M, et al. Debulking or biopsy of malignant glioma in elderly people–a randomised study. Acta Neurochir (Wien) 2003;145(1):5–10.

[25] Janny P, Cure H, Mohr M, et al. Low grade supratentorial astrocytomas. Management and prognostic factors. Cancer 1994;73(7):1937–45.

[26] Leighton C, Fisher B, Bauman G, et al. Supratentorial low-grade glioma in adults: an analysis of prognostic factors and timing of radiation. J Clin Oncol 1997;15(4): 1294–301.

[27] Shibamoto Y, Kitakabu Y, Takahashi M, et al. Supratentorial low-grade astrocytoma. Correlation of computed tomography findings with effect of radiation therapy and prognostic variables. Cancer 1993;72(1):190–5.

[28] Berger MS, Deliganis AV, Dobbins J, et al. The effect of extent of resection on recurrence in patients with low grade cerebral hemisphere gliomas. Cancer 1994;74(6):1784–91.

[29] Claus EB, Horlacher A, Hsu L, et al. Survival rates in patients with low-grade glioma after intraoperative magnetic resonance image guidance. Cancer 2005;103(6):1227–33.

[30] Yeh SA, Ho JT, Lui CC, et al. Treatment outcomes and prognostic factors in patients with supratentorial low-grade gliomas. Br J Radiol 2005;78(927):230–5.

[31] Keles GE, Lamborn KR, Berger MS. Low-grade hemispheric gliomas in adults: a critical review of extent of resection as a factor influencing outcome. J Neurosurg 2001; 95(5):735–45.

[32] Karim AB, Maat B, Hatlevoll R, et al. A randomized trial on dose-response in radiation therapy of low-grade cerebral glioma: European Organization for Research and Treatment of Cancer (EORTC) Study 22844. Int J Radiat Oncol Biol Phys 1996;36(3): 549–56.

[33] Shaw E, Arusell R, Scheithauer B, et al. Prospective randomized trial of low- versus high-dose radiation therapy in adults with supratentorial low-grade glioma: initial report of a North Central Cancer Treatment Group/Radiation Therapy Oncology Group/Eastern Cooperative Oncology Group study. J Clin Oncol 2002;20(9):2267–76.

[34] Karim AB, Afra D, Cornu P, et al. Randomized trial on the efficacy of radiotherapy for cerebral low-grade glioma in the adult: European Organization for Research and Treatment of Cancer Study 22845 with the Medical Research Council study BRO4: an interim analysis. Int J Radiat Oncol Biol Phys 2002;52(2):316–24.

[35] van den Bent MJ, Afra D, de Witte O, et al. Long-term efficacy of early versus delayed radiotherapy for low-grade astrocytoma and oligodendroglioma in adults: the EORTC 22845 randomised trial. Lancet 2005;366(9490):985–90.

[36] Heimans JJ, Taphoorn MJ. Impact of brain tumour treatment on quality of life. J Neurol 2002;249(8):955–60.

[37] Meyers CA, Brown PD. Role and relevance of neurocognitive assessment in clinical trials of patients with CNS tumors. J Clin Oncol 2006;24(8):1305–9.

[38] Armstrong TS, Mendoza TR, Gring I, et al. Validation of the M.D., Anderson Symptom Inventory Brain Tumor Module (MDASI-BT). J Neurooncol 2006; in press.

[39] Shaw EG, Berkey B, Coons SW, et al. Recurrence following neurosurgeon-defined gross total resection of adult supratentorial low-grade glioma. Submitted for publication 2007.

[40] Eyre HJ, Crowley JJ, Townsend JJ, et al. A randomized trial of radiotherapy versus radiotherapy plus CCNU for incompletely resected low-grade gliomas: a Southwest Oncology Group study. J Neurosurg 1993;78(6):909–14.

[41] Buckner JC, Gesme D Jr, O'Fallon JR, et al. Phase II trial of procarbazine, lomustine, and vincristine as initial therapy for patients with low-grade oligodendroglioma or oligoastrocytoma: efficacy and associations with chromosomal abnormalities. J Clin Oncol 2003;21(2): 251–5.

[42] Soffietti R, Ruda R, Bradac GB, et al. PCV chemotherapy for recurrent oligodendrogliomas and oligoastrocytomas. Neurosurgery 1998;43(5):1066–73.

[43] Quinn JA, Reardon DA, Friedman AH, et al. Phase II trial of temozolomide in patients with progressive low-grade glioma. J Clin Oncol 2003;21(4):646–51.

[44] Pace A, Vidiri A, Galie E, et al. Temozolomide chemotherapy for progressive low-grade glioma: clinical benefits and radiological response. Ann Oncol 2003;14(12):1722–6.

[45] van den Bent MJ, Chinot O, Boogerd W, et al. Second-line chemotherapy with temozolomide in recurrent oligodendroglioma after PCV (procarbazine, lomustine and vincristine) chemotherapy: EORTC Brain Tumor Group phase II study 26972. Ann Oncol 2003; 14(4):599–602.

[46] Lang FF, Gilbert MR. Diffusely infiltrative low-grade gliomas in adults. J Clin Oncol 2006; 24(8):1236–45.

[47] Hoang-Xuan K, Capelle L, Kujas M, et al. Temozolomide as initial treatment for adults with low-grade oligodendrogliomas or oligoastrocytomas and correlation with chromosome 1p deletions. J Clin Oncol 2004;22(15):3133–8.

[48] Brada M, Viviers L, Abson C, et al. Phase II study of primary temozolomide chemotherapy in patients with WHO grade II gliomas. Ann Oncol 2003;14(12):1715–21.

[49] Hegi ME, Diserens AC, Gorlia T, et al. MGMT gene silencing and benefit from temozolomide in glioblastoma. N Engl J Med 2005;352(10):997–1003.

[50] Everhard S, Kaloshi G, Criniere E, et al. MGMT methylation: a marker of response to temozolomide in low-grade gliomas. Ann Neurol 2006;60(6):740–3.

[51] Stupp R, Mason WP, van den Bent MJ, et al. Radiotherapy plus concomitant and adjuvant temozolomide for glioblastoma. N Engl J Med 2005;352(10):987–96.

[52] Chamberlain MC, Glantz MJ, Chalmers L, et al. Early necrosis following concurrent Temodar and radiotherapy in patients with glioblastoma. J Neurooncol 2007;82(1): 81–3.

ELSEVIER
SAUNDERS

NEUROLOGIC
CLINICS

Neurol Clin 25 (2007) 1089–1109

# Anaplastic Oligodendroglioma and Oligoastrocytoma

Martin J. van den Bent, MD

*Neuro-Oncology Unit, Daniel den Hoed Cancer Clinic/Erasmus University Medical Center,
PO Box 5201, 3008AE Rotterdam, the Netherlands*

Until approximately 15 years ago, the diagnosis of an oligodendroglioma (OD) was merely as a pathologic entity. The only clinical relevant meaning of this histologic diagnosis was the observation that the prognosis of OD was in general better than that of astrocytic tumors of similar grade. This changed with the recognition of the marked sensitivity to procarbazine, CCNU, and vincristine (PCV) chemotherapy of these tumors, although the best timing of chemotherapy still is unclear [1,2]. A major leap forward was the identification of the combined loss of the short arm of chromosome 1 (1p) and the long arm of chromosome 19 (19q) as the typical genetic lesions of OD, followed by the recognition these 1p/19q codeleted tumors that, in particular, have an excellent response to chemotherapy [3–5]. This 1p/19q codeletion is an early event in the tumorigenesis of OD, mediated by an unbalanced translocation of 19p to 1q:der(1;19)(p10;q10) [6,7]. ODs with this combined loss of 1p/19q not only have a better response to chemotherapy but also have a more indolent clinical behavior and a longer-lasting response to radiotherapy (RT). These observations have led to the current tendency to consider 1p/19q loss low-grade and anaplastic OD (AOD) a separate biologic entity, at least within clinical trials [5,8].

For many years, it has been standard practice to distinguish between low-grade tumors and high-grade tumors. Because low-grade and high-grade tumors carry a different prognosis, this separation is a clinically relevant distinction, but also it is an artificial distinction based on subjective histologic criteria. As a consequence, significant interobserver variation in the grading of OD is the rule. Combined 1p/19q loss low-grade oligodendroglial tumors may have more in common with their anaplastic counterparts than with low-grade astrocytoma. From this perspective, it is questionable if in

*E-mail address:* m.vandenbent@erasmusmc.nl

textbooks low-grade OD should be lumped together with low-grade astrocytoma or with their anaplastic counterparts.

The histologic distinction between pure ODs, mixed oligoastrocytoma, and astrocytoma is subjective, which raises fundamental discussions on the classification of anaplastic oligoastrocytoma (AOA) with necrosis and glioblastoma with oligodendroglial morphology. At present, it is unclear what clinical significance, if any, should be given to the presence of some oligodendroglial elements in these otherwise high-grade astrocytic tumors. Despite ongoing attempts to classify oligodendroglial tumors and grade III glial tumors according to their genetics, the new WHO classification continues to classify these tumors according to their histologic appearance.

## Incidence, clinical presentation, localization

Oligodendroglioma and mixed oligoastrocytoma constitute 5% to 20% of all glial tumors. They predominantly are a tumor of adulthood, with a peak incidence between the fourth and sixth decades of life. Low-grade OD tends to arise in slightly younger patients. Although low-grade OD, in particular, may have a median survival time of more than 10 years, the outcome almost invariably is fatal. Thus, these tumors never should be considered benign.

Most ODs arise in the white matter of cerebral hemispheres, predominantly in the frontal lobes. They can arise, however, throughout the CNS, including infratentorial sites and the spinal cord. Similarly to other astrocytoma, OD tend to remain localized to the CNS. Extra-CNS metastases (especially bone metastases) are described but this is rare and occurs occasionally in patients at later stages of the disease. Leptomeningeal spread is far from rare, but this usually does not develop until the time of recurrence.

The presenting signs and symptoms of OD are unspecific, and depend on the localization and progression of the tumor. They may present with seizures, cognitive deficits, or focal deficits. Low-grade ODs tend to present with seizures, whereas patients who have high-grade tumors often present with focal deficits, increased intracranial pressure or cognitive deficits early in the course of their disease.

## Pathology and genetics

Findings that the majority of ODs are characterized by combined loss of 1p/19q and that this deletion defines a specific subgroup of OD has altered the approach toward these tumors significantly. Table 1 summarizes the differences between tumors with and without combined 1p1/19q loss.

### Histology

Like all diffuse glioma, OD and AOD infiltrate brain tissue diffusely but, in contrast to astrocytoma, areas of remarkable sharp borders with surrounding brain tissue often can be found. The current WHO definition of

Table 1
Clinical, genetic, and radiologic features of oligodendroglioma with and without 1p/19q clodeletion

| | 1p/19q loss | No 1p/19q loss |
|---|---|---|
| Histologic features | In particular, classical oligodendroglial morphology | Presence of astrocytic elements |
| Localization | (Bi)frontal, parietal, occipital | Temporal, deep basal ganglia, diencephalon |
| MRI features | More indistinct borders and mixed signal intensity on T1- and T2-weighted images | Homogeneous T1 and T2 signal intensity, distinct borders |
| Behavior | Often presentation with indolent tumors and seizures only | More rapid clinical progression |
| Enhancement on MRI | Diffuse, patchy | Ring enhancement, necrosis |
| Genetic alterations | 1p/19q loss, in anaplastic tumors p16 deletions | p53 mutations, EGFR amplification, 10 and 10q loss |
| Responsiveness to chemotherapy | 80%–100% of tumors responding, with relatively long duration of response | Less frequent objective response and of shorter duration |
| Median survival in anaplastic tumors | More than 6–7 years | Median 2–3 years |

OD is "a well-differentiated, diffusely infiltrating tumor of adults, typically located in the cerebral hemispheres and composed predominantly of cells morphologically resembling oligodendroglia" [9]. Histologically, low-grade ODs are characterized by uniformly round to oval cells with round nuclei and bland chromatin. The cell density usually is low to moderate. The morphology of these cells often is referred to as the "fried egg appearance" because of a perinuclear halo. A delicate network of branching blood vessels (chicken-wire pattern) also is indicative of low-grade OD. The WHO definition for AOD is "An oligodendroglioma with focal or diffuse histological features of malignancy and a less favorable prognosis" (Fig. 1). Over time, ODs gradually become more anaplastic and evolve from low-grade, "well-differentiated" glioma into high-grade glioma with anaplastic features (high cell density, mitosis, nuclear atypia, microvascular proliferation, and necrosis). Because these morphologic changes that are characteristic of high-grade glioma appear gradually within a glioma, the exact delineation of low- and high-grade oligodendroglioma or AOD is unclear. ODs also may present as anaplastic tumors, without clinically manifest low-grade precursor lesion. No specific immunohistochemical markers for ODs exist. ODs may exhibit sparse glial fibrillary acidic protein (GFAP) staining, which usually is the result of the presence of reactive astrocytes. Occasionally, central neurocytomas, ependymoma, and pilocytic astrocytomas may resemble oligodendroglial tumors.

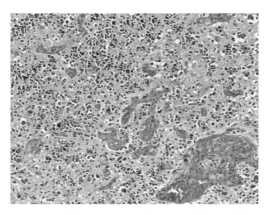

Fig. 1. AOD, with tumor cells with a perinuclear halo, rounded hyperchromatic nuclei, cellular atypia, high cellularity, and extensive endothelial proliferation.

By definition, mixed oligoastrocytoma tumors have morphologic characteristics of astrocytic tumors and pure ODs (Fig. 2). These tumors generally are associated with oligodendroglial foci and gemistocytic astrocytic components mixed within the same region of the tumor. Unlike pure ODs, oligoastrocytomas typically have areas that are GFAP positive. This staining pattern may be the result of the astrocytic component of the tumor but also may be the result of reactive astrocytes. There are no widely accepted histologic criteria as to how much oligodendroglial elements need to be present in a predominantly astrocytic lesion before a tumor may be called oligoastrocytoma. Recent European Organization for Research and Treatment of Cancer (EORTC) and Radiation Therapy Oncology Group

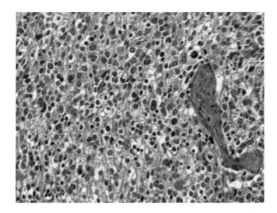

Fig. 2. AOA. Glial tumor with high cellularity, endothelial proliferation, and areas of either cells with rounded nuceli and a perinuclear halo or cells with a predominant astrocytic morphology.

(RTOG) trials used as arbitrary cut-off points the presence of more than 25% oligodendroglial elements, but these scores are subject to interobserver variation [10]. It has been proposed to distinguish between mixed AOA without necrosis and those with necrosis (mixed AOA grade 3 and 4, grade 4 still having a better prognosis compared with GBM) [11]. An ongoing controversy is the existence of glioblastoma with oligodendroglial morphology and how this relates to mixed AOA with necrosis. Many of these tumors have a GBM-like similar clinical behavior and have molecular profiles lesions encountered in GBM. The delineation between these entities and also whether or not that distinction has any clinical significance is unclear. Only a few of those GBMs with OD features and AOA with necrosis have 1p/19q loss, and many have genetic lesions associated with high-grade astrocytic tumors, such as EGFR amplification and 10q loss.

The histologic criteria for distinguishing ODs from astrocytoma also are subjective and prone to interobserver variability. The recognition in the 1990s of the sensitivity to chemotherapy of AOD and AOA resulted in a widening of the histologic criteria for OD, with emphasis on other histologic features, such as microgemistocytes, gliofibrillary oligodendrocytes, and protoplasmic astrocytes [12]. The presence of these features also were considered as suggestive of the tumor being of oligodendroglial origin. These changes in criteria for OD led to in increase of oligodendroglial tumors from approximately 5% of all glial tumors to approximately 20% [12]. With the recognition that combined 1p/19q loss correlates with a favorable clinical outcome and the finding that 1p/19q loss ODs usually are tumors with classical OD morphology, the pendulum is swinging back and pathologists today are less inclined to make the diagnosis of OD in the absence of typical OD features. It would be erroneous, however, to consider only those ODs with 1p/19q loss as true OD.

## Genetics

The most frequent chromosomal lesions in classical OD are the combined allelic losses of 1p and 19q, occurring in 60% to 90% of OD [3,11,13,14]. This combined 1p/19q loss is mediated by an unbalanced translocation of 19p to 1q. Most likely, a centrosomal or pericentrosomal translocation of chromosome 1 and 19 results in two derative chromosomes der(1;19)(p10;q10) and der(1;19)(q10;p10), after which the derative chromosome with the short arm of 1 and the long arm of 19 is lost [6,7]. A possible explanation for this translocation is the strong homology of the centromeric regions of chromosomes 1 and 19, although that by itself does not explain why combined 1p/19q loss is not observed in more cancers. Typically, the loss of 1p/19q is retained at the time of progression, regardless of morphologic changes, emphasizing that 1p/19q loss is an early genetic event [15].

AODs usually have additional chromosomal deletions; in particular, loss of heterozygosity for 9p or deletion of the CDKN2A gene (p16) occurs in

33% to 50% of AOD and deletions on chromosome 10 occur in 19% to 25% of cases [15,16]. Polysomies are more frequent in high-grade tumors [15].

*Genetics and pathology*

Codeletion of 1p/19q is more frequent in oligodendroglial tumors with a classical histologic appearance (perinuclear halo, chicken-wire vascular pattern) compared with tumors with an atypical oligodendroglial appearance [5]. It occurs in 61% to 89% of AOD but in only 14% to 20% in patients who have AOA [11,17]. In mixed oligoastrocytoma with predominant oligodendroglial morphology, the percentage of tumors showing 1p/19q loss already dropped to 39%, emphasizing that even the presence of minor astrocytic elements reduces the chance of finding 1p/19q loss significantly [15]. Still, some atypical ODs have 1p/19q codeletions and some typical OD tumors do not show 1p/19q loss. But, as a rule, in low-grade and in high-grade OD with atypical features, other chromosomal abnormalities are found, which typically are associated with astrocytoma and which usually are mutually exclusive with 1p/19q codeletion (eg, *TP53* mutations, EGFR amplification, 10q loss, and *PTEN* mutations) [15,18–21]. This suggests that these tumors are derived from different precursor cells. It often now is assumed that mixed tumors represent oligodendroglial tumors with 1p/19q loss or tumors with genetic changes consistent with an astrocytic lineage [19].

This hypothesis is supported by the marked differences in outcome and prognosis, with an improved outcome in the presence of 1p/19q loss and with poor survival in AOD with the loss of 10q or the amplification of EFGR [20]. The presence of 10q loss or EGFR amplification in pure AOD is sufficiently rare to suggest an alternate diagnosis (eg, small cell glioblastoma) [15]. AOAs seem to constitute not a fixed class of tumors, rather a continuum between pure OD and astrocytoma.

*Genetics and tumor localization*

1p/19q loss OD tumors often are more localized in the frontal, occipital, and parietal lobe, whereas tumors in the insular region, temporal lobes, and diencephalon are less likely to show 1p/19q loss [17,22,23]. This adds support to the notion that the 1p/19q codeleted tumors are derived from different precursor cells.

**Diagnosis**

On MRI, low-grade ODs show increased signal intensity on T2-weighted images without enhancement (Fig. 3) [24]. On CT, these tumors appear as low-density masses with no enhancement and may exhibit calcifications. The presence of calcification is suggestive (and may be more frequent in 1p/19q loss tumors) but not specific for OD (Fig. 4) [25]. On MRI or CT, most AODs are characterized by enhancement, which is presumed to be

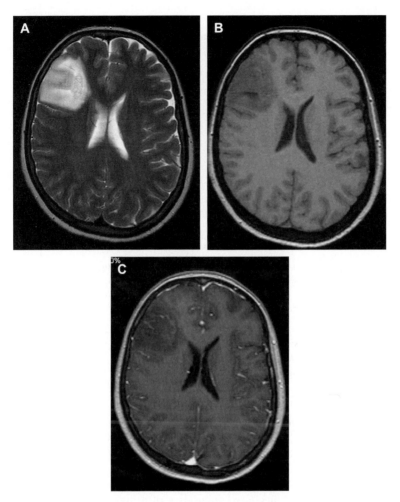

Fig. 3. A 30-year-old female underwent MRI for atypical headache, showing a lesion with distinct borders and high signal intensity on T2-weighted images (*A*), and a low signal intensity on T1-weighted images (*B*) and without contrast enhancement (*C*). The lesion shows some signal heterogeneity on T1 and T2. At surgery a 1p/19q loss low-grade OD was diagnosed.

the macroscopic equivalent of microvascular proliferation. The absence of enhancement, however, does not rule out the possibility of an anaplastic tumor and, vice versa, some contrast enhancement has been observed in low-grade ODs [25]. The pattern of enhancement of 1p/19q codeleted tumors may be different: more patchy and homogeneous, in contrast to ring-like enhancement with necrosis resembling the enhancement typically seen in GBM for tumors without 1p/19q deletion. In addition, 1p/19q loss OD more often seems to have indistinct borders and a mixed signal intensity on T1- and T2-weighted images, in contrast to tumors without 1p/19q codeletion. OD

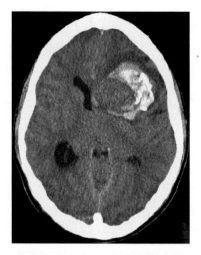

Fig. 4. A 21-year-old man who had a long history of headache developed a sudden onset hemi-plegia. CT scan shows a left frontal hemorrhage, with evidence of calcifications and edema, sug-gestive of a hemorrhage in a tumor. At surgery an anaplastic OD was removed, showing 1p/19q loss.

without 1p/19q loss more often has a distinct border and a uniform signal on T1- and T2-weighted images (see Table 1) [25,26].

None of these imaging findings is specific, however, and for the definitive diagnosis, microscopic examination of tumor tissue remains mandatory (Fig. 5). In view of the significant interobserver variation with respect to the histologic diagnosis of OD, however, this remains a clinical challenge. Moreover, especially in biopsied patients, a sample error easily may lead to the misclassification or undergrading of a brain tumor. For the final di-agnosis and tumor grade, the neuroimaging characteristics, therefore, should be taken into consideration, during which process the presence of en-hancement should be considered suggestive of a high-grade tumor.

For all tumors with oligodendroglial morphology, the assessment of 1p and 19q loss should be considered. This can be done by a variety of tech-niques (fluorescent in situ hybridization, loss of heterozygosity, or compar-ative genome hybridization). Care should be taken that the loss of the entire short arm of chromosome 1 is assessed, and not the partial 1p deletions that are observed mainly in high-grade astrocytic tumors. These partial losses are not associated with 19q loss and carry a poor prognostic significance [27]. In high-grade oligoastrocytomas or in atypical AOD, assessment of EGFR amplification and loss of 10 or 10q can be considered, which may identify tumors with poor prognosis and suggest a different, nonoligodendroglial diagnosis [15,28].

There is no need for routine specific staging procedures (such as craniospi-nal axis imaging of cerebrospinal fluid cytology) in newly diagnosed patients. In patients who have recurrent disease, the presence of leptomeningeal spread

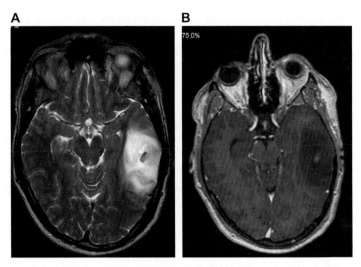

Fig. 5. A 30-year-old man developed seizures, an MRI scan showed a left temporal high T2 signal intensity lesion with somewhat indistinct borders (*A*) and a small enhancing area on T1-weighted images (*B*). At surgery an AOA was found, without 1p/19q loss.

may alter treatment options, and this, therefore, should be taken into account. In the majority of cases, leptomeningeal spread readily is recognized by the presence of distant tumor nodules along the ventricles and so forth. Occasionally, these may not be enhancing, under which circumstances T2-weighted images may be more sensitive for this diagnosis.

## Prognosis

### Histology

Pure oligodendroglial tumors have a better prognosis than astrocytic tumors of the same grade; the prognosis of mixed oligoastrocytoma is in-between these histologies [11]. Most likely, this is the result of underlying genetic lesions (in particular the absence or presence of 1p/19q codeletion [see discussion later]) Despite the relatively favorable clinical prognosis of OD, the outcome ultimately is fatal for virtually all patients.

### Tumor grade

Patients who have low-grade OD (WHO grade II) have a median survival of 10 to 17 years and a 5-year survival rate of approximately 75% [29,30]. Overall survival in patients who have low-grade OD or oligoastrocytoma is longer compared with patients who have low-grade astrocytoma (13 versus 7.5 years, $P = .003$). Patients who have AOD have a substantially worse prognosis, with reported median survivals of 4 to 5 years and a 5-year survival rate of only approximately 40% [31]. The presence of necrosis and endothelial proliferation are poor prognostic factors but this, in particular, may be true for mixed AOA and not for AOD [11]. This subset of mixed AOA and necrosis may have a median survival, which is in the range of GBM [32].

*Genotype*

The presence or absence of combined loss of 1p and 19q is the most important prognostic factor for oligodendroglial tumors [14,33,34]. In one study with limited follow-up, median survival for low-grade OD or oligoastrocytoma was 11.9 years for patients who had 1p/19q codeletion and 10.3 years for patients without the deletion [7]. The median overall survival in anaplastic oligodendroglial tumors without 1p/19q loss is 2 to 3 years but more than 6 to 7 years in tumors with combined 1p and 19q loss. 1p/19q codeleted tumors more likely respond to chemotherapy and have a longer progression-free survival after RT or chemotherapy [34–36]. Furthermore, ODs with 1p/19q loss tend to have a more indolent behavior before initiation of treatment compared with tumors without 1p/19q loss [5,8]. The presence of the unbalanced der(1;19)(p10;q10) translocation may have more prognostic significance that 1p/19q codeletion [7].

*Tumor grade and genetics*

Some evidence exists that the prognostic impact of 1p/19q loss is applicable mainly in tumors with classical AOD morphology but not in oligodendroglial tumors with atypical features or in mixed AOA [11,17]. The presence of other chromosomal aberrations account for these differences in outcome. It also points to a persistent role of classical histology, emphasizing that the proper understanding of the genetics of oligodendroglial tumors requires information on the histology.

*Clinical characteristics*

Clinical prognostic factors are, in particular, the age of patients and the performance status, with elderly patients and patients in a poor condition (functional deficits) doing less well.

**Treatment**

Until recently, most randomized phase III trials of glial tumors included astrocytic and oligodendroglial tumors, the exception being the American and European randomized studies on (neo)adjuvant PCV chemotherapy in anaplastic oligodendroglial tumors [33,34]. Current studies distinguish between patients who have and who do not have 1p/19q loss, but it will take many years before results are available. All data on RT in anaplastic oligodendroglial tumors are derived from retrospective surveys, with inherent pitfalls. Many prospective but uncontrolled single arm studies on chemotherapy in recurrent oligodendroglial tumors are available, mostly on PCV and temozolomide (TMZ) chemotherapy.

*The wait-and-see policy in low-grade oligodendroglial tumors*

The best treatment policy for young patients who have presumed low-grade gliomas, including ODs presenting with seizures only, constitutes an ongoing controversy. As many of these patients may remain stable for a protracted period of time without any treatment, many physicians tend to defer treatment until clinical or radiologic progression. Many of these patients harbor low-grade OD. Advocates of early treatment point to the possibility of an anaplastic lesion that is observed in up to 30% of patients who have unenhancing low-grade glioma-like lesions. They recommend, therefore, always obtaining histologic proof of the nature of the lesion [37]. There is general consensus that patients who have enhancing lesions, lesions with mass effect, focal signs, or symptoms or signs of increased intracranial pressure require treatment without further delay.

An important rationale for the deferral of RT is the concern for late RT-induced cognitive decline. The contribution of RT to delayed cognitive deficits is an unresolved issue, however, with many opinions but limited data. A case-control study has shown that having a brain tumor and the use of antiepileptic drugs are associated to cognitive deficits in patients who have low-grade glioma, whereas the role of RT in the pathogenesis of these deficits is less clear [38,39].

**Surgery**

Surgery serves three goals: verification of the nature of the lesion, relief of signs and symptoms in patients suffering from a lesion with mass effect, and improvement of the prognosis. The relevance of the first two generally are acknowledged, but so far no trial has given evidence beyond reasonable doubt that extensive surgery improves survival compared with less extensive resections. All available data on extent of resection in oligodendroglial tumors come from retrospective studies or from post-hoc analyses. A drawback of those uncontrolled studies is that superficial and small tumors are more likely to undergo an extensive resection. In contrast, deep-seated lesions, large tumors, or tumors with involvement of midline structures, which may hold a worse prognosis regardless of the extent of resection, never will undergo near-complete resections [40].

One uncontrolled study found that complete resection in low-grade OD is associated with long disease-free intervals [41]. Both randomized studies on PCV chemotherapy in anaplastic oligodendroglial tumors observed an association between extent of resection and survival [33,34]. In view of these and similar studies, it is considered standard treatment to resect a tumor as extensively and as safely as possible whenever it is decided to start treatment. In young patients who have seizures only and a low-grade OD, having undergone an extensive resection, a wait-and-see policy with further treatment at the time of progression can be followed (especially in the presence of 1p/19q loss). In patients who have focal deficits, with lesions with mass effect or with anaplastic tumors, further adjuvant treatment (RT or chemotherapy) is recommended.

### Radiotherapy

No prospective randomized trials on the role of RT in OD or AOD are available.

#### Low-grade oligodendroglioma

RT induces clear responses in low-grade glioma [42]. A large study of early versus delayed RT in patients who had low-grade glioma observed an improved progression-free survival after early RT but no increase in overall survival [43]. No histology-based subgroup analysis of this study is available. Until controlled, randomized studies are conducted, a prudent approach in young patients who have low-grade OD and who have undergone a complete or almost complete resection in good clinical condition may be to observe the patients and withhold RT until progression. In contrast, patients who have large, unresectable, or incompletely resected tumors; focal deficits; anaplastic tumors; or enhancing lesions should be treated, including RT, without delay. For low-grade gliomas, 50- to 54 Gy-RT in fractions of 1.8 Gy should be given; a higher cumulative dosage does not improve outcome and may increase toxicity [42,44].

### Anaplastic oligodendroglioma and anaplastic oligoastrocytoma

Randomized trials in high-grade gliomas have demonstrated that adjuvant RT provides significant yet modest improvements in survival [45]. No trial specifically addresses RT in AOD. In high-grade OD, 60 to 65 Gy in 30 to 35 fractions should be given. Some retrospective studies support postoperative RT in patients who have OD [46,47]. Others found survival benefit of RT in patients who have OD, mainly in the subgroup of patients who have neurologic deficit or for whom surgery was limited to biopsy or partial surgery. Other studies report no benefit of postoperative RT in the treatment of OD [30,48–50]. AODs with 1p/19q loss have a superior outcome after RT compared with those without 1p/19q loss.

### Chemotherapy

#### MGMT gene and alkyltransfease

The responsiveness of AOD to chemotherapy was established in trials of recurrent tumors. The initial studies investigated the PCV regimen, with more recent studies focusing on TMZ. No clear explanation is available yet for the favorable response of AOD compared with astrocytic tumors. There are indications that the nuclear enzyme, alkyltransferase, which mediates at least a part of the cell resistance to alkylating and methylating agents, is expressed less in OD and perhaps even more so in 1p/19q codeleted tumors [51]. MGMT expression can be silenced by *MGMT* promoter gene methylation, which was reported in 47% of low-grade OD, without a correlation with 1p/19q codeletion [52]. Other studies did find a correlation between 1p/19q codeletion and *MGMT* promoter methylation, which was observed in up to 80% to 90% of 1p/19q codeleted tumors [53–55]. *MGMT* promoter gene methylation occurs in only 50% of GBM; most likely, this event alone does not account for the entire difference in sensitivity to chemotherapy between astrocytic tumors and OD or the increased sensitivity in 1p/19q loss tumors.

### The procarbazine, CCNU, and vincristine schedule

Cairncross and McDonald were the first to demonstrate the sensitivity of AOD to chemotherapy. They observed favorable responses in recurrent AOD treated with chemotherapy consisting of PCV chemotherapy. Approximately two thirds of patients who have recurrent AOD after prior RT have either a complete response (CR) or partial response (PR) to PCV chemotherapy. The time to progression in these patients is in general 12 to 18 months but occasionally much longer than 24 months [1,2,56]. Because of the cumulative hematologic toxicity and gastrointestinal side effects associated with PCV chemotherapy, most patients do not tolerate the six cycles, which usually are intended. The intensified PCV-I regimen seems to be of similar activity but was found considerably more toxic (especially hematologic and general side effects, including malaise and weight loss) [2,57]. In the absence of better results, this regimen cannot be recommended. Several studies suggest that AO may be less responsive, most likely related to the low frequency of combined 1p/19q loss in OA.

### Temozolomide

The reported response rate of recurrent OD after failure to RT to first-line TMZ varied between 46% and 55%, with 12 months' progression-free survival between 40% and 50% and median progression-free survival of 10 to 12 months [55,58]. Objective responses are more frequent and of longer duration in patients who have combined 1p/19q loss, with 60% to 82% of tumors responding [59]. These response rates seem modest compared with historic PCV trials, in which virtually all patients who had 1p/19q loss responded [4,5].

### Which regimen to prefer?

No formal comparison between PCV and TMZ in recurrent OD is available. A major advantage of TMZ is the good tolerability, with, in general, modest myelosuppression and usually easily controlled nausea and vomiting as its major side effects. In this respect, TMZ compares favorably to the PCV regimen, and TMZ constitutes a clear alternative for the PCV regimen. The better tolerability and the ease of administration of TMZ compared with PCV has made TMZ the drug of first choice for most institutions.

*Second-line treatment with procarbazine, CCNU, and vincristine or temozolomide*

Most trials of recurrent OD after prior chemotherapy with PCV (either given adjuvant or at first recurrence) observed objective response rates (PR and CR) of approximately 25%, with 30% to 50% and 10% to 30% of patients free from progression at 6 and 12 months, respectively [58,60,61]. A fourth trial predominantly selected patients who had responded favorably to PCV (response rate to first-line PCV: 83%) [62]. In this trial, the objective response rate to TMZ was 44%, with 50% and 25% of patients free from progression at 6 and 12 months. Second-line PCV after failure to TMZ included a response in only 17%; still, 50% of patients were free from progression at 6 months (and 21% at 12 months) [63]. Occasionally, patients who do not respond to the one regimen are responsive to the other. The relatively poor response rates, however, even in 1p/19q loss OD to second-line chemotherapy (and regardless of the sequence chosen, TMZ first or PCV first), shows that for further improvement of outcome other therapies needs to be developed.

*Other agents*

Only a few other agents (in particular, paclitaxel, CPT-11, carboplatin, and etoposide plus cisplatin) have been investigated for second-line chemotherapy in patients who have AOD. Except for the small numbers investigated with cisplatin and etoposide, with 4 of 10 patients responding, the response rates are low (in the 10% to 15% range), with one third of patients free from progression at 6 months and virtually all patients progressing at 12 months. A drawback of some of these agents (paclitaxel and CPT-11) is their metabolization through the CYP3A4 cytochrome, which implies that their metabolism may have been induced by enzyme-inducing antiepileptic agents. This enzyme induction limits the role in glial tumors of these and other cytotoxic agents metabolized through the CYP 3A4 pathway (but also may have affected the observed activity in the trials discussed previously). One trial of PCV chemotherapy followed by an autologous bone marrow transplantation after a myeloablative procedure with melphalan proved too toxic, without clearly producing superior results. Despite the upregulation of platelet-derived growth factor (PDGF), signaling pathways in most ODs, the PDGF-receptor tyrosine kinase inhibitor, imatinib, did not show any activity in recurrent OD or AOD/AOA [64].

*Adjuvant chemotherapy in newly diagnosed anaplastic oligoastrocytoma and anaplastic oligodendroglioma*

The two prospective randomized controlled trials in anaplastic oligodendroglial tumors have shown that compared with PCV given at the time or recurrence, (neo)adjuvant PCV chemotherapy does not increase overall survival, although it does increase progression-free survival (Table 2). The first of these trials, RTOG 94-02, randomized patients to either four cycles of upfront intensified PCV chemotherapy followed by RT to a dose of 60 Gy or to RT only [33]. The second trial (EORTC 26951) randomized patients to 60 Gy RT followed by six cycles adjuvant PCV or to 60 Gy RT only [34]. Table 2 summarizes progression-free survival and overall survival in these studies. In both trials, the majority of patients randomized to the RT arm received PCV at progression, which most likely explains the increased progression-free survival without increased overall survival. Because of this, these trials investigated early (adjuvant) versus delayed (at the time of progression) PCV chemotherapy. Even in the 1p/19q loss subgroup analysis, no overall survival benefit of early (either adjuvant or neoadjuvant) PCV could be demonstrated. Table 2 summarizes the outcome in patients who had and who did not have combined 1p/19q loss in both trials.

This finding is somewhat contradictory to the observed survival benefit after combined chemoirradation with TMZ in GBM, especially in tumors with a methylated *MGMT* gene promoter [65,66]. The current clinical question is whether or not this treatment also should be used for AOD and AOA. A particular element here is that anaplastic tumors with combined

Table 2
Median survival and 5-year overall survival (%) according to combined 1p/19q loss status in European Organization for Research and Treatment of Cancer 26,951 and Radiation Therapy Oncology Group 9402, on (neo)adjuvant procarbazine, CCNU, and vincristine chemotherapy in anaplastic oligodendroglial tumors

| | Overall survival | | | |
|---|---|---|---|---|
| | Median (months) | | 5 year (%) | |
| Chromosomal loss | RT/PCV | RT | RT/PCV | RT |
| Combined 1p/19q loss | | | | |
| EORTC | NR | NR | 74 [57, 85] | 75 [55, 87] |
| RTOG | NR | NR (5.4, NA) | 72 [54, 83] | 66 [50, 78] |
| No combined 1p/19q loss | | | | |
| EORTC | 25.2 [18.9, 42.6] | 21.4 [17.6, 30.0] | 34 [24, 43] | 28 [19, 36] |
| RTOG | 2.7 [2.0, 5.5] | 2.8 [1.9, 4.4] | 37 [24, 50] | 31 [19, 45] |

Between brackets: 95% CI.
*Data from* Cairncross JG, Berkey B, Shaw E, et al. Phase III trial of chemotherapy plus radiotherapy (RT) versus RT alone for pure and mixed anaplastic oligodendroglioma (RTOG 9402): an intergroup trial by the RTOG, NCCTG, SWOG, NCI CTG and ECOG. J Clin Oncol 2006;24:2707–14; and van den Bent MJ, Carpentier AF, Brandes AA, et al. Adjuvant PCV improves progression free survival but not overall survival in newly diagnosed anaplastic oligodendrogliomas and oligoastrocytomas: a randomized EORTC phase III trial. J Clin Oncol 2006;24:2715–22.

1p/19q loss have a medium survival over 6 to 7 years; hence, late neurotoxicities of a combined radiochemotherapy approach potentially is an issue. This clearly is less so for tumors without 1p/19q loss, but here the benefit of the combined regimen also is not proved. Current studies are investigating the role of combined chemoirradiation in anaplastic oligodendroglial tumors, with separate trials for tumors with and without combined 1p/19q loss. In view of the outcome of the PCV trials, the relevance of any adjuvant chemotherapy given after the end of RT is at least unclear.

*Upfront chemotherapy in newly diagnosed anaplastic oligodendroglioma*

The chemosensitivity of OD has made upfront chemotherapy strategies (with or without subsequent RT) increasingly popular. The major rationale for upfront chemotherapy is the wish to defer RT. A few medium-sized and uncontrolled studies are available, in particular using TMZ. One showed, in a young population (median age 42 years of age) and 81% of patients having a Karnofsky Performance Status score of 90/100, a median progression-free survival of 27 months with a 1-week on/1-week off regimen [67]. A small trial of upfront TMZ chemotherapy also shows a short time to progression (8 months) in patients who did not have 1p loss, in contrast to all seven patients who had 1p loss who were still free from progression at 24 months [68]. In a phase 2 trial of 69 patients who had newly diagnosed anaplastic or aggressive OD, the intensive PCV regimen was followed by high-dose thiotepa with autologous stem cell rescue, without RT. The median progression-free survival in the 39 patients who received the autologous stem cell procedure is 78 months, and median overall survival has not been reached. Eighteen patients (46%) have relapsed [69]. In view of the patient selection and the absence of a control arm, final conclusions are difficult to draw, and many patients who have AOD have similar survival without such intensive treatments. The trial shows, however, that prolonged progression-free survival without initial RT is possible.

In the North American randomized study of neoadjuvant PCV, progression-free survival of upfront chemotherapy followed by RT for non–1p/19q codeleted tumors was similar to treatment with RT only [33]. It is tempting to speculate that the limited sensitivity to PCV chemotherapy of tumors without combined 1p/19q loss explains the absence of benefit in terms of progression-free survival. Advocates of upfront chemotherapy strategies should realize that historical trials have shown the superior efficacy of RT compared with chemotherapy in malignant glioma [45,70]. Although the upfront chemotherapy approach may be appealing, in the absence of randomized trials, the clinical benefits of this approach are not defined. The clinical significance of the adverse effects of focal RT have not been demonstrated in larger prospective trials, and the choice for chemotherapy or RT may come down to exchanging local side effects of a short series of RT for systemic side effects of (expensive) chemotherapy of 1-year's duration. It seems prudent to limit upfront chemotherapy with deferred RT to patients who have 1p/19q code-leted tumors. It also is unclear whether or not, in the presence of a favorable response to upfront chemotherapy, RT should be withheld.

### Upfront chemotherapy in low-grade oligodendroglioma

The clinical data on the use of chemotherapy in low-grade OD are lim-ited, but they suggest these tumors are as sensitive as their anaplastic coun-terparts [57,71]. One issue is that the neuroradiologic response often is less spectacular than in anaplastic tumors, because these tumors are nonenhanc-ing. Often, only a stabilization of disease is observed, with some decrease in mass effect and an improved seizure control. The PCV schedule and TMZ are effective [72–75]. Evidence suggests that 1p/19q codeleted tumors re-spond better longer [73,75]. Even tumors without loss of 1p/19q and mixed oligoastrocytoma may respond. Especially in large OD lesions (oligo-dendroglial "gliomatosis cerebri"), this may be considered in an individual-ized manner to avoid whole-brain RT in patients who have a favorable prognosis for long-term, disease-free survival. Whether or not this also is useful in patients who have smaller lesions and are candidates for RT with limited fields may be more a matter of side effects. It is at least ques-tionable whether or not it is rational to try to avoid limited-field RT of small brain lesions delivered by modern irradiation techniques by replacement with prolonged systemic chemotherapy. An ongoing EORTC trial compares involved-field RT to a continuous low-dose schedule TMZ in newly diag-nosed low-grade glioma, including low-grade OD.

### References

[1] Cairncross G, Macdonald D, Ludwin S, et al. Chemotherapy for anaplastic oligodendro-glioma. J Clin Oncol 1994;12:2013–21.

[2] van den Bent MJ, Kros JM, Heimans JJ, et al. Response rate and prognostic factors of re-current oligodendroglioma treated with procarbazine, CCNU and vincristine chemother-apy. Neurology 1998;51:1140–5.

[3] Smith JS, Alderete B, Minn Y, et al. Localization of common deletion regions on 1p and 19q in human gliomas and their association with histological subtype. Oncogene 1999;18:4144–52.

[4] Cairncross JG, Ueki K, Zlatescu MC, et al. Specific genetic predictors of chemotherapeutic response and survival in patients with anaplastic oligodendrogliomas. J Natl Cancer Inst 1998;90:1473–9.

[5] van den Bent MJ, Looijenga LHJ, Langenberg K, et al. Chromosomal anomalies in oligo-dendroglial tumors are correlated with clinical features. Cancer 2003;97:1276–84.

[6] Griffin CA, Burger P, Morsberger L, et al. Identification of der(1;19)(q10;p10) in five oligo-dendrogliomas suggests mechanism of concurrent 1p and 19q loss. J Neuropathol Exp Neurol 2006;65(10):988–94.

[7] Jenkins RB, Blair H, Ballman KV, et al. A t(1;19)(q10;p10) mediates the combined deletions of 1p and 19q and predicts a better prognosis of patients with oligodendroglioma. Cancer Res 2006;66(20):9852–61.

[8] Walker C, du Plessis DG, Joyce KA, et al. Molecular pathology and clinical characteristics of oligodendroglial neoplasms. Ann Neurol 2005;57(6):855–65.

[9] Reifenberger G, Kros JM, Burger P, et al. Oligodendroglioma. In: Kleihues P, Cavenee WK, editors. World Health Organization classification of tumours. Pathology and genetics of tumours of the nervous system. Lyon (MI): IARC Press; 2000. p. 55–70.

[10] Krouwer HGJ, van Duinen SG, Kamphorst W, et al. Oligoastrocytomas: a clinicopathological study of 52 cases. J Neurooncol 1997;33:223–38.

[11] Miller CR, Dunham CP, Scheithauer BW, et al. Significance of necrosis in grading of oligodendroglial neoplasms: a clinicopathologic and genetic study of newly diagnosed high-grade gliomas. J Clin Oncol 2006;24(34):5419–26.

[12] Coons SW, Johnson PC, Scheithauer BW, et al. Improving diagnostic accuracy and interobserver concordance in the classification and grading of primary gliomas. Cancer 1997;79: 1381–91.

[13] Reifenberger J, Reifenberger G, Liu L, et al. Molecular genetic analsysis of oligodendroglial tumors shows preferential allelic deletions on 19q and 1p. Am J Pathol 1994;145:1175–90.

[14] Smith JS, Perry A, Borell TJ, et al. Alterations of chromosome arms 1p and 19q as predictors of survival in oligodendrogliomas, astrocytoma, and mixed oligoastrocytomas. J Clin Oncol 2000;18:636–45.

[15] Fallon KB, Palmer CA, Roth KA, et al. Prognostic value of 1p, 19q, 9p, 10q, and EGFR-FISH analyses in recurrent oligodendrogliomas. J Neuropathol Exp Neurol 2004;63(4): 314–22.

[16] Bigner SH, Matthews MR, Rasheed BKA, et al. Molecular genetic aspects of oligodendrogliomas including analysis by comparative genomic hybridization. Am J Pathol 1999;155: 375–86.

[17] McDonald JM, See SJ, Tremont IW, et al. The prognostic impact of histology and 1p/19q status in anaplastic oligodendroglial tumors. Cancer 2005;104(7):1468–77.

[18] Sasaki H, Zlatescu MC, Betensky RA, et al. Histopathological-molecular genetic correlations in referral pathologist-diagnosed low-grade "oligodendroglioma". J Neuropathol Exp Neurol 2002;61:58–63.

[19] Maintz D, Fiedler K, Koopmann J, et al. Molecular genetic evidence for subtypes of oligoastrocytomas. J Neuropathol Exp Neurol 1997;56:1098–104.

[20] Hoang-Xuan K, Huguet S, Mokhtari K, et al. Molecular heterogeneity of oligodendrogliomas suggests alternative pathways in tumor progression. Neurology 2002;57:1278–81.

[21] Jeuken JWM, Sprenger SHE, Wesseling P, et al. Identification of subgroups of high-grade oligodendroglial tumors by comparative genomic hybridization. J Neuropathol Exp Neurol 1999;58:606–12.

[22] Zlatescu MC, Tehrani Yazdi A, Sasaki H, et al. Tumor location and growth pattern correlate with genetic signature in oligodendroglial neoplasms. Cancer Res 2001;18:6713–5.

[23] Mueller W, Hartmann C, Hoffmann A, et al. Genetic signature of oligoastrocytomas correlates with tumor location and denotes distinct molecular subsets. Am J Pathol 2002;161: 313–9.

[24] Lee Y, van Tassel P. Intracranial oligodendrogliomas: imaging findings in 35 untreated cases. AJR Am J Roentgenol 1989;152:361–9.

[25] Jenkinson MD, du Plessis DG, Smith TS, et al. Histological growth patterns and genotype in oligodendroglial tumours: correlation with MRI features. Brain 2006;129(Pt 7):1884–91.

[26] Megyesi JF, Kachur E, Lee DH, et al. Imaging correlates of molecular signatures in oligodendroglioma. Clin Cancer Res 2004;10:4303–6.

[27] Idbaih A, Marie Y, Pierron G, et al. Two types of chromosome 1p losses with opposite significance in gliomas. Ann Neurol 2005;58(3):483–7.

[28] Dehais C, Laigle-Donadey F, Marie Y, et al. Prognostic stratification of patients with anaplastic gliomas according to genetic profile. Cancer 2006;107(8):1891–7.

[29] Leighton C, Fisher B, Bauman G, et al. Supratentorial low-grade glioma in adults: an analysis of prognostic factors and the timing of radiation. J Clin Oncol 1997;15:1294–301.

[30] Shaw EG, Scheithauer BW, O'Fallon JR, et al. Oligodendrogliomas: the Mayo Clinic experience. J Neurosurg 1992;76:428–34.

[31] Shaw EG, Scheithauer BW, O'Fallon JR. Supratentorial gliomas: a comparative study by grade and histologic type. J Neurooncol 1997;31:273–8.

[32] Kros JM, Troost D, Van Eden CG, et al. Oligodendroglioma: a comparison of two grading systems. Cancer 1988;61:2251–9.

[33] Cairncross JG, Berkey B, Shaw E, et al. Phase III trial of chemotherapy plus radiotherapy (RT) versus RT alone for pure and mixed anaplastic oligodendroglioma (RTOG 9402): an intergroup trial by the RTOG, NCCTG, SWOG, NCI CTG and ECOG. J Clin Oncol 2006;24:2707–14.

[34] van den Bent MJ, Carpentier AF, Brandes AA, et al. Adjuvant PCV improves progression free survival but not overall survival in newly diagnosed anaplastic oligodendrogliomas and oligoastrocytomas: a randomized EORTC phase III trial. J Clin Oncol 2006;24:2715–22.

[35] Ino Y, Betensky RA, Zlatescu MC, et al. Molecular subtypes of anaplastic oligodendroglioma: implications for patient management at diagnosis. Clin Cancer Res 2001;7:839–45.

[36] van den Bent MJ, Chinot O-L, Cairncross JG. Recent developments in the molecular characterization and treatment of oligodendroglial tumors. Neuro Oncol 2003;5:128–38.

[37] Barker FG, Chang CH, Huhn SL, et al. Age and the risk of anaplasia in magnetic resonance-nonenhancing supratentorial cerebral tumors. Cancer 1997;80:936–41.

[38] Klein M, Heimans JJ, Aaronson NK, et al. Effect of radiotherapy and other treatment-related fators on mid-term to long-term cognitive sequelae in low grade gliomas: a comparative study. Lancet 2002;360:1361–8.

[39] Klein M, Fagel S, Taphoorn MJB, et al. Neurocognitive functioning in long-term low-grade glioma survivors: a six year follow-up study [(abstract # O27)Abs]. Neuro-Oncology 2006; 8:302.

[40] Pignatti F, van den Bent MJ, Curran D, et al. Prognostic factors for survival in adult patients with cerebral low-grade glioma. J Clin Oncol 2002;20:2076–84.

[41] Berger MS, Deliganis AV, Dobbins J, et al. The effect of extent of resection on recurrence in patients with low grade cerebral hemisphere gliomas. Cancer 1994;74:1784–91.

[42] Shaw E, Arusell RM, Scheithauer B, et al. A prospective randomized trial of low versus high dose radiation in adults with a supratentorial low grade glioma: initial report of a NCCTG-RTOG-ECOG study. J Clin Oncol 2002;20:2267–76.

[43] van den Bent MJ, Afra D, De Witte O, et al. Long term results of EORTC study 22845: a randomized trial on the efficacy of early versus delayed radiation therapy of low-grade astrocytoma and oligodendroglioma in the adult. Lancet 2005;366:985–90.

[44] Karim ABMF, Maat B, Hatlevoll R, et al. A randomized trial on dose-response in radiation therapy of low grade cerebral glioma: European organization for research and treatment of cancer (EORTC) study 2284. Int J Radiat Oncol Biol Phys 1996;36:549–56.

[45] Walker MD, Alexander E, Hunt WE, et al. Evaluation of BCNU and/or radiotherapy in the treatment of anaplastic gliomas. A cooperative clinical trial. J Neurosurg 1978;49: 333–43.

[46] Gannett DE, Wisbeck WM, Silbergeld DL, et al. The role of postoperative irradiation in the treatment of oligodendroglioma. Int J Radiat Oncol Biol Phys 1994;30:567–73.

[47] Wallner KE, Gonzales M, Sheline GE. Treatment of oligodendrogliomas with or without postoperative irradiation. J Neurosurg 1988;68:684–8.

[48] Celli P, Nofrone I, Palma L, et al. Cerebral oligodendroglioma: prognostic factors and life history. Neurosurgery 1994;35:1018–35.

[49] Bullard DE, Rawlings CE III, Philllips B, et al. Oligodendroglioma. An analysis of the value of radiation therapy. Cancer 1987;60:2179–88.

[50] Nijjar TS, Simpson WJ, Gadalla T, et al. Oligodendroglioma. The princess margaret hospital experience (1958–1984). Cancer 1993;71:4002–6.

[51] Nutt CL, Costello JF, Bambrick LL, et al. O6 methylguanine-DNA methyltransferase in tumors and cells of the oligodendrocyte lineage. Can J Neurol Sci 1995;22:111–5.

[52] Watanabe T, Nakamura M, Kros JM, et al. Phenotype versus genotype correlation in oligodendrogliomas and low-grade diffuse astrocytomas. Acta Neuropathol 2002;103:267–75.

[53] Dong SM, Pang JC, Poon WS, et al. Concurrent hypermethylation of multiple genes is associated with grade of oligodendroglial tumors. J Neuropathol Exp Neurol 2001;60(8): 808–16.

[54] Möllemann M, Wolter M, Felsberg J, et al. Frequent promotor hypermethylation and low expression of the MGMT gene in oligodendroglial tumors. Int J Cancer 2004;113:379–85.

[55] Brandes AA, Tosoni A, Cavallo G, et al. Correlations between O6-methylguanine DNA methyltransferase promoter methylation status, 1p and 19q deletions, and response to temozolomide in anaplastic and recurrent oligodendroglioma: a prospective GICNO study. J Clin Oncol 2006;24(29):4746–53.

[56] Soffietti R, Ruda R, Bradac GB, et al. PCV chemotherapy for recurrent oligodendrogliomas and oligoastrocytomas. Neurosurgery 1998;43:1066–73.

[57] Mason WP, Krol GS, DeAngelis LM. Low-grade oligodendroglioma responds to chemotherapy. Neurology 1996;46:203–7.

[58] van den Bent MJ, Taphoorn MJ, Brandes AA, et al. Phase II study of first-line chemotherapy with temozolomide in recurrent oligodendroglioma: the European Organisation of Research and Treatment of Cancer Brain Tumor Group study 26971. J Clin Oncol 2003;21:2525–8.

[59] Kouwenhoven MC, Kros JM, French PJ, et al. 1p/19q loss within oligodendroglioma is predictive for response to first line temozolomide but not to salvage treatment. Eur J Cancer 2006;42(15):2499–503.

[60] van den Bent MJ, Keime-Guibert F, Brandes AA, et al. Temozolomide chemotherapy in recurrent oligodendroglioma. Neurology 2001;57:340–2.

[61] Constanza A, Borgogne M, Nobile M, et al. Temozolomide in recurrent oligodendroglioma: a phase II study [S66Abs]. Neuro-Oncology 2001;3.

[62] Chinot O, Honore S, Dufour H, et al. Safety and efficacy of temozolomide in patients with recurrent anaplastic oligodendrogliomas after standard radiotherapy and chemotherapy. J Clin Oncol 2001;19:2449–55.

[63] Triebels V, Taphoorn MJB, Brandes AA, et al. Response to 2nd line PCV chemotherapy in recurrent oligodendroglioma after 1st line temozolomide. Neurology 2004;63:904–6.

[64] van den Bent MJ, Brandes AA, van Oosterom AT, et al. Multicentre phase II study of imatinib mesylate (Gleevec) in patients with recurrent glioblastoma: an EORTC NDDG/BTG intergroup study [(abstract # TA-57)Abs]. Neuro-Oncology 2004;6:383.

[65] Stupp R, Mason WP, van den Bent MJ, et al. Radiotherapy plus concomitant and adjuvant temozolomide for glioblastoma. N Engl J Med 2005;352:987–96.

[66] Hegi ME, Diserens A-C, Gorlia T, et al. MGMT gene silencing and benefit from temozolomide in glioblastoma. N Engl J Med 2005;352:997–1003.

[67] Peereboom D, Brewer C, Schiff D, et al. Dose-intense temozolomide in patients with newly diagnosed pure and mixed anaplastic oligodendroglioma: a phase II multicenter study [(abstract #TA-40)Abs]. Neuro-Oncology 2006;8:448.

[68] Taliansky-Aronov A, Bokstein F, Lavon I, et al. Temozolomide treatment for newly diagnosed anaplastic oligodendrogliomas: a clinical efficacy trial. J Neurooncol 2006;79(2): 153–7.

[69] Abrey LE, Childs BH, Paleologos N, et al. High-dose chemotherapy with stem cell rescue as initial therapy for anaplastic oligodendroglioma: long-term follow-up. Neuro Oncol 2006; 8(2):183–8.

[70] Walker MD, Green SB, Byar DP, et al. Randomized comparisons of radiotherapy and nitrosoureas for the treatment of malignant glioma after surgery. N Engl J Med 1980;303:1323–9.

[71] Mason WP, DeAngelis LM. Procarbazine, CCNU, vincristine (PCV) chemotherapy (CT) for benign oligodendroglioma [abstract]. Neurology 1994;44:A262–3.

[72] Brada M, Viviers L, Abson C, et al. Phase II study of primary temozolomide chemotherapy in patients with WHO grade II gliomas. Ann Oncol 2003;14:1715–21.

[73] Hoang-Xuan K, Capelle L, kujas M, et al. Temozolomide as initial treatment for adults with low-grade oligodendrogliomas or oligoastrocytomas and correlation with chromosome 1p deletions. J Clin Oncol 2004;22:3133–8.

[74] Buckner JC, Gesme D, O'Fallon JR, et al. Phase II trial of procarbazine, lomustine, and vincristine as initial therapy for patients with low-grade oligodendroglioma or oligoastrocytoma: efficacy and and associations with chromosomal abnormalities. J Clin Oncol 2003; 21:251–5.

[75] Biemond-ter Stege E, Kros JM, de Bruin HG, et al. Treatment of low grade oligodendroglial tumors with PCV chemotherapy. Cancer 2005;103:802–9.

ELSEVIER
SAUNDERS

Neurol Clin 25 (2007) 1111–1139

NEUROLOGIC
CLINICS

# Diagnosis and Treatment of High-Grade Astrocytoma

Sith Sathornsumetee, MD[a,b,c],
Jeremy N. Rich, MD[d,e,f,g,h], David A. Reardon, MD[e,i,]*

[a]Division of Neurology, The Preston Robert Tisch Brain Tumor Center,
Duke University Medical Center, DUMC 3624, Durham, NC 27710, USA
[b]Division of Neurosurgery, The Preston Robert Tisch Brain Tumor Center,
Duke University Medical Center, DUMC 3624, Durham, NC 27710, USA
[c]Division of Neurology, Department of Medicine, Faculty of Medicine at Siriraj Hospital,
Mahidol University, 10700 Bangkok, Thailand
[d]Department of Medicine, The Preston Robert Tisch Brain Tumor Center,
Duke University Medical Center, DUMC 2900, Durham, NC 27710, USA
[e]Department of Surgery, The Preston Robert Tisch Brain Tumor Center,
Duke University Medical Center, DUMC 2900, Durham, NC 27710, USA
[f]Department of Neurobiology, The Preston Robert Tisch Brain Tumor Center,
Duke University Medical Center, DUMC 2900, Durham, NC 27710, USA
[g]Department of Pharmacology, The Preston Robert Tisch Brain Tumor Center,
Duke University Medical Center, DUMC 2900, Durham, NC 27710, USA
[h]Department of Cancer Biology, The Preston Robert Tisch Brain Tumor Center,
Duke University Medical Center, DUMC 2900, Durham, NC 27710, USA
[i]Department of Pediatrics, The Preston Robert Tisch Brain Tumor Center,
Duke University Medical Center, DUMC 3624, Durham, NC 27710, USA

An estimated 18,500 cases of primary malignant central nervous system (CNS) tumors, representing 1.35% of primary cancers, were diagnosed in the United States in 2006 [1]. Malignant gliomas are the most common primary CNS tumors in adults accounting for 78% of all primary intrinsic malignant CNS tumors [1]. Gliomas are characterized based on histologic similarity to mature glial cells, including astrocytes and oligodendrocytes.

This work was supported by grant no. NS20023, CA11898, and SPORE 1 P20 CA096890 from the National Institutes of Health and additional funding from the Pediatric Brain Tumor Foundation of the United States and the Accelerate Brain Cancer Cure (ABC²) Foundation. J.N.R. is a Damon-Runyon Cancer Research Foundation clinical investigator and a Sidney-Kimmel Foundation scholar.

\* Corresponding author. Preston Robert Tisch Brain Tumor Center, Duke University Medical Center, DUMC 3624, Durham, NC 27710.

*E-mail address:* reard003@mc.duke.edu (D.A. Reardon).

Astrocytomas are the most common type of gliomas. High-grade (malignant) astrocytomas include anaplastic astrocytoma (AA) (World Health Organization [WHO] grade III) and glioblastoma multiforme (GBM) (WHO grade IV). High-grade astrocytomas represent highly lethal cancers that pose great therapeutic challenges. In a population-based study conducted in Switzerland between 1980 and 1994, the survival rate of patients who had newly diagnosed GBM, the most common malignant astrocytoma, was approximately 18% at 1 year and only 3% at 2 years [2]. Despite available state-of-the-art multimodality treatments, the median survival of patients who have GBM is 9 to 12 months, whereas that of AA is 2 to 3 years [3]. Favorable prognostic factors include young age, absent or minimal neurologic signs, complete surgical resection, and good performance status [4]. Current standard-of-care therapies include surgery, radiation, and chemotherapy. Recent elucidation of molecular abnormalities underlying glioma pathogenesis has led to several novel therapeutic approaches, which include molecularly targeted therapy, immunotherapy, and gene therapy. In addition, strategies to enhance delivery of therapeutic agents into the CNS, which include local polymer administration, convection-enhanced delivery (CED), and other novel delivery systems, such as nanoparticles, may increase therapeutic efficacy. This review discusses recent advances in the diagnosis and treatment of malignant astrocytomas.

## Molecular aberrations in malignant astrocytomas

Malignant astrocytomas exhibit characteristics common to other cancers, including self-initiated proliferation, diminished apoptosis, evasion of external growth control and immunosurveillance, tissue invasion, and ability to form and sustain new blood vessels [5,6]. Although malignant astrocytomas are highly invasive, they almost never metastasize outside of the CNS. Malignant astrocytomas genetically are heterogeneous across and within tumors. Common genetic alterations that maintain malignant phenotypes of tumors, however, frequently are found. Low-grade astrocytomas (WHO grade II) often display disruption of tumor suppressor gene TP53 and overexpression of platelet-derived growth factor (PDGF) ligands and receptors. In response to genotoxic stress, the TP53 gene functions to induce cell cycle arrest, apoptosis, and DNA repair. Inactivation of TP53 is associated with abnormal cell division and neoplastic transformation. Progression to anaplastic astrocytoma involves accumulation of other genetic alterations of associated cell cycle regulatory pathways, including deletion or mutations of cyclin-dependent kinase (CKD) inhibitor $p16^{INK4A}$/CDKN2A or the retinoblastoma susceptibility locus 1 (pRB1) and amplification or overexpression of CDK4 and human double minute 2 (HDM2). Transformation to GBM (termed secondary GBM) is associated with deletion of chromosome 10, which includes the tumor suppressor phosphatase and tensin homolog

(PTEN). Most GBMs are diagnosed, however, without antecedent lower-grade tumor—termed primary or de novo GBMs. Primary GBMs occur in older patients compared to secondary GBMs and share some similar genetic abnormalities with secondary GBMs, such as loss of PTEN, deletion or mutation of CDK inhibitors $p16^{INK4A}$ (which shares a locus with $p14^{ARF}$ on chromosome 9), and amplification of HDM2 or CDK4. Additional molecular changes distinguish primary and secondary GBMs [7]. Specifically, molecular analyses have identified epidermal growth factor receptor (EGFR) amplification as exclusive to primary GBMs, whereas TP53 loss is a genetic hallmark of low-grade astrocytoma and secondary GBMs (Fig. 1) [8]. Transcriptional profile analyses have demonstrated common and differential gene expression between primary and secondary GBMs [9]. Primary GBM-associated genes involve stromal and mesenchymal stem cell–like properties, whereas secondary GBM-associated genes commonly involve mitotic cell cycle components [9].

Some of these genetic abnormalities lead to deregulation of signal transduction pathways, a communication network of regulatory molecules within the cell, controlling cellular processes contributing to normal homeostasis and malignancy. For example, amplification or mutation of EGFR can increase activity in the RAS–mitogen-activated protein kinase (MAPK)

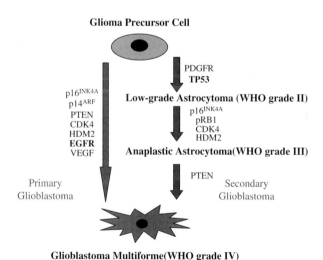

Fig. 1. Molecular alterations in astrocytomas. Secondary GBM can develop from malignant transformation of lower-grade astrocytomas (low-grade astrocytoma [WHO grade II] or anaplastic astrocytoma [WHO grade III]), whereas the more common type, primary GBM, develops without antecedent lower-grade tumors. Genetic analyses reveal common and differential molecular aberrations between primary and secondary GBMs. No single genetic mutation represents malignant astrocytomas indicating the inherent genetic heterogeneity of these tumors. Therapeutic agents targeting only single genetic/molecular pathways are less likely to achieve tumor control in a broad range of patients.

pathway and the phosphatidylinositide-3-kinase (PI3K)/AKT pathway. In addition, PI3K/AKT overactivity may result from loss of PTEN, a negative regulator of PI3K function. Understanding these molecular and genetic abnormalities has led to a rational development of molecular targeted therapies in malignant astrocytoma.

## Diagnosis

Malignant astrocytoma, like other brain tumors, can cause focal or generalized neurologic symptoms and signs. Generalized neurologic symptoms usually are related to increased intracranial pressure, which may include headache, vomiting, and visual abnormalities (papilledema on fundoscopy or diplopia from a sixth-nerve palsy). Focal neurologic abnormalities, such as aphasia, weakness, or numbness, may reflect location of tumor in the CNS. Headache occurs in approximately 50% of patients who have malignant glioma and usually is diffuse but can be localized to the same side of the head as the tumor [10]. Unlike slow-growing low-grade glioma, seizures are not the most common presenting symptom (only 15% to 30%) in malignant glioma [10].

The diagnostic imaging modality of choice for malignant astrocytomas is MRI with contrast administration. CT may not depict lesions in the posterior fossa and may miss small tumors that are not enhanced with contrast agent. Anaplastic astrocytomas usually exhibit hypointense T1- and hyperintense T2-weighted signal abnormality that may include various degrees of contrast enhancement and edema (Fig. 2A, B), whereas MRI of GBMs characteristically demonstrate irregular ring-nodular enhancing lesions with central necrosis and surrounding vasogenic edema (Fig. 2C, D). The tumor frequently tracks into white matter and can spread across the corpus callosum to involve both hemispheres. Positron emission tomography (PET) and magnetic resonance spectroscopy (MRS) can be helpful to distinguish tumor from non-neoplastic processes and to guide the location for biopsy. Imaging findings often are nonspecific, however, and definite diagnosis must be obtained from a histologic examination by biopsy or surgical resection. Anaplastic astrocytoma histologically displays cellular atypia, nuclear pleomorphism, and mitoses, whereas GBM is defined by vascular proliferation or necrosis with frequent pseudopallisading features.

## Treatment of newly diagnosed malignant glioma with temozolomide

After histologic diagnosis of malignant astrocytoma, patients usually undergo multimodality treatments, including surgical resection, radiation, and chemotherapy. Gross or near total resection, if feasible, improves survival significantly [11]. Radiation therapy has been the mainstay treatment for

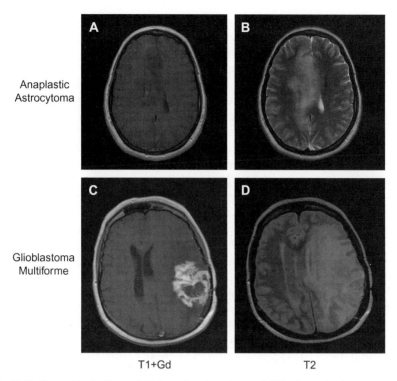

Fig. 2. Radiographic findings of high-grade astrocytomas. MRI of anaplastic astrocytoma (WHO grade III) demonstrates (*A*) hypointense T1-weighted lesion at the bilateral frontal lobes involving the corpus callosum with minimal intratumoral enhancement after gadolinium administration and (*B*) hyperintense T2-weighted abnormality. MRI of glioblastoma multiforme (WHO grade IV) demonstrates (*C*) large, heterogeneous, ring-nodular gadolinium enhancing lesion with central hypointensity at the left frontoparietal area on T1-weighted image with (*D*) extensive surrounding hyperintense T2-weighted abnormality consistent with vasogenic edema.

malignant astrocytoma [12]. It generally is administered in 1.5- to 2-Gy fractions to a total dose of 58 to 60 Gy delivered to a focal field, including the tumor bed or resection cavity with a 2- to 3-cm margin. The role of adjuvant chemotherapy had been limited until recently, when Stupp and colleagues reported that adjunctive temozolomide (TMZ) improved survival of patients who had GBM significantly without degradation in quality of life in a phase III, randomized, controlled trial [13,14]. Therefore, TMZ administered concurrently during external radiation treatment (XRT) and after XRT using adjuvant monthly cycles has become a new standard-of-care treatment of GBM. Several other novel treatments, such as locoregional treatments and targeted therapeutics that are investigational in newly diagnosed malignant astrocytoma, are discussed later.

TMZ (Temodar, Schering-Plough, New Jersey) is an orally available, imidazotetrazine-derived, second-generation, methylating agent [15]. TMZ methylates specific DNA sites—$N^7$ position of guanine, $O^3$ position of adenine, and $O^6$ position of guanine. The $O^6$ position of guanine is a critical site to mediate TMZ toxicity, although it accounts for only 5% to 10% of DNA lesions [15]. Nucleotide mismatch between complementary strands caused by TMZ leads to continuous cycles of futile mismatch repair, which eventually increase DNA double-strand breaks and apoptosis. TMZ has almost 100% oral availability. It readily crosses the blood-brain barrier to achieve a cerebrospinal fluid concentration that is approximately 40% of plasma. TMZ demonstrates dose-linear pharmacokinetics with area under the concentration-time curve increasing in proportion to the dose [15]. The most common adverse effects of TMZ are hematologic toxicity (leucopenia and thrombocytopenia), particularly when administered concurrently with radiation therapy. Severe infections are uncommon and other nonhematologic toxicities, such as nausea, vomiting, constipation, and fatigue, are mild to moderate.

TMZ exhibits broad antitumor activity in various types of CNS tumors (glioma, ependymoma, and medulloblastoma) in subcutaneous and orthotopic xenograft models [16]. Based on the promising initial clinical trial results, TMZ was granted an accelerated approval from the United States Food and Drug Administration (FDA) in 1999 for treatment of nitrosourea-resistant recurrent AA and from the similar agency in Europe for treatment of recurrent AA and GBM. Friedman and colleagues [17] initially reported a 51% radiographic response rate of TMZ in newly diagnosed GBM before radiation therapy. Based on preclinical evidence of synergy, three subsequent studies evaluated the efficacy of TMZ in a concurrent daily dose with XRT, followed by monthly cycles of adjuvant TMZ in patients newly diagnosed with GBM [13,18,19]. A pivotal, randomized, phase III study by the European Organization of Research and Treatment of Cancer (EORTC) and the National Cancer Institute of Canada (NCIC), with a total of 573 patients, demonstrated a 2-year survival rate of 24% for XRT-TMZ (75 mg/m²/day for 42 consecutive days)/TMZ (150–200 mg/m²/day for 5 days every 28 day cycle) group compared with 10% for the XRT group. The median survival was 14.6 months for the XRT-TMZ/TMZ group compared with 12.1 months for the XRT group [13]. Another study conducted by Athanassiou and coworkers [19] used a more intensive, post-XRT adjuvant TMZ regimen (150 mg/m²/day on days 1–5 and days 14–19 of each 28-day cycle) in a total of 110 randomized patients. The median survival was 13.4 months for XRT-TMZ/TMZ group compared with 7.7 months for XRT-alone group. Lower survival rates in both groups in this study reflect the comparatively poorer patient characteristics of the study population. Taken together, results from these trials support the use of TMZ in the treatment regimen of patients who have newly diagnosed GBM. Whether or not the XRT-TMZ/TMZ regimen provides a survival benefit in patients who have newly diagnosed AA remains to be elucidated in randomized clinical trials [20].

Although the addition of TMZ significantly prolongs survival for patients who have GBM, the degree of benefit is modest. Additional strategies to enhance the efficacy of this regimen are needed. Alternative dosing schedules, extended length of therapy, delivery enhancement, addition of agents to prevent or rescue TMZ resistance, and combination with other modalities, such as targeted therapeutics, gene therapy, or immunotherapy, may improve treatment efficacy. Correlative biomarkers to identify patients who are likely to respond to TMZ are critical to stratify patients and optimize TMZ benefit. Several studies have identified a potential biomarker of clinical response to TMZ. $O^6$-alkylguanine-DNA alkyltransferase (AGT) (also termed $O^6$-methylguanine-DNA methyltransferase [MGMT]) is a DNA repair protein that removes alkyl groups from the $O^6$ position of guanine, a critical site for DNA alkylation [21]. AGT functions as a suicidal protein: the reversion of $O^6$-methylguanine to an unmethylated state consumes the protein, triggering new protein production. When TMZ-induced $O^6$-methylguanine is left unrepaired, cells undergo futile DNA replication with eventual apoptosis. Methylation of CpG islands within the *AGT* promoter is an epigenetic silencing factor that decreases AGT activity and thus compromises DNA repair [21]. AGT activity in tumors can be assayed by immunohistochemistry or by a methylation-specific polymerase chain reaction (PCR). Using immunohistochemical detection of AGT, Friedman and colleagues [17] reported a 60% response rate to TMZ among patients who had newly diagnosed GBM and a low level of AGT, compared with only 9% among patients who had high level of AGT. Subsequently, Hegi and colleagues [21] used methylation-specific PCR to study tumor *MGMT* methylation status of patients who had newly diagnosed GBM from the randomized EORTC/NCIC trial. In this study, patients who had a silenced *MGMT* gene had a longer survival when treated with TMZ-XRT/TMZ but not if they received XRT alone. The 2-year survival rate for patients who had a methylated *MGMT* gene promoter increased from 22% for patients receiving only XRT to 46% for patients treated with TMZ-XRT/TMZ. In patients who had an unmethylated *MGMT* promoter, the 2-year survival rates were only 2% and 13%, when treated with XRT or TMZ-XRT/TMZ, respectively [21]. These data also suggest that tumor MGMT status may be an independent prognostic factor in patients who have GBM. Despite the promise of MGMT as a predictive biomarker, prospective randomized studies are required for further validation. Technical considerations, such as sensitivity, specificity, reliability, and reproducibility, of each test must be evaluated. Until such studies are completed and analyzed fully, the use of MGMT expression to determine whether or not to administer TMZ to specific patients is not recommended.

Several approaches have been implemented to overcome TMZ resistance in malignant astrocytoma. Dose-dense and intensified TMZ schedules may be more effective in depleting AGT in a tumor. Clinical trials of alternative schedules of TMZ are ongoing. $O^6$-benzylguanine ($O^6$-BG) is an AGT substrate that inhibits AGT by suicidal inactivation. Preclinical studies demonstrate that the antitumor activity of TMZ is enhanced by $O^6$-BG in an animal model [22]. A phase I trial of intravenous $O^6$-BG alone [23] or in combination with TMZ [24] confirmed that AGT was depleted after $O^6$-BG administration. A phase II trial of TMZ plus $O^6$-BG recently has completed accrual. Another potent AGT inhibitor that has the advantage of being an oral formulation, $O^6$-(4-bromothenyl)-guanine (PaTrin-2), currently is in preclinical development [25]. Resistance of TMZ also is demonstrated in tumor cells deficient in the DNA mismatch repair system, independent from the AGT level. This deficiency leads to intolerance of $O^6$-methylguanine and the ability of the cell to survive despite the presence of persistent DNA damage. Recently, attempts to overcome resistance conferred by mismatch repair deficiency have focused on blocking base excision repair, which differentially repairs the methyl adducts at the $N^3$ adenine and $N^7$ guanine position rather than at the $O^6$ guanine [26]. One of the strategies used to block base excision repair includes the inhibition of a key enzyme, poly (ADP-ribose) polymerase (PARP). Several PARP inhibitors have been developed and are undergoing preclinical and early clinical evaluation [26].

## Management of recurrent malignant astrocytomas

### Diagnosis of recurrence

Most patients who have malignant astrocytoma eventually recur or progress after the multimodality treatment (discussed previously). Interpretation of MRI on recurrence or progression can be difficult after chemoradiation. Although tumor progression usually is evident on MRI as increased contrast enhancement and edema, various treatments, such as high-dose radiation therapy and brachytherapy, may cause similar changes that represent diagnostic challenge. Several imaging modalities, such as MRS [27], diffusion-weighted MRI [28], and PET, may be helpful to distinguish tumor progression from treatment-related effects and also may direct a biopsy to the site of optimal yield. MRS presents an analysis of the presence and ratio of tissue metabolites, such as *N*-acetylaspartate, choline, creatine, and lactate. An elevated choline-to-creatine ratio usually is a signature for tumor metabolites, whereas generalized suppression of all metabolites is consistent with treatment effects. MRS, however, cannot accurately determine an area of mixed necrosis and tumor. Prospective studies are required to establish a direct correlation of MRS findings and histologic diagnosis. Diffusion-weighted MRI measures the apparent diffusion coefficient, which indicates mobility of extracellular water. Diffusion of water may be greater for necrotic tissues in the treatment-related effects than for recurrent tumor.

Therefore, apparent diffusion coefficient ratios of recurrent tumors generally are lower than those of treated brain tissue. Corticosteroids, however, such as dexamethasone, can affect water diffusion in the peritumoral area, which can pose additional interpretation difficulties [29]. Other MRI techniques, such as diffusion-tensor imaging and perfusion MRI, also may be helpful but require further prospective investigation.

[18F] fluorodeoxyglucose (FDG)-PET is another imaging technique used for differentiating tumor recurrence/progression from treatment effects. High uptake of FDG (hypermetabolic) usually is consistent with tumor progression. False-positive results can occur, however, with accumulation of macrophages as a result of treatment effect. In addition, high background activity from adjacent cerebral cortex may add to interpretive difficulties. Several new radiotracers, such as 18F-fluorodeoxythymidine (FLT) and 11C-methionine, have been developed to overcome this challenge [30,31]. If the clinical diagnosis of recurrent/progressive tumor remains unclear, a biopsy guided by findings on these imaging modalities should be considered.

## Treatment of recurrent malignant astrocytoma

On recurrence, treatment may involve repeat resection, focal reirradiation, salvage chemotherapy, and novel targeted therapeutics. Available salvage therapies after progression are ineffective, with 6-month progression-free survival (PFS-6) rates of 15% for GBM and 31% for AA [32]. The median PFS was 9 weeks for GBM and 13 weeks for AA [32]. PFS-6 recently has become a more widely acceptable primary endpoint for phase II trials in malignant gliomas [33].

## Surgical resection

Repeat resection in recurrent malignant astrocytoma may be considered for diagnostic confirmation, symptomatic relief for mass effect/edema, and cytoreduction [34]. Surgical resection may increase survival in selected patients who have recurrent malignant astrocytoma. Symptomatic patients who have large mass effect are likely to achieve benefit from surgery [35]. There is no randomized controlled trial, however, to address the actual survival benefit from repeat resection in patients who have recurrent malignant astrocytomas. In addition, repeat resection may be required in clinical trials using locoregional therapeutics for patients who have recurrent tumors.

## Locoregional therapy

Potential advantages of locoregional therapy include direct delivery of therapeutics without blood-brain barrier penetration and minimized systemic toxicity. In addition, because the majority of malignant astrocytomas recur within 2 cm of the primary tumor site [36], locoregional treatments, such as chemotherapy wafers, high-dose focal (stereotactic) irradiation, radioimmunoconjugates, and conjugated biologic toxins, may improve local tumor control that may translate into better patient outcome.

*Carmustine wafers*

1,3-bis[2-chloroethyl]-1-nitrosourea (BCNU)-impregnated wafers (Gliadel, MGI Pharma, Minnesota) are the first FDA-approved biodegradable wafers (polifeprosan 20) containing carmustine (BCNU) for the treatment of malignant glioma. Two double-blind, randomized, controlled trials demonstrated significant, albeit modest, survival benefits with BCNU wafers in newly diagnosed and recurrent GBMs [37,38]. In a phase III study of 240 patients who had newly diagnosed GBM, BCNU wafer placement after resection followed by radiation therapy was associated with a 2.3-month survival benefit compared with placebo [37]. Furthermore, the survival benefit was maintained up to 3 years after treatment [39]. Similarly, in recurrent GBM, BCNU wafers provided an 8-week prolongation of survival [38]. Cerebrospinal fluid leak and intracranial hypertension, however, were seen more commonly in the BCNU-wafer treated group. Several studies are ongoing to evaluate the efficacy of a higher concentration BCNU polymer preparation, which was shown in a recent phase I study to have a higher maximal tolerated dose than that of the current formulation [40]. Combinations of BCNU wafers with systemically administered agents, such as TMZ [41] or $O^6$-BG [42,43], have demonstrated safety and encouraging efficacy. In addition, this polymer system has been engineered to deliver a wide range of therapeutics, including alternative chemotherapies, radiosensitizers, antiangiogenic agents, and immunomodulators [44].

*Convection-enhanced delivery system*

In addition to local polymer delivery system of therapeutics, CED is another mode of locoregional delivery that has been investigated in malignant astrocytoma. Increased interstitial pressure in glial tumors may limit drug delivery from systemic vasculature and local infusion. CED uses the "pressure-gradient" concept of small volume infusion at high pressure over long periods (3–5 days) to optimize delivery of therapeutics in tumor/surgical bed via stereotactically placed catheters [45]. Various therapeutic agents delivered by CED have been evaluated, including chemotherapies, gene/virus therapy, and ligand-toxin conjugates [45]. Glioma cells commonly express several high-affinity cell surface receptors at greater density than normal surrounding brain cells. The ligands for these receptors can be engineered to specifically deliver toxins or radioisotopes to permit specific tumor cytotoxicity on binding and internalization. Several agents based on this approach include transforming growth factor alpha conjugated with mutated pseudomonas toxin (TP-38, IVAX, Miami, Florida, and Teva Pharmaceuticals, North Wales, Pennsylvania) that binds EGFR [46]; transferrin-CRM107

(TransMID, Xenova, Berkshire, United Kingdom), a transferrin-diphtheria conjugate [47]; interleukin (IL)-4–conjugated pseudomonas exotoxin [48]; and IL-13 conjugated with pseudomonas exotoxin (IL-13–PE38QQR, cintredekin besudotox, NeoPharm, Illinois) [49]. A phase I/II study of cintredekin besudotox in recurrent malignant gliomas demonstrated safety and encouraging efficacy [49]. A recently completed randomized phase III study of cintredekin besudotox versus BCNU wafer (PRECISE trial), however, failed to demonstrate significant difference in survival benefit. Large randomized studies for transferrin-CRM107 in recurrent malignant glioma and cintredekin besudotox in newly diagnosed GBM are ongoing.

*Reirradiation*

Most patients who have recurrent malignant astrocytoma have undergone a full course of external beam radiation therapy. Reirradiation with conventional radiotherapy generally is not recommended because of the lack of clear survival benefit and the high incidence of radiation necrosis [50]. Newer radiation techniques designed to limit normal CNS exposure, such as intensity-modulated radiotherapy, have been evaluated in recurrent malignant glioma with a median survival time of 10.1 months after reirradiation in one study [51].

Stereotactic radiosurgery (SRS) is highly focused radiation, which can be administered as a single fraction or multiple fractions. SRS usually is suitable for brain lesions up to 3 to 4 cm in size. In newly diagnosed GBM, SRS followed by conventional radiotherapy did not improve outcome in a randomized phase III trial [52]. In recurrent GBM, several small studies have demonstrated the promising activity of SRS with a median survival of 10 to 12 months after single-fraction radiosurgery and 7 to 12 months after fractionated radiosurgery [53–57]. Large prospective studies are required to evaluate the efficacy and toxicity of SRS further in recurrent malignant astrocytoma [57].

Temporary brachytherapy with high-activity $^{125}I$ seeds was associated with median survival of 11 to 12 months in recurrent malignant gliomas and with a high rate of symptomatic radiation necrosis [34]. This technique rarely is used at present.

GliaSite Radiation Therapy System (Cytyc, Alpharetta, Georgia) is a novel temporary locoregional radiation technique [58]. GliaSite consists of a silicone spherical balloon catheter and an aqueous radiation source (Iotrex [sodium 3-($^{125}I$)-iodo-4-hydroxybenzenesulfonate]). Two recent independent studies of GliaSite in patients who had recurrent GBM demonstrated median survival of approximately 36 weeks after the treatment [58,59]. Treatment generally was well tolerated, although a few patients from each trial developed symptomatic radiation necrosis.

Radiotoxin and radioimmunotherapy are novel approaches in the treatment of malignant astrocytoma by using radiolabeled toxins or monoclonal antibodies, respectively, to enhance peritumoral radiation delivery. Several tumor targets and antigens have been identified and led to the synthesis of therapeutic radiotoxin- and radioimmunoconjugates. One of the most evaluated targets in malignant astrocytoma is tenascin, an extracellular matrix protein commonly expressed in high-grade gliomas but not in normal brain. In a phase II trial, intracavitary [131]I-labeled monoclonal antibody against tenascin ([131]I-m81C6) administration after resection of newly diagnosed GBM, followed by conventional external-beam radiotherapy and a year of alkylator-based chemotherapy, was associated with the median survival of 79.4 weeks [60]. In general, this therapy was well tolerated; however, 27% of patients developed reversible hematologic toxicity and 15% developed histologically confirmed, treatment-related neurologic toxicity, which was reversible in most cases [60]. A randomized phase II trial of [131]I-m81C6 administration in patients who had newly diagnosed malignant glioma before radiation therapy with concurrent TMZ is ongoing. In addition, [131]I-m81C6 was evaluated in a phase II trial of patients who had recurrent malignant gliomas. With a median follow-up of 172 weeks, 63% and 59% of patients who had GBM and AA tumors were alive at 1 year. Median overall survival for patients who had GBM and AA tumors was 64 and 99 weeks, respectively [61]. Other targets for radioimmunotherapy may include glycoprotein NMB, MRP3, insulin growth factor receptors, and EGFRs [62]. [131]I-TM-601 (TransMolecular, Cambridge, Massachusetts) is a radiolabeled chlorotoxin that recently has demonstrated safety and promising antitumor activity in a phase I trial of recurrent malignant gliomas [63]. A phase II trial of [131]I-TM-601 is in progress.

Other radiation techniques, such as boron-neutron capture therapy and photodynamic therapy, currently are being evaluated in clinical trials.

*Salvage chemotherapy*

As TMZ has become a standard-of-care treatment for newly diagnosed GBM and most neuro-oncologists typically continue monthly TMZ until patients develop clinical or radiographic progression, the role of TMZ monotherapy in recurrent GBM is decreasing. In a study of TMZ (150–200 $mg/m^2$/day for 5 days in 28 day-cycle) for patients who had GBM with first relapse, 5% had a partial response (PR) and 40% had stable disease (SD) with PFS-6 of 21% [64]. In a phase II trial of patients who had TMZ-naïve recurrent GBM, TMZ administered at 75 $mg/m^2$/day for 21 consecutive days each 28-day cycle was associated with a 9% overall response rate with a PFS-6 rate of 30% [65]. In addition, salvage therapy with TMZ may be effective in recurrent malignant glioma patients currently not on TMZ but who had a prior response to TMZ [66]. In recurrent AA, TMZ treatment was associated with 8% complete response (CR), 44% PR, and 44% SD with PFS-6 of 46% [67]. TMZ has been evaluated with other chemotherapies, such as procarbazine, BCNU, irinotecan, etoposide, and topotecan, with modest combinatorial benefit [68–72].

Irinotecan (Camptosar [CPT-11], Pfizer, New York) is a camptothecin derivative that acts as a prodrug that undergoes hydrolysis to an active metabolite SN-38, a potent topoisomerase-I inhibitor [73]. Irinotecan displayed robust antitumor activity against human glioma xenografts [74]; it also demonstrated encouraging clinical activity in an early clinical trial [75]. Several subsequent phase II trials, however, have not shown survival benefits in patients who have recurrent malignant glioma [76,77]. Combinations of irinotecan with other chemotherapies or targeted agents have been explored. In a recently published phase I trial of irinotecan plus TMZ in recurrent malignant glioma, the combination was safe and well tolerated. The overall radiographic response was 14% with the median time-to-progression of 54.9 weeks in recurrent GBM [70]. Several phase II trials of irinotecan plus TMZ are ongoing. More recently, irinotecan has undergone clinical evaluation in combination with bevacizumab (Avastin, Genentech, South San Francisco, California), a humanized monoclonal antibody to vascular endothelial growth factor (VEGF). This combination demonstrated a remarkable radiographic response rate of 63% with PFS-6 of 32% for GBM and 61% for recurrent anaplastic gliomas [78]. The contribution of irinotecan to this regimen is unknown. A multicenter randomized phase II trial of bevacizumab versus bevacizumab plus irinotecan in recurrent GBM is ongoing to confirm the single-center data and to address the contribution of each agent to antitumor efficacy.

Other chemotherapeutic agents, such as gemcitabine, oxaliplatin, and etoposide, are under clinical investigation in malignant glioma. High-dose chemotherapy with stem cell rescue [79] and intra-arterial chemotherapy [80] have demonstrated some activity in recurrent malignant glioma. Prospective randomized trials are required, however, to confirm efficacy and evaluate toxicity of these approaches further.

## Molecularly targeted therapy

Despite the genetic heterogeneity of malignant astrocytoma, common molecular alterations often are found in signal transduction pathways, a communication network of regulatory molecules within the cell, that control cellular processes contributing to normal homeostasis and malignancy. These cellular processes are regulated by several growth factors, hormones, and cytokines. Most receptors for growth factor pathways (such as epidermal growth factor [EGF], PDGF, and VEGF) are associated with a tyrosine kinase and, therefore, share common mechanisms of pathway activation. Overexpression or mutations of receptors and intracellular downstream effectors have been identified in malignant gliomas, leading to constitutive activation of signaling pathways, resulting in uncontrolled cellular proliferation, survival, invasion, and secretion of angiogenic factors (Fig. 3). New treatments have been developed to target molecules in these signaling pathways with the goal to increase specific efficacy and minimize toxicity.

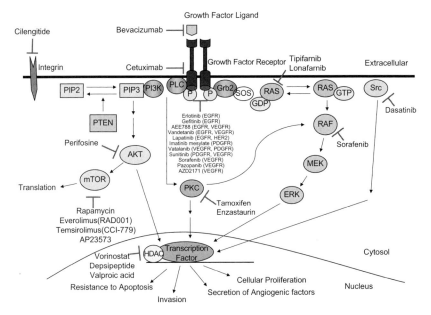

Fig. 3. Signal transduction pathways in malignant astrocytomas and targeted therapeutics. Malignant astrocytoma cells and associated endothelial cells often have constitutive activation of the pathways of several growth factor receptors, such as EGFR, VEGFR, and PDGFR. Each growth factor family consists of several members for which cognate receptors are transmembrane glycoproteins associated with protein-tyrosine kinase activity. Ligand binding to receptors induces receptor dimerization and phosphorylation (P). This receptor activation permits the binding of adaptor proteins, such as growth factor receptor-bound 2 (Grb2)/son of sevenless (SOS), and induces the activity of many intracellular signal transduction pathways that regulate gene transcription of essential cellular proteins contributing to malignancy. Several points in these cascades are the targets of therapies in development for malignant astrocytoma, some of which are shown. Signaling molecules might include RAS, RAF, MEK, ERK, PI3K, AKT, mTOR, and PKC. Several points in these cascades are the targets of therapies in development for malignant gliomas, some of which are shown. GDP, guanine diphosphate; $PIP_2$, phosphatidylinositol (4,5) bisphosphate; $PIP_3$, phosphatidylinositol (3,4,5) trisphosphate; PLC, phospholipase C.

## Inhibition of growth factor receptor

Relevant growth factors in malignant gliomas include EGF, PDGF, VEGF, insulin-like growth factor, fibroblast growth factor, and hepatocyte growth factor/scatter factor. In high-grade astrocytoma, several of these receptors (eg, EGFR) are overexpressed or mutated, leading to an upregulation of downstream signaling pathways. Kinase inhibitors of these receptors have been developed in clinical trials of malignant glioma.

## Epidermal growth factor receptor

EGFR is amplified in approximately 50% of GBMs and is overexpressed in many malignant gliomas independent of amplification status [81]. In addition, the frequent overexpression of several EGFR mutants, including EGFRvIII, suggests that EGFR is a key factor in tumorigenesis and provides a rationale for the use of EGFR targeted therapies in these patients [82]. Two kinase inhibitors of EGFR, erlotinib (Tarceva [OSI-774], Genentech, San Francisco, California) and gefitinib (Iressa [ZD1839], AstraZeneca, Wilmington, Delaware), have been tested in malignant gliomas. In a phase II trial of gefitinib for patients who had recurrent GBM, the median event-free survival was only 8.1 weeks and no radiographic responses were observed, although 9 of the 53 patients (17%) remained progression free for at least 6 months [83]. In a published phase I trial, erlotinib as monotherapy or in combination with TMZ demonstrated a 14% PR rate and a PFS-6 of 11% [84]. Other phase II trials of erlotinib have demonstrated a PR rate of 6% to 25% with modest impact on PFS or overall survival rates. [85,86] Therefore, erlotinib seems more effective against malignant gliomas than gefitinib in terms of radiographic response rate, but both have no clear impact on survival. Activating EGFR kinase region mutations linked to clinical efficacy in lung cancer have not been observed in human glioma specimens [87–89]. Two recent studies elegantly demonstrated that high expression of wild-type EGFR and low levels of phosphorylated AKT/protein kinase B in one study [90] and coexpression of EGFRvIII and wild-type PTEN in another study [91] were associated with increased radiographic response to EGFR kinase inhibitors (erlotinib and gefitinib), although the durability of responses noted generally was limited. These findings may serve as a rationale to stratify patients in future clinical trials involving EGFR-targeted therapy, although more data are needed to confirm the predictive value of these biomarkers.

*Platelet-derived growth factor receptor*

PDGF and its cognate receptors, PDGFRs, are important in tumor growth and angiogenesis of gliomas. Imatinib mesylate (Gleevec [STI571], Novartis Pharmaceuticals, East Hanover, New Jersey), an inhibitor of PDGFR, c-kit, and bcr-abl kinases, exhibited antiglioma activity in preclinical studies [92]. Imatinib monotherapy, however, has failed to show significant clinical benefits in several phase I/II trials [93]. Nonetheless, imatinib mesylate in combination with hydroxyurea has demonstrated encouraging antitumor efficacy in a patient series [94], which subsequently was confirmed by a phase II study [95]. In this trial of 33 patients who had recurrent GBMs, the radiographic response rate was 9% with PFS-6 of 27% [95]. An additional study confirmed the antitumor activity of this regimen in some patients who had recurrent grade 3 malignant glioma [96]. The mechanism of combinatorial effects of imatinib and hydroxyurea is unclear. Given the encouraging results of imatinib mesylate plus hydroxyurea, several combinations of imatinib mesylate with other chemotherapies, such as TMZ, are under clinical investigation [97].

*Vascular endothelial growth factor receptor*

Malignant gliomas display striking vascularity with high expression of VEGF, a key growth factor for new blood vessel formation (neoangiogenesis). In addition to targeting VEGF ligands with a neutralizing monoclonal antibody bevacizumab (as described previously), kinase inhibitors disrupting VEGF receptors have been developed in preclinical and clinical trials for malignant astrocytoma. Vatalanib (PTK787/ZK222584; Novartis), a kinase inhibitor of VEGFR and PDGFR, has demonstrated modest efficacy in multicenter phase I/II trials either alone [98] or in combination with chemotherapy [99]. Recently, a pilot study of AZD2171 (AstraZeneca), a pan-VEGFR inhibitor, has demonstrated encouraging antiangiogenic efficacy in patients who have GBM [100]. A phase II clinical trial of AZD2171 in recurrent GBM is ongoing, and a phase III trial is planned.

*Inhibition of intracellular effectors*

After growth factor receptor activation, effector molecules, such as RAS, phosphatidylinositide-3-kinase (PI3K), and phospholipase C (PLC), are recruited to the cell membrane. Most gliomas are associated with either activation of these effector molecules or inactivating mutations of the negative regulators of these kinases, such as PTEN in the PI3K pathway. Sequential activation by phosphorylation of intracellular effectors along signal transduction pathways relays important information to regulate cellular processes contributing to malignancy. Crucial intracellular mediators in oncogenic pathways include RAF, mitogen-activated protein extracellular regulated kinase (MEK), extracellular regulated kinase (ERK) (also termed MAPK), AKT, and mammalian target of rapamycin (mTOR). A variety of inhibitors of these intracellular effectors have been developed in preclinical and clinical studies of malignant gliomas (see Fig. 3; Table 1).

*RAS/RAF/mitogen-activated protein extracellular regulated kinase/ extracellular regulated kinase pathways*

The RAS superfamily of genes encodes small guanine triphosphate (GTP)-binding proteins that regulate many cellular functions, such as proliferation, differentiation, cytoskeletal organization, protein trafficking, and the secretion of angiogenic factors [101]. Gliomas rarely express oncogenic RAS mutations; however, they often have increased RAS activity because of mutation or amplification of upstream growth factor receptors [102]. Farnesylation is the rate-limiting step in RAS maturation; therefore, several farnesyltransferase inhibitors (FTIs) have undergone clinical evaluation as a RAS targeted therapy. Two FTIs, tipifarnib (Zarnestra [R115777], Johnson & Johnson, New Brunswick, New Jersey), and lonafarnib (Sarasar [SCH66336], Schering-Plough, Kenilworth, New Jersey), have been developed. A phase I/II study of tipifarnib in recurrent malignant gliomas demonstrated PFS-6 of 9% in recurrent WHO grade III gliomas and 12% in recurrent GBMs [103]. In a phase I trial of TMZ plus lonafarnib, 27% of patients who had prior TMZ failure had a PR and the estimated PFS-6 was 33% [104]. Downstream of RAS lies the RAF-MEK-ERK pathway, an important signaling cascade. Activation of ERK is associated with poor outcome in patients who have GBM patients [105]. Clinical trials of sorafenib (Nexavar, Bayer, West Haven, Connecticut, and Onyx, Emeryville, California), an inhibitor of RAF/VEGFR-2, in combination with several other targeted agents are ongoing.

*Phosphatidylinositide-3-kinase/AKT/ mammalian target of rapamycin pathways*

PI3K pathways regulate several malignant phenotypes, including antiapoptosis, cell growth, and proliferation [101]. Activation of PI3K pathways is associated with poor prognosis in patients who have glioma [106]. Loss of PTEN is a common genetic feature in GBM that leads to constitutive activation of PI3K pathways. Activated PI3K phosphorylates several downstream effectors including AKT. Inhibitors of PI3K and AKT have undergone preclinical evaluation with encouraging results [107]. Perifosine (Keryx Biopharmaceuticals, New York, New York), an oral AKT and AMPK inhibitor, is undergoing clinical evaluation in malignant gliomas.

mTOR is downstream from AKT and can be activated by not only AKT but also RAS pathways. Rapamycin (sirolimus [Rapamune], Wyeth, Collegeville, Pennsylvania) and its synthesized analogs, temsirolimus (CCI-779, Wyeth), everolimus (RAD001, Novartis), and AP23573 (Ariad Pharmaceuticals, Cambridge, Massachusetts), have been evaluated in clinical trials of malignant gliomas. Two recent phase II studies of temsirolimus in recurrent GBMs have been reported [108,109]. In a study by the North Central Cancer Treatment Group trial, radiographic improvement was evident in 36% of patients [108]. This radiographic improvement did not translate, however, into a survival benefit as measured by a PFS-6 of only 7.8%. Similarly, the North American Brain Tumor Consortium (NABTC) trial demonstrated 5% PR and PFS-6 of only 2.5% [109].

*Protein kinase C pathways*

Protein kinase C (PKC) is a serine/threonine kinase that regulates cell proliferation, invasion and angiogenesis. The PKC-β inhibitor with activity against glycogen synthase kinase-3β, enzastaurin (LY317615, Eli-Lilly, Indianapolis, Indiana), has demonstrated activity against glioma xenografts [110] and has shown promising clinical efficacy in a phase II trial of recurrent malignant gliomas with a 29% radiographic response rate [111]. A multicentered phase III trial of enzastaurin versus lomustine, however, recently was discontinued because of failure to achieve a survival benefit.

*Multitargeted kinase inhibitors*

In clinical trials thus far, single-targeted kinase inhibitors have been associated with modest responses in unselected patients who have malignant gliomas (see Table 1). These failures may result from limited CNS delivery;

Table 1
Selected clinical trials of molecularly targeted therapy in high-grade astrocytomas

| Targets | Agent | Phase | Comments |
|---|---|---|---|
| EGFR | Gefitinib | II | Recurrent GBM (first relapse): no radiographic response; PFS-6: 17% |
| | Erlotinib ± TMZ | I/II | Recurrent MG: 6%–25% PR; PFS-6 10%–20% |
| | Erlotinib + XRT | I | Newly diagnosed GBM: MTD not reached; median TTP: 26 weeks |
| | Cetuximab | II | Recurrent GBM: ongoing |
| PDGFR | Imatinib mesylate | I/II | Recurrent GBM: PFS-6: 3% |
| | | | Recurrent AA: PFS-6: 10% |
| | Imatinib mesylate + hydroxyurea | II | Recurrent GBM: PFS-6: 27%; 9% PR; 42% SD |
| VEGFR | Vatalanib (± TMZ or lomustine) | I/II | Recurrent GBM: 4% PR; 66% SD; TTP: 12–16 weeks |
| | Pazopanib (+ lapatinib) | I | Recurrent MG: ongoing |
| | AZD2171 | I/II | Recurrent GBM: ongoing |
| VEGF | Bevacizumab + irinotecan | II | Recurrent MG: 63% CR + PR PFS-6 GBM 32%; AA 61% |
| | Bevacizumab versus bevacizumab + irinotecan | II | Recurrent MG: ongoing |
| RAS (farnesyltransferase) | Tipifarnib | I/II | Recurrent GBM: PFS-6: 12% |
| | | | Recurrent AA: PFS-6: 9% |
| | Lonafarnib + TMZ | I | Recurrent GBM: 27% PR; PFS-6: 33% |
| RAF (+VEGFR) | Sorafenib (+ tipifarnib, temsirolimus, or erlotinib) | I/II | Recurrent MG: ongoing |
| AKT | Perifosine | II | Recurrent MG: ongoing |
| mTOR | Sirolimus + gefitinib | I | Recurrent MG: MTD identified; 6% PR; 38% SD |
| | Everolimus + AEE788 | I | Recurrent GBM: ongoing |
| | Everolimus + gefitinib | I | Recurrent GBM: 10% PR; median overall survival 6.5 months |

| | | | |
|---|---|---|---|
| PKC-β | Temsirolimus | I/II | Recurrent GBM: radiographic response: 5%–36%; PFS-6: 2.5%–7.8% |
| | Temsirolimus + erlotinib | I/II | Recurrent GBM: ongoing |
| | AP23573 | I (with surgery) | Target validation with in vivo inhibition of mTOR; no radiographic response |
| | Enzastaurin | II | Recurrent GBM: 22% PR; 5% SD Recurrent AA: 24% PR; 13% SD |
| | Enzastaurin versus lomustine | III | Recurrent MG: ongoing |
| Proteasome | Bortezomib | I/II | Recurrent MG: ongoing |
| Integrins | Cilengitide | I | Recurrent MG: MTD not reached; 4% CR; 6% PR; 8% SD |
| Src, bcr-abl | Dasatinib | I/II | Recurrent MG: planned |
| HDAC | Vorinostat | II | Recurrent GBM: completed |
| | Vorinostat + TMZ | I | MG: ongoing |
| | Depsipeptide | I/II | Recurrent MG: ongoing |
| | Valproic acid (+ XRT/TMZ) | II | Newly diagnosed MG: ongoing |
| EGFR, VEGFR | AEE788 | I | Recurrent GBM: completed |
| | Vandetanib | I/II | Recurrent MG: ongoing |
| EGFR, HER2 | Lapatinib | II | Recurrent GBM: ongoing |
| VEGFR, PDGFR | Sunitinib | I/II | Recurrent GBM: planned |

*Abbreviations:* MG, malignant glioma; MTD, maximum tolerated dose; TTP, time to progression.

altered pharmacokinetic metabolism; pharmacokinetic interactions, particularly with hepatic cytochrome-P450–inducing antiepileptic agents; inadequate intratumoral concentration resulting from active efflux multidrug transporters; and the existence of multiple parallel or compensatory pathways and genetic heterogeneity across and within the tumor. Some cancers, such as chronic myeloid leukemia and gastrointestinal stromal tumor, greatly depend on nonredundant single pathways (so-called "oncogene addiction") for maintaining their malignancy. Targeted signal inhibitors, such as imatinib monotherapy [112,113], have been remarkably successful against such malignancies. In such cancers, these pathways provide an Achilles heel as a target for therapy [114].

Several strategies have been developed to improve the efficacy of targeted therapies in more genetically complex tumors, such as malignant glioma [115]. One such approach includes targeting multiple signal transduction pathways with multitargeted kinase inhibitors. AEE788 (Novartis) is a dual EGFR and VEGFR-2 inhibitor with efficacy against GBM in a preclinical study [116]. A phase I/II study of AEE788 in recurrent malignant glioma recently has been performed. Treatment with vandetanib (ZD6474, Zactima, AstraZeneca), another inhibitor of EGFR/VEGFR-2, in murine intracranial glioma xenografts, was associated with survival prolongation [117]. A phase I/II trial of vandetanib in malignant gliomas is ongoing. Sunitinib malate (Sutent [SU11248], Pfizer), an inhibitor of VEGFR-2, PDGFR, c-KIT, and FMS-like tyrosine kinase (FLT)-3, has activity against a subcutaneous malignant glioma xenograft [118]. A phase II study of sunitinib malate in malignant gliomas is underway.

*Miscellaneous*

Several other molecular targets are candidates for development of novel therapy in malignant astrocytoma. Src kinase is a multifunctional, intracellular tyrosine kinase that regulates cellular proliferation, survival, motility, and angiogenesis. Dasatinib (BMS-354,825, Bristol-Myers-Squibb, New York, New York), a dual inhibitor of src and bcr-abl kinases, is undergoing clinical evaluation in malignant glioma.

Integrins are cell adhesion molecules important in glioma cell migration and angiogenesis. Cilengitide (EMD121974, EMD Pharmaceuticals, Durham, North Carolina), an intravenous inhibitor of $\alpha_v\beta_3$ and $\alpha_v\beta_5$ integrins, demonstrated preclinical efficacy against malignant glioma [119]. A phase I trial of cilengitide in recurrent malignant gliomas by the New Approaches to Brain Tumor Therapy (NABTT) has been completed with no dose-limiting toxicities and an encouraging 10% radiographic response rate [120]. Phase II trials of cilengitide monotherapy in recurrent GBM and cilengitide with radiation therapy in newly diagnosed GBM are ongoing.

Histone deacetylase (HDAC) inhibitors induce cell-cycle arrest and apoptosis in cancer cells [121]. Pretreatment with an HDAC inhibitor, suberoylanilide hydroxamic acid (SAHA [vorinostat], Aton Pharma, Tarry-town, New York), can sensitize glioma cells to radiation and chemotherapy [122]. Clinical trials of vorinostat in recurrent malignant glioma are ongoing. Another HDAC inhibitor, depsipeptide (FK228, Gloucester Pharmaceuticals, Cambridge, Massachusetts), has demonstrated preclinical efficacy in GBM [123]. A phase I/II study of depsipeptide in recurrent malignant gliomas is ongoing within the NABTC.

The ubiquitin-proteasome system is important in regulating cell-cycle proteins to balance cell proliferation and apoptosis [124]. Disruption of the temporal degradation of these regulatory molecules by proteasome inhibitors can induce cell growth arrest and apoptosis. A proteasome inhibitor bortezomib (Velcade [PS-341], Millennium Pharmaceuticals, Cambridge, Massachusetts), induced cell-cycle arrest and apoptosis in glioma cell lines [125]. A phase I/II study of bortezomib in malignant gliomas is ongoing within the NABTT [126].

## Combination therapy and multimodality treatment

Targeting multiple signaling pathways or even different targets in the same pathway, through combination therapy, may increase treatment efficacy of molecularly targeted agents. A strategy to determine the most promising combinations is important, as the number of therapeutic combination essentially is limitless [127]. In addition, proper administration sequencing of each drug may be important to avoid negative interactions; for instance, some agents might require cells to be cycling to induce apoptosis, whereas others only may induce cell-cycle arrest [128]. As the most common molecular alterations in GBM involve activation of EGFR and/or PI3K pathway (by loss of PTEN), several combination studies have focused on dual-targeting EGFR and downstream effectors in the PI3K pathways, such as mTOR. Three independent preclinical studies have demonstrated combinatorial benefits of EGFR kinase inhibitors and mTOR inhibitors [116,129,130]. A recent phase I trial of gefitinib plus sirolimus in recurrent malignant gliomas demonstrated safety and tolerability with encouraging antitumor activity [131]. Several clinical trials based on this principle of combining EGFR and mTOR inhibitors are ongoing.

Combinations of molecularly targeted agents and radiation therapy or chemotherapy may offer synergistic or at least additive antitumor efficacy [132,133]. Carefully designing clinical trials of such multimodality treatments is important. The sequencing and timing of drug administration in relation to radiation treatment is crucial because there is differential efficacy in an animal study [134].

## Other novel approaches

Several cutting-edge therapeutic approaches for malignant gliomas have been developed in the past few decades. These experimental therapies, which include gene/virus therapy [135], cell-based and stem cell therapy [136], and immunotherapy have demonstrated promise in preclinical and early clinical studies. This topic is beyond the scope of this review, however. Further evaluation of these approaches is warranted.

## Summary and future direction

Treatment of high-grade astrocytoma has remained one of the most challenging fields in cancer therapy. Standard-of-care treatments include resection, radiation therapy, and adjuvant chemotherapy. TMZ, a new standard chemotherapy, has marked a new era of therapy in neuro-oncology by extending the survival of patients who have newly diagnosed GBM in combination with radiotherapy. Several strategies are being considered to improve the efficacy of TMZ, as more is understood about mechanisms of response and resistance. Tumor-AGT status is a potential correlative biomarker for TMZ response. If validated prospectively, it may identify optimal patient subsets for TMZ therapy. The fundamental challenges of limited therapeutic delivery and molecular/genetic heterogeneity of tumors need to be overcome to improve patient outcome. Locoregional therapeutics and molecularly targeted agents represent new promising approaches for malignant astrocytoma treatment. Most targeted agents of growth and survival pathways, when administered as monotherapies, have failed to achieve a survival benefit in unselected glioma patient populations. Targeting multiple signaling pathways by multitargeted kinase inhibitors or combinations of single-targeted kinase inhibitors may increase treatment efficacy. Several other strategies have been developed to improve effectiveness of targeted therapeutics, which may include genomic or network analyses to identify new targets and promising combinations, more predictive preclinical models for drug testing, improved therapeutic delivery systems, pharmacokinetic and pharmacodynamic or biomarker studies, and novel clinical trial designs and endpoints. Identification of correlative biomarkers eventually will lead to rational "individualized" targeted therapy based on molecular or genetic signatures of tumors from each patient [137].

More recently, identification of cancer stem cells in glioblastomas has generated a paradigm shift in neuro-oncology research [138]. These stem cell–like glioblastoma cells play important roles in promoting angiogenesis [139] and mediating resistance to radiation [140]. As the molecular and genetic abnormalities of cancer stem cells undergo vigorous investigation, targeted therapies aiming at these cells simultaneously will be developed [141,142].

## References

[1] CBTRUS. Statistical report: primary brain tumors in the United States, 1997–2001. Chicago: Central Brain Tumor Registry of the United States (CBTRUS); 2006.

[2] Ohgaki H, Dessen P, Jourde B, et al. Genetic pathways to glioblastoma: a population-based study. Cancer Res 2004;64(19):6892–9.

[3] Scott CB, Scarantino C, Urtasun R, et al. Validation and predictive power of Radiation Therapy Oncology Group (RTOG) recursive partitioning analysis classes for malignant glioma patients: a report using RTOG 90-06. Int J Radiat Oncol Biol Phys 1998;40(1):51–5.

[4] Behin A, Hoang-Xuan K, Carpentier AF, et al. Primary brain tumours in adults. Lancet 2003;361(9354):323–31.

[5] Reardon DA, Rich JN, Friedman HS, et al. Recent advances in the treatment of malignant astrocytoma. J Clin Oncol 2006;24(8):1253–65.

[6] Sathornsumetee S, Rich JN. New treatment strategies for malignant gliomas. Expert Rev Anticancer Ther 2006;6(7):1087–104.

[7] Houillier C, Lejeune J, Benouaich-Amiel A, et al. Prognostic impact of molecular markers in a series of 220 primary glioblastomas. Cancer 2006;106(10):2218–23.

[8] Kleihues P, Ohgaki H. Primary and secondary glioblastomas: from concept to clinical diagnosis. Neuro Oncol 1999;1:44–51.

[9] Tso CL, Freije WA, Day A, et al. Distinct transcription profiles of primary and secondary glioblastoma subgroups. Cancer Res 2006;66:159–67.

[10] DeAngelis LM. Brain tumors. N Engl J Med 2001;344(2):114–23.

[11] Lacroix M, Abi-Said D, Fourney DR, et al. A multivariate analysis of 416 patients with glioblastoma multiforme: prognosis, extent of resection, and survival. J Neurosurg 2001;95(2):190–8.

[12] Walker MD, Green SB, Byar DP, et al. Randomized comparisons of radiotherapy and nitrosoureas for the treatment of malignant glioma after surgery. N Engl J Med 1980;303(23):1323–9.

[13] Stupp R, Mason WP, van den Bent MJ, et al. Radiotherapy plus concomitant and adjuvant temozolomide for glioblastoma. N Engl J Med 2005;352(10):987–96.

[14] Taphoorn MJ, Stupp R, Coens C, et al. Health-related quality of life in patients with glioblastoma: a randomised controlled trial. Lancet Oncol 2005;6(12):937–44.

[15] Mutter N, Stupp R. Temozolomide: a milestone in neuro-oncology and beyond? Expert Rev Anticancer Ther 2006;6(8):1187–204.

[16] Friedman HS, Dolan ME, Pegg AE, et al. Activity of temozolomide in the treatment of central nervous system tumor xenografts. Cancer Res 1995;55(13):2853–7.

[17] Friedman HS, McLendon RE, Kerby T, et al. DNA mismatch repair and O6-alkylguanine-DNA alkyltransferase analysis and response to Temodal in newly diagnosed malignant glioma. J Clin Oncol 1998;16(12):3851–7.

[18] Stupp R, Dietrich PY, Ostermann Kraljevic S, et al. Promising survival for patients with newly diagnosed glioblastoma multiforme treated with concomitant radiation plus temozolomide followed by adjuvant temozolomide. J Clin Oncol 2002;20(5):1375–82.

[19] Athanassiou H, Synodinou M, Maragoudakis E, et al. Randomized phase II study of temozolomide and radiotherapy compared with radiotherapy alone in newly diagnosed glioblastoma multiforme. J Clin Oncol 2005;23(10):2372–7.

[20] Siker ML, Chakravarti A, Mehta MP. Should concomitant and adjuvant treatment with temozolomide be used as standard therapy in patients with anaplastic glioma? Crit Rev Oncol Hematol 2006;60(2):99–111.

[21] Hegi ME, Diserens AC, Gorlia T, et al. MGMT gene silencing and benefit from temozolomide in glioblastoma. N Engl J Med 2005;352:997–1003.

[22] Friedman HS, Dolan ME, Moschel RC, et al. Enhancement of nitrosourea activity in medulloblastoma and glioblastoma multiforme. J Natl Cancer Inst 1992;84(24):1926–31.

[23] Friedman HS, Kokkinakis DM, Pluda J, et al. Phase I trial of O6-benzylguanine for patients undergoing surgery for malignant glioma. J Clin Oncol 1998;16:3570–5.

[24] Quinn JA, Desjardins A, Weingart J, et al. Phase I trial of temozolomide plus O6-benzylguanine for patients with recurrent or progressive malignant glioma. J Clin Oncol 2005;23:7178–87.

[25] Clemons M, Kelly J, Watson AJ, et al. O6-(4-bromothenyl)guanine reverses temozolomide resistance in human breast tumour MCF-7 cells and xenografts. Br J Cancer 2005;93: 1152–6.

[26] Cheng CL, Johnson SP, Keir ST, et al. Poly(ADP-ribose) polymerase-1 inhibition reverses temozolomide resistance in a DNA mismatch repair-deficient malignant glioma xenograft. Mol Cancer Ther 2005;4:1364–8.

[27] Hollingworth W, Medina LS, Lenkinski RE, et al. A systematic literature review of magnetic resonance spectroscopy for the characterization of brain tumors. AJNR Am J Neuroradiol 2006;27(7):1404–11.

[28] Asao C, Korogi Y, Kitajima M, et al. Diffusion-weighted imaging of radiation-induced brain injury for differentiation from tumor recurrence. AJNR Am J Neuroradiol 2005; 26(6):1455–60.

[29] Bastin ME, Carpenter TK, Armitage PA, et al. Effects of dexamethasone on cerebral perfusion and water diffusion in patients with high-grade glioma. AJNR Am J Neuroradiol 2006;27(2):402–8.

[30] Saga T, Kawashima H, Araki N, et al. Evaluation of primary brain tumors with FLT-PET: usefulness and limitations. Clin Nucl Med 2006;31(12):774–80.

[31] Tsuyuguchi N, Takami T, Sunada I, et al. Methionine positron emission tomography for differentiation of recurrent brain tumor and radiation necrosis after stereotactic radiosurgery–in malignant glioma. Ann Nucl Med 2004;18(4):291–6.

[32] Wong ET, Hess KR, Gleason MJ, et al. Outcomes and prognostic factors in recurrent glioma patients enrolled onto phase II clinical trials. J Clin Oncol 1999;17(8):2572–8.

[33] Ballman KV, Buckner JC, Brown PD, et al. The relationship between six-month progression-free survival and 12-month overall survival end points for phase II trials in patients with glioblastoma multiforme. Neuro Oncol 2007;9(1):29–38.

[34] Butowski NA, Sneed PK, Chang SM. Diagnosis and treatment of recurrent high-grade astrocytoma. J Clin Oncol 2006;24(8):1273–80.

[35] Guyotat J, Signorelli F, Frappaz D, et al. Is reoperation for recurrence of glioblastoma justified? Oncol Rep 2000;7(4):899–904.

[36] Wallner KE, Galicich JH, Krol G, et al. Patterns of failure following treatment for glioblastoma multiforme and anaplastic astrocytoma. Int J Radiat Oncol Biol Phys 1989;16(6): 1405–9.

[37] Westphal M, Hilt DC, Bortey E, et al. A phase 3 trial of local chemotherapy with biodegradable carmustine (BCNU) wafers (Gliadel wafers) in patients with primary malignant glioma. Neuro Oncol 2003;5(2):79–88.

[38] Brem H, Piantadosi S, Burger PC, et al. Placebo-controlled trial of safety and efficacy of intraoperative controlled delivery by biodegradable polymers of chemotherapy for recurrent gliomas. The Polymer-brain Tumor Treatment Group. Lancet 1995;345(8956): 1008–12.

[39] Westphal M, Ram Z, Riddle V, et al. On behalf of the Executive Committee of the Gliadel Study Group. Gliadel wafer in initial surgery for malignant glioma: long-term follow-up of a multicenter controlled trial. Acta Neurochir (Wien) 2006;148(3):269–75.

[40] Olivi A, Grossman SA, Tatter S, et al. Dose escalation of carmustine in surgically implanted polymers in patients with recurrent malignant glioma: a New Approaches to Brain Tumor Therapy CNS Consortium trial. J Clin Oncol 2003;21(9):1845–9.

[41] Gururangan S, Cokgor L, Rich JN, et al. Phase I study of Gliadel wafers plus temozolomide in adults with recurrent supratentorial high-grade gliomas. Neuro Oncol 2001;3(4): 246–50.

[42] Quinn JA, Vredenburgh JJ, Rich JN, et al. Phase II trial of Gliadel plus O6-benzylguanine (O6-BG) for patients with recurrent glioblastoma multiforme. J Clin Oncol 2006;24(18S): 1568.

[43] Weingart J, Grossmn ST, Carson KA, et al. Phase I trial of Polifeprosan 20 with carmustine implant plus continuous infusion of intravenous O6-benzylguanine in adults with recurrent

malignant glioma: New Approaches to Brain Tumor Therapy CNS Consortium trial. J Clin Oncol 2007;25:399–404.

[44] Guerin C, Olivi A, Weingart JD, et al. Recent advances in brain tumor therapy: local intracerebral drug delivery by polymers. Invest New Drugs 2004;22(1):27–37.

[45] Vogelbaum MA. Convection enhanced delivery for treating brain tumors and selected neurological disorders: symposium review. J Neurooncol 2007;83(1):97–109.

[46] Sampson JH, Akabani G, Archer GE, et al. Progress report of a phase I study of the intracerebral microinfusion of a recombinant chimeric protein composed of transforming growth factor (TGF)-alpha and a mutated form of the Pseudomonas exotoxin termed PE-38 (TP-38) for the treatment of malignant brain tumors. J Neurooncol 2003;65:27–35.

[47] Weaver M, Laske DW. Transferrin receptor ligand-targeted toxin conjugate (Tf-CRM107) for therapy of malignant gliomas. J Neurooncol 2003;65:3–13.

[48] Weber F, Asher A, Bucholz R, et al. Safety, tolerability, and tumor response of IL4-Pseudomonas exotoxin (NBI-3001) in patients with recurrent malignant glioma. J Neurooncol 2003;64:125–37.

[49] Prados M, Kunwar S, Lang FF, et al. Final results of phase I/II studies of IL-13-PE38QQR administered intratumorally (IT) and/or peritumorally (PT) via convection-enhanced delivery (CED) in patients undergoing tumor resection for recurrent malignant glioma. J Clin Oncol 2005;23(Suppl 115S):1506.

[50] Bauman GS, Sneed PK, Wara WM, et al. Reirradiation of primary CNS tumors. Int J Radiat Oncol Biol Phys 1996;36(2):433–41.

[51] Voynov G, Kaufman S, Hong T, et al. Treatment of recurrent malignant gliomas with stereotactic intensity modulated radiation therapy. Am J Clin Oncol 2002;25(6):606–11.

[52] Souhami L, Seiferheld W, Brachman D, et al. Randomized comparison of stereotactic radiosurgery followed by conventional radiotherapy with carmustine to conventional radiotherapy with carmustine for patients with glioblastoma multiforme: report of Radiation Therapy Oncology Group 93-05 protocol. Int J Radiat Oncol Biol Phys 2004;60(3): 853–60.

[53] Shrieve DC, Alexander E 3rd, Wen PY, et al. Comparison of stereotactic radiosurgery and brachytherapy in the treatment of recurrent glioblastoma multiforme. Neurosurgery 1995; 36(2):275–82.

[54] Cho KH, Hall WA, Gerbi BJ, et al. Single dose versus fractionated stereotactic radiotherapy for recurrent high-grade gliomas. Int J Radiat Oncol Biol Phys 1999;45(5):1133–41.

[55] Combs SE, Widmer V, Thilmann C, et al. Stereotactic radiosurgery (SRS): treatment option for recurrent glioblastoma multiforme (GBM). Cancer 2005;104(10):2168–73.

[56] Combs SE, Thilmann C, Edler L, et al. Efficacy of fractionated stereotactic reirradiation in recurrent gliomas: long-term results in 172 patients treated in a single institution. J Clin Oncol 2005;23(34):8863–9.

[57] Tsao MN, Mehta MP, Whelan TJ, et al. The American Society for Therapeutic Radiology and Oncology (ASTRO) evidence-based review of the role of radiosurgery for malignant glioma. Int J Radiat Oncol Biol Phys 2005;63(1):47–55.

[58] Chan TA, Weingart JD, Parisi M, et al. Treatment of recurrent glioblastoma multiforme with GliaSite brachytherapy. Int J Radiat Oncol Biol Phys 2005;62:1133–9.

[59] Gabayan AJ, Green SB, Sanan A, et al. GliaSite brachytherapy for treatment of recurrent malignant gliomas: a retrospective multi-institutional analysis. Neurosurgery 2006;58: 701–9.

[60] Reardon DA, Akabani G, Coleman RE, et al. Phase II trial of murine (131)I-labeled antitenascin monoclonal antibody 81C6 administered into surgically created resection cavities of patients with newly diagnosed malignant gliomas. J Clin Oncol 2002;20:1389–97.

[61] Reardon DA, Akabani G, Coleman RE, et al. Salvage radioimmunotherapy with murine iodine-131-labeled antitenascin monoclonal antibody 81C6 for patients with recurrent primary and metastatic malignant brain tumors: phase II study results. J Clin Oncol 2006;24: 115–22.

[62] Boskovitz A, Wikstrand CJ, Kuan CT, et al. Monoclonal antibodies for brain tumour treatment. Expert Opin Biol Ther 2004;4(9):1453–71.

[63] Mamelak AN, Rosenfeld S, Bucholz R, et al. Phase I single-dose study of intracavitary-administered iodine-131-TM-601 in adults with recurrent high-grade glioma. J Clin Oncol 2006;24:3644–50.

[64] Yung WK, Albright RE, Olson J, et al. A phase II study of temozolomide vs. procarbazine in patients with glioblastoma multiforme at first relapse. Br J Cancer 2000;83(5): 588–93.

[65] Brandes AA, Tosoni A, Cavallo G, et al. Temozolomide 3 weeks on and 1 week off as first-line therapy for recurrent glioblastoma: phase II study from gruppo italiano cooperativo di neuro-oncologia (GICNO). Br J Cancer 2006;95(9):1155–60.

[66] Franceschi E, Omuro AM, Lassman AB, et al. Salvage temozolomide for prior temozolomide responders. Cancer 2005;104(11):2473–6.

[67] Yung WK, Prados MD, Yaya-Tur R, et al. Multicenter phase II trial of temozolomide in patients with anaplastic astrocytoma or anaplastic oligoastrocytoma at first relapse. Temodal Brain Tumor Group. J Clin Oncol 1999;17(9):2762–71.

[68] Newlands ES, Foster T, Zaknoen S. Phase I study of temozolomide (TMZ) combined with procarbazine (PCB) in patients with gliomas. Br J Cancer 2003;89:248–51.

[69] Prados MD, Yung WK, Fine HA, et al. Phase II study of BCNU and temozolomide for recurrent glioblastoma multiforme: North American Brain Tumor Consortium Study. Neuro Oncol 2004;6:33–7.

[70] Reardon DA, Quinn JA, Rich JN, et al. Phase I trial of irinotecan plus temozolomide in adults with recurrent malignant glioma. Cancer 2005;104:1478–86.

[71] Yung WKA, Lieberman FS, Wen P, et al. Combination of temozolomide (TMZ) and irinotecan (CPT-11) showed enhanced activity for recurrent malignant gliomas: a North American Brain Tumor Consortium (NABTC) phase II study. J Clin Oncol 2005;23:119S.

[72] Korones DN, Benita-Weiss M, Coyle TE, et al. Phase I study of temozolomide and escalating doses of oral etoposide for adults with recurrent malignant glioma. Cancer 2003;97: 1963–8.

[73] Friedman HS, Keir ST, Houghton PJ. The emerging role of irinotecan (CPT-11) in the treatment of malignant glioma in brain tumors. Cancer 2003;97(9 Suppl):2359–62.

[74] Houghton PJ, Cheshire PJ, Hallman JD 2nd, et al. Efficacy of topoisomerase I inhibitors, topotecan and irinotecan, administered at low dose levels in protracted schedules to mice bearing xenografts of human tumors. Cancer Chemother Pharmacol 1995;36:393–403.

[75] Friedman HS, Petros WP, Friedman AH, et al. Irinotecan therapy in adults with recurrent or progressive malignant glioma. J Clin Oncol 1999;17:1516–25.

[76] Batchelor TT, Gilbert MR, Supko JG, et al. Phase 2 study of weekly irinotecan in adults with recurrent malignant glioma: final report of NABTT 97-11. Neuro Oncol 2004;6: 21–7.

[77] Prados MD, Lamborn K, Yung WK, et al. A phase 2 trial of irinotecan (CPT-11) in patients with recurrent malignant glioma: a North American Brain Tumor Consortium study. Neuro Oncol 2006;8(2):189–93.

[78] Vredenburgh JJ, Desjardins A, Herndon JE, et al. Phase II trial of bevacizumab in combination with irinotecan for patients with recurrent malignant gliomas. Clin Cancer Res 2007; 13(4):1253–9.

[79] Durando X, Lemaire JJ, Tortochaux J, et al. High-dose BCNU followed by autologous hematopoietic stem cell transplantation in supratentorial high-grade malignant gliomas: a retrospective analysis of 114 patients. Bone Marrow Transplant 2003;31(7):559–64.

[80] Madajewicz S, Chowhan N, Tfayli A, et al. Therapy for patients with high grade astrocytoma using intraarterial chemotherapy and radiation therapy. Cancer 2000;88:2350–6.

[81] Ekstrand AJ, James CD, Cavenee WK, et al. Genes for epidermal growth factor receptor, transforming growth factor alpha, and epidermal growth factor and their expression in human gliomas in vivo. Cancer Res 1991;51(8):2164–72.

[82] Kuan CT, Wikstrand CJ, Bigner DD. EGF mutant receptor vIII as a molecular target in cancer therapy. Endocr Relat Cancer 2001;8:83–96.

[83] Rich JN, Reardon DA, Peery T, et al. Phase II trial of gefitinib in recurrent glioblastoma. J Clin Oncol 2004;22:133–42.

[84] Prados MD, Lamborn KR, Chang S, et al. Phase 1 study of erlotinib HCl alone and combined with temozolomide in patients with stable or recurrent malignant glioma. Neuro Oncol 2006;8(1):67–78.

[85] Vogelbaum MA, Peereboom D, Stevens G, et al. Phase II trial of EGFR tyrosine kinase inhibitor erlotinib for single agent therapy of recurrent glioblastoma multiforme: interim results. J Clin Oncol 2004;22:1558a.

[86] Raizer JJ, Abrey LE, Wen P, et al. Phase II trial of erlotinib (OSI-779) in patients (pts) with recurrent malignant gliomas (MG) not on EIAEDs. J Clin Oncol 2004;22:1502a.

[87] Rich JN, Rasheed BK, Yan H. EGFR mutations and sensitivity to gefitinib. N Engl J Med 2004;351(12):1260–1.

[88] Marie Y, Carpentier AF, Omuro AM, et al. EGFR tyrosine kinase domain mutations in human gliomas. Neurology 2005;64(8):1444–5.

[89] Lassman AB, Rossi MR, Raizer JJ, et al. Molecular study of malignant gliomas treated with epidermal growth factor receptor inhibitors: tissue analysis from North American Brain Tumor Consortium Trials 01-03 and 00-01. Clin Cancer Res 2005; 11(21):7841–50.

[90] Haas-Kogan DA, Prados MD, Tihan T, et al. Epidermal growth factor receptor, protein kinase B/Akt, and glioma response to erlotinib. J Natl Cancer Inst 2005;97:880–7.

[91] Mellinghoff IK, Wang MY, Vivanco I, et al. Molecular determinants of the response of glioblastomas to EGFR kinase inhibitors. N Engl J Med 2005;353:2012–24.

[92] Kilic T, Alberta JA, Zdunek PR, et al. Intracranial inhibition of platelet-derived growth factor-mediated glioblastoma cell growth by an orally active kinase inhibitor of the 2-phenylaminopyrimidine class. Cancer Res 2000;60:5143–50.

[93] Wen PY, Yung WK, Lamborn KR, et al. Phase I/II study of imatinib mesylate for recurrent malignant gliomas: North American Brain Tumor Consortium Study 99-08. Clin Cancer Res 2006;12(16):4899–907.

[94] Dresemann G. Imatinib and hydroxyurea in pretreated progressive glioblastoma multiforme: a patient series. Ann Oncol 2005;16:1702–8.

[95] Reardon DA, Egorin MJ, Quinn JA, et al. Phase 2 study of imatinib mesylate plus hydroxyurea in adults with recurrent glioblastoma multiforme. J Clin Oncol 2005;23: 9359–68.

[96] Desjardins A, Quinn JA, Vredenburgh JJ, et al. Phase II study of imatinib mesylate and hydroxyurea for recurrent grade III malignant gliomas. J Neurooncol 2007;83(1):53–60, [epub ahead of print].

[97] Sathornsumetee S, Reardon DA, Quinn JA, et al. An update on Phase I of dose-escalating imatinib mesylate plus standard-dosed temozolomide for the treatment of patients with malignant glioma. J Clin Oncol 2006;24(18S):1560.

[98] Conrad C, Friedman H, Reardon D, et al. A phase I/II trial of single-agent PTK 787/ZK 222584 (PTK/ZK), a novel, oral angiogenesis inhibitor, in patients with recurrent glioblastoma multiforme (GBM). J Clin Oncol 2004;22:110S–1512S.

[99] Reardon D, Friedman H, Yung WKA, et al. A phase I/II trial of PTK787/ZK 222584 (PTK/ZK), a novel, oral angiogenesis inhibitor, in combination with either temozolomide or lomustine for patients with recurrent glioblastoma multiforme (GBM). J Clin Oncol 2004;22:110S–1513S.

[100] Batchelor TT, Sorensen AG, di Tomaso E, et al. AZD2171, a pan-VEGF receptor tyrosine kinase inhibitor, normalizes tumor vasculature and alleviates edema in glioblastoma patients. Cancer Cell 2007;11(1):83–95.

[101] Shaw RJ, Cantley LC. Ras, PI(3)K and mTOR signalling controls tumour cell growth. Nature 2006;441:424–30.

[102] Knobbe CB, Reifenberger J, Reifenberger G. Mutation analysis of the Ras pathway genes NRAS, HRAS, KRAS and BRAF in glioblastomas. Acta Neuropathol (Berl) 2004;108: 467–70.

[103] Cloughesy TF, Wen PY, Robins HI, et al. Phase II trial of tipifarnib in patients with recurrent malignant glioma either receiving or not receiving enzyme-inducing antiepileptic drugs: a North American Brain Tumor Consortium Study. J Clin Oncol 2006;24(22): 3651–6.

[104] Gilbert MR, Gaupp P, Lin V, et al. A Phase I study of temozolomide (TMZ) and the farnesyltransferase inhibitor (FTI), lonafarnib (Sarasar, SCH66336) in recurrent glioblastoma. J Clin Oncol 2006;24:1556.

[105] Pelloski CE, Lin E, Zhang L, et al. Prognostic associations of activated mitogen-activated protein kinase and Akt pathways in glioblastoma. Clin Cancer Res 2006;12(13):3935–41.

[106] Chakravarti A, Zhai G, Suzuki Y, et al. The prognostic significance of phosphatidylinositol 3-kinase pathway activation in human gliomas. J Clin Oncol 2004;22:1926–33.

[107] Momota H, Nerio E, Holland EC. Perifosine inhibits multiple signaling pathways in glial progenitors and cooperates with temozolomide to arrest cell proliferation in gliomas in vivo. Cancer Res 2005;65:7429–35.

[108] Galanis E, Buckner JC, Maurer MJ, et al. Phase II trial of temsirolimus (CCI-779) in recurrent glioblastoma multiforme: a North Central Cancer Treatment Group Study. J Clin Oncol 2005;23:5294–304.

[109] Chang SM, Wen P, Cloughesy T, et al. Phase II study of CCI-779 in patients with recurrent glioblastoma multiforme. Invest New Drugs 2005;23(4):357–61.

[110] Graff JR, McNulty AM, Hanna KR, et al. The protein kinase Cbeta-selective inhibitor, Enzastaurin (LY317615.HCl), suppresses signaling through the AKT pathway, induces apoptosis, and suppresses growth of human colon cancer and glioblastoma xenografts. Cancer Res 2005;65:7462–9.

[111] Fine HA, Kim L, Royce C, et al. Results from phase II trial of enzastaurin (LY317615) in patients with recurrent high grade gliomas. J Clin Oncol 2005;23(16S):1504.

[112] Druker BJ, Talpaz M, Resta DJ, et al. Efficacy and safety of a specific inhibitor of the BCR-ABL tyrosine kinase in chronic myeloid leukemia. N Engl J Med 2001;344:1031–7.

[113] Demetri GD, von Mehren M, Blanke CD, et al. Efficacy and safety of imatinib mesylate in advanced gastrointestinal stromal tumors. N Engl J Med 2002;347(7):472–80.

[114] Weinstein IB. Cancer. Addiction to oncogenes—the Achilles heal of cancer. Science 2002; 297:63–4.

[115] Wen PY, Kesari S, Drappatz J. Malignant gliomas: strategies to increase the effectiveness of targeted molecular treatment. Expert Rev Anticancer Ther 2006;6(5):733–54.

[116] Goudar RK, Shi Q, Hjelmeland MD, et al. Combination therapy of inhibitors of epidermal growth factor receptor/vascular endothelial growth factor receptor 2 (AEE788) and the mammalian target of rapamycin (RAD001) offers improved glioblastoma tumor growth inhibition. Mol Cancer Ther 2005;4:101–12.

[117] Rich JN, Sathornsumetee S, Keir ST, et al. ZD6474, a novel tyrosine kinase inhibitor of vascular endothelial growth factor receptor and epidermal growth factor receptor, inhibits tumor growth of multiple nervous system tumors. Clin Cancer Res 2005;11:8145–57.

[118] Schueneman AJ, Himmelfarb E, Geng L, et al. SU11248 maintenance therapy prevents tumor regrowth after fractionated irradiation of murine tumor models. Cancer Res 2003; 63:4009–16.

[119] MacDonald TJ, Taga T, Shimada H, et al. Preferential susceptibility of brain tumors to the antiangiogenic effects of an alpha(v) integrin antagonist. Neurosurgery 2001;48:151–7.

[120] Nabors LB, Rosenfeld SS, Mikkelsen T, et al. NABTT 9911: a phase I trial of EMD 121974 for treatment of patients with recurrent malignant gliomas. Neuro Oncol 2004;6:379.

[121] Conley BA, Wright JJ, Kummar S. Targeting epigenetic abnormalities with histone deacetylase inhibitors. Cancer 2006;107:832–40.

[122] Chinnaiyan P, Vallabhaneni G, Armstrong E, et al. Modulation of radiation response by histone deacetylase inhibition. Int J Radiat Oncol Biol Phys 2005;62:223–9.

[123] Sawa H, Murakami H, Kumagai M, et al. Histone deacetylase inhibitor, FK228, induces apoptosis and suppresses cell proliferation of human glioblastoma cells in vitro and in vivo. Acta Neuropathol (Berl) 2004;107(6):523–31.

[124] Mani A, Gelmann EP. The ubiquitin-proteasome pathway and its role in cancer. J Clin Oncol 2005;23:4776–89.

[125] Yin D, Zhou H, Kumagai T, et al. Proteasome inhibitor PS-341 causes cell growth arrest and apoptosis in human glioblastoma multiforme (GBM). Oncogene 2005;24:344–54.

[126] Phuphanich S, Supko J, Carson KA, et al. Phase I trial of bortezomib in adults with recurrent malignant glioma. J Clin Oncol 2006;24:1567.

[127] Dancey JE, Chen HX. Strategies for optimizing combinations of molecularly targeted anticancer agents. Nat Rev Drug Discov 2006;5:649–59.

[128] Rich JN, Bigner DD. Development of novel targeted therapies in the treatment of malignant glioma. Nat Rev Drug Discov 2004;3(5):430–46.

[129] Rao RD, Mladek AC, Lamont JD, et al. Disruption of parallel and converging signaling pathways contributes to the synergistic antitumor effects of simultaneous mTOR and EGFR inhibition in GBM cells. Neoplasia 2005;7:921–9.

[130] Wang MY, Lu KV, Zhu S, et al. Mammalian target of rapamycin inhibition promotes response to epidermal growth factor receptor kinase inhibitors in PTEN-deficient and PTEN-intact glioblastoma cells. Cancer Res 2006;66(16):7864–9.

[131] Reardon DA, Quinn JA, Vredenburgh JJ, et al. A phase I study of gefitinib plus rapamycin in recurrent glioblatoma multiforme. Clin Cancer Res 2006;12:860–8.

[132] Chakravarti A, Chakladar A, Delaney MA, et al. The epidermal growth factor receptor pathway mediates resistance to sequential administration of radiation and chemotherapy in primary human glioblastoma cells in a RAS-dependent manner. Cancer Res 2002;62: 4307–15.

[133] Damiano V, Melisi D, Bianco C, et al. Cooperative antitumor effect of multitargeted kinase inhibitor ZD6474 and ionizing radiation in glioblastoma. Clin Cancer Res 2005;11: 5639–44.

[134] Williams KJ, Telfer BA, Brave S, et al. ZD6474, a potent inhibitor of vascular endothelial growth factor signaling, combined with radiotherapy: schedule-dependent enhancement of antitumor activity. Clin Cancer Res 2004;10:8587–93.

[135] Lesniak MS. Gene therapy for malignant glioma. Expert Rev Neurother 2006;6(4):479–88.

[136] Terzis AJ, Niclou SP, Rajcevic U, et al. Cell therapies for glioblastoma. Expert Opin Biol Ther 2006;6(8):739–49.

[137] Potti A, Dressman HK, Bild A, et al. Genomic signatures to guide the use of chemotherapeutics. Nat Med 2006;12:1294–300.

[138] Singh SK, Hawkins C, Clarke ID, et al. Identification of human brain tumour initiating cells. Nature 2004;432:396–401.

[139] Bao S, Wu Q, Sathornsumetee S, et al. Stem cell-like glioma cells promote tumor angiogenesis through vascular endothelial growth factor. Cancer Res 2006;66:7843–8.

[140] Bao S, Wu Q, McLendon RE, et al. Glioma stem cells promote radioresistance by preferential activation of the DNA damage response. Nature 2006;444:756–60.

[141] Piccirillo SG, Reynolds BA, Zanetti N, et al. Bone morphogenetic proteins inhibit the tumorigenic potential of human brain tumour-initiating cells. Nature 2006;444(7120): 761–5.

[142] Pellegatta S, Poliani PL, Corno D, et al. Neurospheres enriched in cancer stem-like cells are highly effective in eliciting a dendritic cell-mediated immune response against malignant gliomas. Cancer Res 2006;66(21):10247–52.

NEUROLOGIC
CLINICS

Neurol Clin 25 (2007) 1141–1171

# Novel Therapies for Malignant Gliomas

Robert Cavaliere, MD[a],*, Patrick Y. Wen, MD[b],
David Schiff, MD[c]

[a]Division of Neuro-Oncology, Ohio State University, 463 Means Hall, 1654 Upham Drive,
Columbus, OH 43210, USA
[b]Center For Neuro-Oncology, Dana-Farber/Brigham and Women's Cancer Center,
SW430D, 44 Binney Street, Boston, MA 02115, USA
[c]Neuro-Oncology Center, University of Virginia Health Science Center,
Box 800432, Charlottesville, VA 22908-0432, USA

The blood-brain barrier effectively separates systemic circulation from the central nervous system (CNS), thereby creating a sanctuary within the CNS. As a result of the blood-brain barrier, large hydrophilic agents are excluded from the CNS. Yet it is recognized that the blood-brain barrier is "leaky" within tumors, thereby allowing the entry of agents that may otherwise have been excluded. Alternative mechanisms of drug delivery are being used to facilitate blood-brain barrier penetration. Agents are available that readily penetrate the blood-brain barrier. Subtypes of gliomas are now recognized as being chemosensitive. Consequently, interest in chemotherapy has increased and has become an active field of research for neuro-oncologists.

The last decade has also seen burgeoning interest in the use of novel therapies to treat high-grade gliomas, and a surfeit of theoretically promising agents and delivery strategies. Insight into the molecular biology of gliomas has increased our awareness of the mechanisms of tumor development and progression and resistance to treatment. Consequently, agents have been developed to undermine these abnormalities specifically. In addition, markers of response have allowed us to tailor treatment to specific tumors. As our understanding of treatment resistance increases, agents to sensitize tumors to available therapies are also being developed.

* Corresponding author.
E-mail address: robert.cavaliere@osumc.edu (R. Cavaliere).

## Cytotoxic chemotherapy

*Nitrosoureas*

Alkylating agents, including carmustine (BCNU) and lomustine (CCNU), have long been standard agents in the management of high-grade gliomas. These lipophilic agents, which readily penetrate the blood-brain barrier, act by forming DNA adducts that ultimately are converted into DNA cross-links. An early phase III clinical trial of radiotherapy with or without BCNU in patients who had glioblastoma (GBM) failed to demonstrate statistically significant improvements in median survival. Eighteen-month survival increased by almost 50%, however [1]. Subsequent studies of BCNU in primarily astrocytic tumors have been inconclusive [2]. Meta-analysis of the available data suggests nitrosoureas have modest activity against high-grade gliomas [3,4]. As such, until recently BCNU was commonly used in the adjuvant setting following radiotherapy or at the time of tumor recurrence. A recent phase II study of BCNU in patients who had recurrent GBM following surgery and radiotherapy demonstrated a median time to progression and 6-month progression-free survival of 13.3 weeks and 17.5%, respectively. Six evaluable patients (15%) had a partial response, and the 6-month overall survival was 55% [5].

CCNU, usually in combination with procarbazine and vincristine (commonly referred to as PCV), has been used routinely to manage oligodendroglial tumors. These tumors have been recognized as more chemosensitive than their astrocytic counterparts. It was recently recognized that in the presence of deletions of chromosomes 1p and 19q, oligodendrogliomas were exquisitely sensitive to chemotherapy. Two large randomized studies were reported in which patients who had oligodendroglial tumors were treated with radiotherapy with or without PCV. The Radiation Therapy Oncology Group (RTOG) randomized patients who had anaplastic oligodendroglial tumors to radiotherapy with or without preradiation, dose-intensive PCV [6]. Overall survival was similar between the two groups, although progression-free survival was longer among those treated with PCV (2.6 versus 1.7 years). Similar results were reported in a second phase III randomized study by the European Organization for Research and Treatment of Cancer (EORTC) [7]. In this study, patients who had oligodendroglial tumors were randomized to either radiotherapy alone or adjuvant standard PCV following radiotherapy. Once again, overall survival was similar between the two groups, although progression-free survival was prolonged among those randomized to PCV. A critical observation in both studies was that 1p/19q status was a more important predictor of outcome than treatment assignment (Table 1) [6,7]. The relative impact of tumor progression or treatment toxicity on quality of life was not assessed. Similar studies assessing the efficacy of temozolomide in patients who have

Table 1
The impact of 1p and 19q deletions on response to treatment and outcome in newly diagnosed, high-grade oligodendroglial tumors

|  | PCV/RT | RT alone |
| --- | --- | --- |
| RTOG phase III study [7] | | |
| Overall survival | | |
|   Combined 1p/19 deletion | NR | 6.6 y |
|   No combined deletion | 2.7 y | 2.8 y |
| Progression-free survival | | |
|   Combined 1p/19 deletion | NR | 2.6 y |
|   No combined deletion | 1.4 y | 1.0 y |
| EORTC phase III study [6] | | |
| Overall survival | | |
|   Combined 1p/19 deletion | NR | NR |
|   No combined deletion | 25.2 mo | 21.4 mo |
| Progression-free survival | | |
|   Combined 1p/19 deletion | NR | 62.2 mo |
|   No combined deletion | 15.3 mo | 8.9 mo |

*Abbreviations:* NR, not reached; RT, radiation therapy.

oligodendroglial tumors are ongoing in Europe and North America. Several treatment paradigms will be explored, including the relative impact of radiotherapy and chemotherapy and 1p/19q status.

*Temozolomide*

Temozolomide, an oral methylating agent with excellent bioavailability, is spontaneously hydrolyzed to its active metabolite at physiologic pH. The active metabolite, which readily penetrates the CNS, methylates DNA at the O6 and N7 positions of guanine and the N3 position of adenine. The cytotoxicity of temozolomide has been attributed to the O6 adduct, which, during replication, is incorrectly paired with thymine. This incorrect pairing leads to activation of the mismatch repair system, which removes the incorrectly paired base without correcting the underlying adduct. Consequently, thymidine is preferentially reinserted. Repetitive, futile attempts by the mismatch repair system to repair the DNA ultimately lead to cell death.

In a large EORTC phase III randomized study of patients who had newly diagnosed GBM, patients were randomized to radiotherapy with or without concomitant daily temozolomide ($75mg/m^2$ daily for the duration of radiotherapy). Those patients randomized to chemotherapy also received 6 months of adjuvant temozolomide ($200mg/m^2$ on days 1 through 5 of a 28-day cycle). The addition of temozolomide to radiotherapy improved median survival from 12.1 to 14.6 months. Two-year survival improved from 10.4% to 26.5%. Treatment was well tolerated, with grade 3 and

4 toxicity occurring in less than 10% of patients [8]. This study led to Food and Drug Administration approval of temozolomide for patients who have newly diagnosed GBM.

The optimal duration of adjuvant temozolomide following radiotherapy remains unknown. In the EORTC trial, six cycles of adjuvant temozolomide were administered following radiotherapy. Yet it is common practice in the United States to continue temozolomide for a longer duration. One study found that progression-free survival was shorter among patients who received 12 to 18 cycles of temozolomide and discontinued treatment in the absence of tumor progression than for patients who received temozolomide for more than 19 cycles [9]. In a retrospective review of 128 patients who received at least 12 cycles of temozolomide, grade III or IV thrombocytopenia, leukopenia, gastrointestinal toxicity, and infections occurred in 10%, 7%, 5%, and 4% of patients, respectively, suggesting that prolonged treatment is well tolerated [10]. Rare reports, however, linking temozolomide to myelodysplastic syndrome suggests a causative association [11,12].

Alternative temozolomide schedules are being evaluated. Daily administration of low doses of chemotherapy, referred to as metronomic dosing, has several theoretic advantages over standard dosing. Such schedules may deplete alkylguanine-alkyl transferase (AGT) in tumor cells, thereby overcoming tumor resistance (see later discussion). This finding was demonstrated in the peripheral mononuclear cells of patients treated with protracted schedules of temozolomide [13]. More frequent exposure of cells to chemotherapy may induce injury that would otherwise be repaired during chemotherapy breaks. In addition, such regimens may inhibit angiogenesis, a common feature in high-grade gliomas. Tumor-associated endothelial cells are genetically normal and therefore less likely to develop chemo-resistance than tumor cells; in addition, they have a significantly greater proliferative index than normal endothelial cells elsewhere in the body. Furthermore, tumor-associated endothelial cells are readily accessible to systemic therapy. Kim and colleagues [14] noted a significant decrease in microvessel density in mice treated with protracted schedules of temozolomide, compared with those treated with standard schedules. In addition, metronomic temozolomide dosing significantly inhibited tumor growth and induced apoptosis in otherwise temozolomide-resistant tumors. Metronomic temozolomide has not been explored extensively in patients who have GBM. In a pilot study of metronomic temozolomide in 12 patients who had recurrent GBM previously treated with radiotherapy and standard temozolomide, progression-free survival was 12 months. Two patients had partial radiographic responses and five had stable disease. No grade III/IV toxicity occurred [15]. Brandes and colleagues [16] treated 33 chemo-naïve GBM patients with temozolomide on days 1 through 21 of a 28-day cycle. The radiographic response rate was 9%, with an additional 51% having stable disease, and 6-month progression-free survival was 30%. No correlation was found between *methylguanine methyltransferase* (*MGMT*) promoter methylation (see later discussion) and radiographic response, progression-free survival, and overall survival. Protracted temozolomide schedules may, however, be associated with a higher rate of cumulative lymphopenia, occurring in 12% of early cycles and 91% of later cycles. Twenty-seven percent of patients developed grade III or IV lymphopenia during the study period, which was associated with a higher rate of infections (including one fatal fungal pneumonia). In addition, the study had a higher rate of treatment interruptions compared with standard schedules, and 10% of patients refused to continue treatment. The investigators suggested that, in the absence of superiority data, such protracted schedules should be reserved for clinical trials [17].

In a single-institution, retrospective review of patients treated with the current standard regimen, grade III/IV thrombocytopenia occurred in 19% of patients, of which 80% of cases were attributed to protracted temozolomide. The median duration of grade III/IV thrombocytopenia was 32 days. Four percent of patients required biweekly transfusions for over 6 months. Seventeen percent of patients discontinued treatment because of temozolomide [18].

An alternative, dose-intense, weekly alternating regimen, in which temozolomide is administered at 150 mg/m$^2$ on days 1 through 7 and 15 through 21 of a 28-day cycle, has also been considered. Comparatively, drug exposure is 2.1 fold greater than the standard 5-day regimen. In a small phase II study of patients who had recurrent GBM previously treated with radiation therapy (43% also received nontemozolomide chemotherapy), the radiographic response rate was 9.5%. Median progression-free survival was 21 weeks and 6-month progression-free survival was 48%, which compares favorably with standard temozolomide in a similar setting. Treatment was well tolerated, with mainly hematologic toxicity [19]. Currently, the RTOG is conducting a phase III trial (RTOG 0525) randomizing patients who had newly diagnosed GBM to either standard-dosed or protracted (21 consecutive days of a 28-day cycle) adjuvant temozolomide following radiotherapy.

*Chemotherapy resistance*

Resistance to treatment remains a major barrier to effective therapy. AGT is a DNA repair protein encoded by the *MGMT* gene on chromosome 10. It effectively removes alkyl groups from the O6 position of guanine, thereby reversing the cytotoxic lesion incorporated onto DNA by nitrosourea and temozolomide. Preclinical and clinical studies have linked increased cellular AGT to alkylator resistance [20–23]. Epigenetic silencing of *MGMT* by promoter methylation is associated with loss of *MGMT* expression (and consequently less cellular AGT), diminished DNA repair, and increased tumor chemosensitivity [24]. Among 36 patients who had newly diagnosed GBM treated with temozolomide, the response rate was 60% and 9.1% among those with tumors in which less than or greater than 20% of cell stained for AGT, respectively [20]. Other studies have shown a similar inverse relationship between tumoral AGT levels and radiographic response rate and overall survival in patients who had high-grade gliomas treated with BCNU and temozolomide [21–23]. Response to temozolomide and overall survival has also been shown to correlate with *MGMT* promoter methylation status [23,25]. Median survival among patients who had methylated tumors was 18.2 months, compared with 12.2 months among those whose tumors were not methylated. The *MGMT* promoter methylation status was a more significant predictor of outcome than treatment assignment in the EORTC randomized study (Table 2) [25].

Several strategies to overcome AGT-mediated chemotherapy resistance are under investigation. Preclinical data suggest that inhibition of AGT may sensitize otherwise resistant tumor cell lines to BCNU and temozolomide [26]. O6-benzylguanine (O6BG), an AGT substrate that irreversibly inhibits this enzyme, has been shown to deplete AGT in high-grade gliomas when administered to patients before surgery [27]. In a phase I study, however, myelosuppression necessitated significant dosage reductions of BCNU when combined with O6BG [28]. A subsequent phase II study evaluating this combination in patients who had recurrent high-grade glioma previously treated with BCNU reported very limited activity; only 5 of 18 patients achieved stable disease [29]. Similar results were encountered when this combination was used in patients who had soft tissue sarcomas and advanced melanoma [30,31]. In addition to myelotoxicity, lung injury was greater among mice treated with O6BG and BCNU, compared with BCNU alone [32]. Myelosuppression was the dose-limiting toxicity when a single dose of temozolomide was administered following treatment with O6BG [33]. In a phase III study of patients who had newly diagnosed GBM, the addition of O6BG to radiotherapy and BCNU did not improve overall and progression-free survival. Furthermore, toxicity, primarily hematologic, was significantly greater in the experimental arm [34].

Table 2
Median overall and 2-year survival among patients treated with radiotherapy with or without temozolomide according to *methylguanine methyltransferase* promoter status

| *MGMT* promoter status | Radiotherapy | Radiotherapy + temozolomide |
|---|---|---|
| Overall survival (mo) | | |
| Hypomethylated | 11.8 | 12.7 |
| Hypermethylated | 15.3 | 21.7 |
| 2-y survival (%) | | |
| Hypomethylated | <2.0 | 13.8 |
| Hypermethylated | 22.7 | 46.0 |

*Data from* Stupp R, Mason WP, van den Bent MJ, et al. Radiotherapy plus concomitant and adjuvant temozolomide for glioblastoma. N Engl J Med 2005;352(10):987–96.

Dose-limiting myelosuppression necessitated a greater than 50% dosage reduction of temozolomide when administered to children on a standard schedule with O6BG [35]. A phase II study of this combination is ongoing. Alternatively, systemic O6BG infusions combined with BCNU-impregnated wafers placed within the surgical cavity has been shown to be safe, without any systemic toxicity [36]. Another approach involves transfecting peripheral blood stem cells with a mutated *MGMT* that encodes an O6BG-resistant AGT. Subsequent treatment with O6BG and temozolomide in escalating doses may select for the resistant stem cells, thereby allowing for dose-intensification of temozolomide while minimizing myelosuppression. Preclinical studies were encouraging and pilot studies are ongoing [37,38].

The cytotoxicity of temozolomide has been attributed mainly to the O6 adduct. In addition to detoxification of DNA by AGT, the functional mismatch repair system is required for O6-methyl–mediated toxicity [39,40]. Less is known about the significance of the other more prevalent adducts that temozolomide induces (N7 of guanine and N3 of adenine). The base excision repair system efficiently repairs N-methyl adducts. During the initial step, the damaged base is removed by N-methyl-purine-DNA glycosylase, after which the DNA is cut at the abasic site by endonucleases. Subsequently, poly (ADP-ribose) polymerase (PARP) binds to and is activated by the DNA strand break. A cascade of events is initiated that culminates in the removal of the temozolomide-induced adducts and religation of DNA. PARP inhibitors, including INO-001, AG-14,361, and GPI-15,427, have been shown to enhance toxicity against neoplastic cells in the preclinical setting [41–43]. In particular, the strand breaks induced by the endonucleases are not ligated, culminating in cell death. In preclinical studies, PARP inhibitors have enhanced temozolomide-induced cytotoxicity; additionally, they are effective in cells with a dysfunctional mismatch repair system and proficient AGT [43]. Phase I studies combining PARP inhibitors with temozolomide are planned.

*Irinotecan*

Irinotecan, a water-soluble camptothecin derivative that inhibits topoisomerase I, is currently approved for patients who have metastatic colon and rectal cancer. Topoisomerase I binds to DNA as part of a cleavable complex that ultimately leads to single strand breaks. The complex and the single strand breaks are short-lived, and, ultimately, the double-strand integrity of DNA is restored. Camptothecin derivatives bind to and stabilize the cleavable complex, thereby preventing the religation of DNA. Cell death occurs when the replication fork encounters the cleavable complex. Although irinotecan itself is a weak topoisomerase inhibitor, it undergoes hepatic deesterification to an active lipophilic metabolite, SN-38. This metabolite is subsequently conjugated by uridine-diphosphoglucuronosyl transferase to form a less active metabolite, SN-38G.

Irinotecan has been studied extensively in patients who have recurrent high-grade glioma. Friedman and colleagues [44] reported a control rate of 70%, including a 17% response rate among patients who had recurrent GBM treated with irinotecan monotherapy weekly for 4 weeks followed by 2 weeks off. Median time to progression was 18 weeks. In contrast, a second phase II study reported that all patients had progressive disease within 6 weeks of initiating therapy [45]. The results of several other phase II studies confirmed only limited activity of single agent irinotecan in patients who had high-grade glioma, with disease control rates (including response rates and stable disease) of 10% to 48% and a median time to progression of 6 to 12 weeks [46–50]. However, phase I studies in patients receiving cytochrome P450–inducing anticonvulsants have reported the maximum tolerated dose of irinotecan to be increased 2 to 3.5 fold [51,52]. Unfortunately, even when accounting for irinotecan pharmacokinetics, its activity when administered as monotherapy is disappointing [49,50].

Irinotecan has also been evaluated in combination with other agents. Preclinical studies have shown that irinotecan and alkylating agents (which have different mechanisms of action and dose-limiting toxicities), including BCNU and temozolomide, have synergistic activity when administered together [53,54]. Furthermore, the enhanced cytotoxicity is schedule dependent and requires the administration of the alkylating agent before irinotecan [55]. Although the mechanism is unknown, it is thought that the enhanced cytotoxicity of the combination results from the presence of the O6 adduct before irinotecan exposure [55]. Pourquier and colleagues [56] demonstrated that incorporation of O6 methyl adducts immediately downstream of the topoisomerase I cleavage site resulted in an 8 to 10 fold increase in the formation of reversible cleavage complexes. Consequently, such cells are more sensitive to topoisomerase inhibitors that act by stabilizing the cleavable complexes. Removal of the O6 adduct by AGT abrogated the formation of the cleavable complexes [56].

Although a phase I study of BCNU and irinotecan in recurrent high-grade glioma demonstrated the combination to be well tolerated [57], a phase II study failed to confirm the synergistic activity of the combination. Among patients who had newly diagnosed and recurrent GBM, radiographic response rates (including partial and complete responses) were 11% each. Median time to progression of patients who had recurrent GBM was only 11.3 weeks [58]. A second study of this combination in patients who had recurrent GBM demonstrated similar results, with 21% achieving a partial radiographic response. Six-month progression-free survival and median time to progression were 30% and 17 weeks, respectively [59]. Both studies reported diarrhea to be among the most common side effects. In addition, pulmonary toxicity was noted in fewer than 10% of patients. A phase I study of temozolomide plus irinotecan in patients who had recurrent high-grade gliomas reported that both drugs can be administered safely at full doses without significant toxicity. The radiographic response rate was 14%, of whom one third had complete responses. Patients who had GBM had a median time to progression of 11.4 weeks [60]. In a small phase II study including 18 patients who had GBM, 5 patients had a radiographic response rate, including 2 complete responses. An additional 10 patients had stable disease. Median progression-free and 6-month progression-free survival were 22 weeks and 39%, respectively [61]. Additional phase II studies assessing temozolomide and irinotecan in the adjuvant setting following radiotherapy and at the time of tumor recurrence are ongoing.

Studies of other topoisomerase I inhibitors such as gimatecan, edotecarin, and karenitecin have show only minimal activity. Novel chemotherapeutic agents that can penetrate the blood-brain barrier, such as the anthracycline derivative RTA744, are currently in clinical trials.

## Molecular chemotherapy

Advances in our understanding of the molecular biology of gliomas have led to the development and application of agents that target proteins known to be overexpressed in gliomas, which theoretically permits selectively attacking causative abnormalities present in tumors cells, avoiding systemic toxicity. In addition, this treatment can be tailored to specific tumors based on detected molecular abnormalities. Several targets have been characterized, including tyrosine kinase receptors (TKR) and their intracellular effectors.

## Tyrosine kinase receptors

TKR, a broad group of receptors with similar molecular biology, are transmembrane proteins that contain an extracellular ligand-binding domain, an intracellular tyrosine kinase (TK) domain, and a transmembrane anchoring segment. Following ligand binding to the extracellular domain, homo- and heterodimeric complexes form, activating the intracelaular TK domains. Subsequently, intracellular proteins are phosphorylated and secondary signaling cascades, including the Ras-Raf-mitogen activated protein kinase (MAPK) and phosphatidylinositol-3-kinase (PI3K)/Akt pathways, are activated. Ultimately, gene transcription is modulated. Among the glioma-relevant receptor subtypes are the epidermal growth factor receptor (EGFR, erbB1), the platelet-derived growth factor receptor (PDGFR), the vascular endothelial growth factor receptor (VEGFR), and c-Met, the receptor for hepatocyte growth factor/scatter factor. These receptors and their ligands are overexpressed or mutated to varying extents on tumor cells and supportive tissue in malignant gliomas. Consequently, overactivation leads to aberrant intracellular signaling and tumor development or progression. Several drugs targeting these receptors and their intracellular effectors have been developed and are undergoing clinical evaluation (Table 3).

*Epidermal growth factor receptor*

Aberrant EGFR signaling is common in GBM; it occurs in approximately 50% of tumors, usually as a result of gene amplification. Additionally, EGFR gene mutations have been detected in as many as 75% of tumors with gene amplification. The most common mutation, referred to as the vIII mutant, is the loss of the coding sequence for amino acids 6-273. The resulting protein, present in 40% to 67% of EGFR-amplified tumors, lacks the extracellular ligand-binding domain, and has constitutive, ligand-independent activity. In its presence, cell proliferation and invasiveness are enhanced, apoptosis is inhibited, and tumor cells are resistant to chemo- and radiotherapeutics [62].

*Phosphatidylinositol-3-kinase/Akt/phosphatase and tensin pathway*

The PI3K/Akt pathway is one of several pathways that transduce signals from the cell membrane to the nucleus. It is commonly overexpressed in high-grade gliomas, either by excessive upstream stimulation (eg, EGFR overactivation) or downstream dysregulation. PI3K phosphorylation initiates a cascade of events that culminates in phosphorylation and activation of Akt. This enzyme subsequently phosphorylates several substrates that modulate genetic expression. One particular target, mammalian target of rapamycin (mTOR), plays a central role in cell survival and proliferation. The *phosphatase and tensin (PTEN)* suppressor gene located on chromosome 10 encodes a lipid phosphatase that inhibits this crucial pathway by removing phosphate groups from key intracellular signaling molecules. *PTEN* mutations, which occur in 30% to 40% of GBM, and deletions of chromosome 10, result in constitutive activation of the PI3K/Akt pathway. Such mutations have been associated with treatment resistance and a more aggressive phenotype [63].

The high incidence of EGFR and PIK3/Akt pathway dysregulation and its association with an aggressive phenotype make EGFR and PIK3/Akt pathway targeting attractive. Several lines of evidence support EGFR antagonism as a potential therapeutic [64,65]. Gefitinib (Iressa) and erlotinib (Tarceva), small-molecule, EGFR-specific TK inhibitors, compete with adenosine triphosphate at the intracellular catalytic site. Preclinical evidence suggests that both agents have activity against malignant gliomas. In addition, both agents synergize with radiotherapy and other pharmacologic agents [66–68]. Erlotinib was shown in preclinical studies to have activity against tumors bearing the vIII variant. In addition, long-term erlotinib exposure may decrease EGFRvIII expression [69]. Erlotinib and gefitinib undergo metabolism through CYP3A4. Consequently, concomitant usage of

Table 3
Selected targeted molecular agents in malignant gliomas

| Target | Molecular agent |
|---|---|
| Receptor tyrosine kinases | |
| EGFR | ATP-binding site inhibitors |
| | Erlotinib (OSI-774, Tarveca) |
| | Gefitinib (ZD1839, Iressa) |
| | Lapatinib (GW572016, Tykerb) |
| | Monoclonal antibodies |
| | Cetuximab (C225, Erbitux) |
| | h-R3 (nimotuzumab, TheraCIM, TheraLOC) |
| | $^{125}$I-MAb 425 |
| | mAb 806 (EGFRvIII monoclonal antibody) |
| | Fusion proteins |
| | TP-38 (TGF-$\alpha$/pseudomonas exotoxin) |
| PDGFR | ATP-binding site inhibitors |
| | Imatinib mesylate (STI-571, Gleevec) |
| | MLN518 |
| | Dasatinib (Sprycel®) |
| VEGFR | ATP-binding site inhibitors |
| | AEE788 |
| | AZD2171 |
| | Pazopanib (GW786034) |
| | Sorafenib (BAY439006, Nexavar) |
| | Sunitinib (SU11248, Sutent) |
| | Vandetanib (ZD6474, Zactima) |
| | Vatalanib (PTK787/ZK222584) |
| | Monoclonal antibody targeting VEGF |
| | Bevacizumab (Avastin) |
| | Soluble decoy receptor |
| | VEGF (VEGF-Trap) |
| IGFR | ATP-binding site inhibitors |
| | AG1024[a] |
| | NVP-TAE226[a] |
| c-Met | ATP-binding site inhibitors |
| | PHA66572[a] |
| | XL880 |
| | Monoclonal antibody targeting SF/HGF |
| | AMG 102 |
| Notch | Gamma secretase inhibitor |
| | MK 0752 |
| FGFR | ATP-binding site inhibitors |
| | 5'-methylthioadenosine (MTA)[a] |
| | TKI258[a] |
| | XL999[a] |
| Nonreceptor tyrosine kinases | |
| Src | ATP-binding site inhibitors |
| | Dasatinib (BMS-354,825) |
| FAK | ATP-binding site inhibitors |
| | NVP-TAE226[a] |
| Serine-threonine kinases | |
| Ras | Farnesyltransferase inhibitors |
| | Lonafarnib (SCH66336, Sarasar) |
| | Tipifarnib (R115777, Zarnestra) |

(continued on next page)

Table 3 (*continued*)

| Target | Molecular agent |
|---|---|
| Raf | ATP-binding site inhibitors |
| | Sorafenib (BAY439006, Nexavar) |
| MEK | Noncompetitive ATP-binding site inhibitors |
| | AZD6244[a] |
| | PD0325901[a] |
| PI3K | ATP-binding site inhibitors |
| | PI-103[a] |
| | BEZ235[a] |
| | PX-866[a] |
| Akt | Alkylphospholipid inhibitor |
| | Perifosine |
| mTOR | Small molecule inhibitors |
| | AP23573 |
| | Everolimus (RAD001) |
| | Temsirolimus (CCI-779) |
| | Sirolimus (Rapamycin; Rapamune) |
| PKC-β | ATP-binding site inhibitors |
| | Enzastaurin (LY317615) |
| TGF-βR | Antisense oligonucleotide to TGF-β |
| | AP 12,009 (specific for TGF-β) |
| CDK | ATP-binding site inhibitors |
| | Flavopiridol[a] |
| | UCN-01[a] |
| Multiple targets | |
| Multiple kinases | ATP-binding site multikinase inhibitors (targets) |
| | AEE788 (EGFR and VEGFR) |
| | AZD2171 (pan-VEGFR) |
| | Dasatinib (Src, Abl, VEGFR, PDGFR, and Flt-3) |
| | Imatinib (Abl, c-Kit and PDGFR) |
| | Lapatinib (EGFR and HER2) |
| | MLN518 (PDGFR, Flt-3, and c-Kit) |
| | NVP-TAE226 (FAK and IGF-IR)[a] |
| | Pazopanib (VEGFR, PDGFR and c-Kit) |
| | PI-103 (PI3K, mTORC1 and mTORC2)[a] |
| | Sorafenib (Raf, VEGFR-2, -3, PDGFR, Flt-3 and c-Kit) |
| | Sunitinib (VEGFR2, PDGFR, c-Kit and Flt-3) |
| | TKI258 (FGFR, VEGFR, PDGFR, Flt-3)[a] |
| | Vandetanib (EGFR and VEGFR2) |
| | Vatalanib (VEGFR and PDGFR) |
| | XL880 (c-Met, RON, VEGFR, PDGFR, Tie-2)[a] |
| | XL999 (FGFR, VEGFR, PDGFR, Flt-3)[a] |
| Chaperones | HSP90 inhibitors |
| | 17-allylaminogeldanamycin (17-AAG)[a] |
| | IPI-504[a] |

*Abbreviations:* ATP, adenosine triphosphate; CDK, cyclin-dependent kinase; FAK, focal adhesion kinase; FGFR, fibroblast growth factor receptor; HER2, human epidermal growth factor receptor 2; HSP90, heat-shock protein 90; IGF-IR, insulin growth factor I-receptor; IGFR, insulin-like growth factor receptor; MEK, mitogen activated protein (MAPK) kinase; mTOR, mammalian target of rapamycin; PKC, protein kinase C; RON, recepteur d'origine nantais; SF/HGF, scatter factor/hepatocyte growth factor; TGF, transforming growth factor.

[a] Not yet in clinical trials in gliomas.

*Adapted from* Chi A, Wen PY. Inhibiting kinases in malignant gliomas. Expert Opinion Ther Tar 2007;11(4):473–96; with permission.

enzyme-inducing anticonvulsants may accelerate degradation of these agents. The degree to which erlotinib and gefitinib penetrate the blood-brain barrier remains uncertain, although case reports suggest modest CNS and tumor penetration at previously demonstrated active concentrations [70,71].

Several studies have explored gefitinib in patients who have GBM. Rich and colleagues [72] treated 57 patients who had recurrent GBM with daily gefitinib. Six-month event-free and median event-free survival were 13% and 8.1 weeks, respectively. Of the 11 patients who had assessable disease, none had a radiographic response. Among 96 newly diagnosed GBM patients who were at least stable following radiotherapy, gefitinib did not improve overall or progression-free survival, compared with historical controls [73]. Expression of wild-type or mutant EGFR did not correlate with outcome, although the occurrence of diarrhea was associated with better overall survival in both studies.

EGFR dysregulation may contribute to the radioresistance of high-grade gliomas. EGFRvIII expression and wild-type EGFR overexpression are linked to radioresistance [74,75]. Furthermore, preclinical models suggest that radiotherapy may induce EGFR autophosphorylation and activation [76]. Antagonism of EGFR and its downstream effectors may reverse this phenomenon and sensitize cells to radiotherapy [67,74,76,77]. To exploit this, clinical trials have combined EGFR inhibitors with radiotherapy in high-grade glioma patients. In a phase I/II study of patients who had newly diagnosed high-grade glioma, the combination of gefitinib and radiotherapy was well tolerated. However, median overall survival was only 11 months and progression-free survival was 5.1 months, similar to historical controls [78]. In a phase I study of patients who had newly diagnosed GBM treated simultaneously with radiotherapy, temozolomide, and erlotinib, toxicity was significant (including three probable treatment-related deaths) and efficacy limited (median progression-free survival of 3.6 months) [79]. However, in another phase I study, erlotinib was administered concomitantly with radiotherapy after a 1-week run-in period of daily erlotinib. The combination was well tolerated, with 6 of 9 patients achieving stable disease in each group of patients who were or were not on enzyme-inducing anticonvulsants. Patients in the higher dose levels had longer overall survival than those who received lower dose levels, although the patient population was small [80].

Dysregulation of PI3K/Akt pathway and its association with tumor progression and development have led to the development of agents specifically targeting this pathway. Sirolimus (rapamycin) and its analogs, temsirolimus (CCI-779) and everolimus (RAD-001), form a complex with mTOR, thereby blocking its activity. In doing so, the downstream activation of PIK3/Akt effectors is reduced. These agents may reverse the overactivity associated with PTEN-deleted tumors. A phase II study of 41 patients who had recurrent GBM treated with temsirolimus monotherapy had two partial responses and 20 patients who had stable disease. Median time to progression and 6-month progression-free survival were short, however, at 9 weeks and 2.5%, respectively [81]. A second study of temsirolimus in recurrent GBM reported similar results: radiographic disease "regression" in 36% of patients with short median time to progression and 6-month progression-free survival (2.3 months and 7.8%, respectively). Neuroimaging response and p70s6 kinase phosphorylation showed a significant association in baseline tumors [82]. Temsirolimus is currently undergoing study in various combinations, including with temozolomide and with sorafenib.

The identification of markers of response to treatment with EGFR inhibitors is a critical step in evaluating the efficacy of these agents. In clinical trials, response to EGFR inhibitors is independent of the degree of amplification of EGFR [83]. EGFR mutations associated with TK inhibitor response in lung cancer (mutations in the kinase domain) are not present in malignant gliomas [84]. Favorable response to EGFR inhibitors has, however, been associated with the presence of the EGFRvIII mutant. Mellinghoff and colleagues [85] reviewed the molecular profiles of GBM treated with erlotinib and gefitinib at two institutions. They found that EGFRvIII-expressing tumors were more responsive to treatment than those without this mutated receptor. Furthermore, the enhanced sensitivity was present only in the presence of functional *PTEN*. If, however, *PTEN* function is lost, tumors become resistant to EGFR inhibitors. Akt-dependent and independent mechanisms underlie the loss of sensitivity to EGFR inhibitors. The greatest likelihood of a response to EGFR inhibitors occurred with coexpression of EGFRvIII and PTEN. Similarly, Haas-Kogan and colleagues [86] noted that the levels of phosphorylated Akt were the strongest predictors of response to erlotinib. Rich and colleagues [72], however, did not find EGFRvIII-expressing GBM to be more sensitive to gefitinib in their study. Lassman and colleagues [87] analyzed the tumor tissue of patients obtained while on treatment with EGFR inhibitors. The study showed no association between response to therapy and EGFR gene amplification or protein expression, the presence of mutations (although none of the analyzed tumors had the EGFRvIII variant), changes in EGFR phosphorylation, or downstream signaling. Steady-state concentrations of erlotinib and its active metabolite in tumor were low, possibly suggesting that drug penetration was low in the cases analyzed.

The emerging data that suggest that loss of *PTEN* function may contribute to resistance to EGFR inhibitors have prompted studies combining inhibitors of mTOR and EGFR [88]. In a retrospective review of 28 pretreated patients who had GBM treated with either erlotinib or gefitinib plus sirolimus, 19% and 50% of patients had a partial response or stable disease, respectively, and 6-month progression-free survival was 25% [89]. Wen and colleagues [90] combined erlotinib and temsirolimus in a phase I study that demonstrated significant rash and mucositis; efficacy results have not yet been reported. The combination of gefitinib and sirolimus was well tolerated in a phase I study of patients who had recurrent high-grade glioma, with a "tumor control" rate of 44% [91]. Two minor responses and a 6-month progression-free survival of 16.6% were reported in a study of 18 patients who had recurrent GBM treated with gefitinib and sirolimus [92]. Gefitinib and everolimus were combined in a phase I/II study of 19 heavily pretreated patients who had recurrent GBM, and the response rate was 32%. An additional 16% had stable disease. Median progression-free survival was only 2.6 months [93]. Studies evaluating the effectiveness and tolerability of this approach are ongoing.

*Platelet-derived growth factor receptor and vascular endothelial growth factor receptor*

Platelet-derived growth factor (PDGF) and vascular endothelial growth factor (VEGF) systems, both of which are overexpressed in gliomas, play a significant role in the development and progression of gliomas. These two intertwined systems are overexpressed predominantly in the stroma of tumors, where their actions predominate. In particular, they contribute to neoangiogenesis, a defining feature of high-grade gliomas. Pericytes, whose homeostasis is regulated in significant part by signaling thorough the PDGF system, are thought to provide endothelial cells with crucial survival signals. Consequently, antagonism of this system results in significant disruption of the normal vascular development [94–97]. In gliomas, PDGFR are located predominantly on endothelial cells, smooth muscle cells, and pericytes, whereas their expression is limited on tumor cells and in normal brain vasculature [98]. Coexpression of PDGFR and PDGF leads to the formation of autocrine loops and the activation of intracellular signal cascades, including Ras/Raf/MAPK, PI3K/Akt, and phospholipase C (PLC)/protein kinase C (PKC) pathways [99–102]. Several lines of evidence support the role of the autocrine loops on the gliomagenesis [101,103–106]. The PDGF system has been linked to neoangiogenesis, a common feature in gliomas [98,101,106,107]. Furthermore, in preclinical studies, interruption of the autocrine loop results had antitumor effects [108–113]. The most notable changes occur within the stroma of tumors [114,115]. Indirectly, PDGF influences the tumor environment by stimulating VEGF in stromal cells (vide infra) [107,116]. Thus, the impact of PDGF is mediated through VEGF-dependent and VEGF-independent mechanisms [107,116,117].

An emerging theory is that PDGF overexpression in tumor cells acts in a paracrine fashion to stimulate VEGF expression (thereby creating VEGF autocrine loops) in tumor endothelial cells, thus increasing endothelial cell proliferation and migration [107,118]. Also, PDGF acts directly on pericytes, which play an essential role in blood vessel development and maturation [107]. This mechanism occurs independent of VEGF.

It is well known that VEGF mRNA and protein are increased in gliomas [119]. Although VEGF expression is present in gliomas of all grades, it is more intense in tumors of higher grade [120]. VEGF expression correlates with tumor vascularity and tumorigenicity, is present in tumor cells and blood vessels around areas of necrosis, and is most prominent in glomeruloid capillaries. It is not present in the endothelium of normal brain [120,121]. VEGF is upregulated in gliomas through various mechanisms. Perhaps the most potent stimulant of VEGF expression is hypoxia, which leads to stabilization of the hypoxia-inducible factor that binds to the hypoxia response element within the VEGF promoter. Consequently, VEGF gene transcription is increased. In addition, hypoxia leads to increased stability of VEGF mRNA [122]. VEGF expression may also be increased in the presence of dysfunctional p53, a common aberration in gliomas [123,124]. Increased expression of VEGF may also occur by way of overactivation of PI3K, resulting from excessive stimulation from upstream TKR or aberrant regulation of the cascade, as occurs with PTEN mutations [125,126]. Both phenomena are known to occur in gliomas. VEGF may contribute to a malignant phenotype because it is a potent endothelial cell mitogen and chemotactant. In addition, VEGF induces the expression of several genes involved in extracellular matrix degradation, including urokinase and tissue plasminogen activators. Antagonism of the VEGF/VEGFR system by monoclonal antibodies, antisense sequences, induction of dominant negative mutants, or TK inhibition has been shown to inhibit tumorigenicity in glioma in in vivo and in vitro experiments [127–131].

The most extensively studied PDGFR inhibitor is imatinib mesylate (Gleevec), a selective receptor TK inhibitor. Of 34 patients who had recurrent GBM, 2 patients had partial responses and 5 had stable disease. Among 21 patients who had grade III gliomas, no patients had radiographic responses and only 5 patients had stable disease. Six-month progression-free survival was 3% and 10% among patients who had GBM and grade III gliomas, respectively. Although toxicity was low, five patients had intratumoral hemorrhage [132]. Similar disappointing results were reported in a second phase II study [133]. Imatinib has also been evaluated in combination with hydroxyurea. Among 30 patients who had recurrent GBM treated with this combination, 6 patients had radiographic responses, including one complete response. An additional 11 patients had stable disease. Six-month progression-free survival was 32% [134]. In a second phase II study of imatinib mesylate and hydroxyurea in patients who had recurrent GBM, radiographic response and stable disease rate were 9% and 42%, respectively. Six-month progression-free survival was 27% [135]. Several explanations have been offered for the apparent synergistic activity of this combination, including facilitating CNS penetration by efflux pump inhibition; reducing interstitial pressure, thereby improving chemotherapy delivery to tumor cells; and imatinib-mediated inhibition of DNA repair, which enhances hydroxyurea cytotoxicity. Given the promising activity of the imatinib/hydroxyurea combination, additional study is warranted. Similar to EGFR inhibitors, imatinib is CYP3A metabolized, and interaction with enzyme-inducing anticonvulsants must be considered [135].

Anti-VEGF strategies have recently assumed increasing importance in glioblastoma. Bevacizumab, a monoclonal immunoglobulin (Ig)G antibody that binds to and inhibits human VEGF-A, is the agent furthest along in malignant gliomas studies. In most studies, bevacizumab has been used in combination with irinotecan (Fig. 1). Among 21 patients who had malignant gliomas treated with this combination, 9 had a radiographic partial response (including 1 complete response) and 11 had stable disease [136]. A subsequent phase II study reported a 63% response rate, far exceeding historical controls. Six-month progression-free survival was 38% [137]. Similar encouraging results were reported in another smaller study [138]. Larger, multi-institutional studies of this regimen are ongoing. VEGF Trap (aflibercept), a soluble hybrid receptor composed of the VEGFR-1 second immunoglobulin (Ig) domain fused to the third VEGFR-2 immunoglobulin domain, binds and depletes circulating VEGF with greater potency than bevacizumab. Clinical trials of this agent in recurrent gliomas are in progress.

Targeting the VEGFR also holds promise. A recent phase II clinical trial used the oral, pan-VEGF TK inhibitor AZD2171 (cediranib) in recurrent/progressive glioblastoma [139]. Nine of 16 patients had radiographic partial responses (56%) and an additional 3 patients had minor responses (tumor shrinkage from 25% to 50%) (Fig. 2). The median progression-free survival of 16 weeks compared favorably with historical controls. Dynamic contrast-enhanced MR studies demonstrated that the agent had a rapid effect on vascular permeability and routinely improved vasogenic edema, often permitting a reduction in concomitant corticosteroids. Future planned studies of AZD2171 include its incorporation into

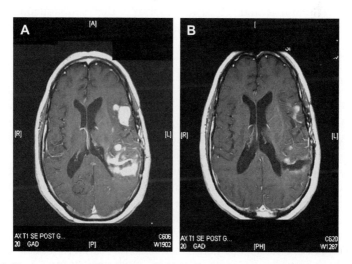

Fig. 1. A 44-year-old man with recurrent glioblastoma (*A*) treated with bevacizumab and irinotecan, showing marked reduction in enhancement after 4 weeks of therapy (*B*).

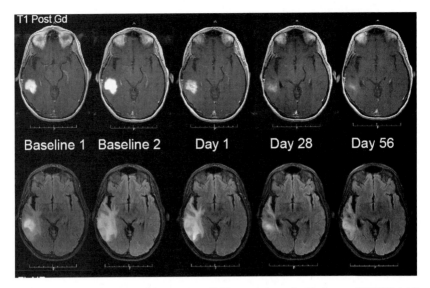

Fig. 2. A 47-year-old woman with recurrent glioblastoma treated with the pan-VEGFR inhibitor AZD2171, showing marked reduction of T1-contrast enhancement (*upper row*) and peritumoral edema on FLAIR images (*lower row*) over 56 days. Gd, gadolinium.

initial glioblastoma therapy with temozolomide and radiotherapy, and a phase III trial comparing AZD2171 alone and in combination with CCNU to CCNU alone. Multi-TK inhibitors, including sunitinib malate, vatalanib, and pazopanib (PDGFR and VEGFR inhibitors), sorafenib (Raf kinase and VEGFR/PDGFR inhibitor), and vandetanib (ZD6474) and AEE788 (EGFR and VEGFR inhibitors), that simultaneously target multiple TKR including VEGFR are also being studied in high-grade gliomas.

## Ras pathway and farnesyltransferase inhibitors

Ras is a G-protein that localizes to the inner surface of the plasma membrane. In its inactive form, ras is bound to guanine diphosphate. Upon ligand binding of certain receptors (including EGFR), guanine diphosphate is converted to guanine triphosphate, resulting in ras activation. Consequently, several downstream effectors are stimulated, including mitogen-activated protein kinase and protein kinase C. Before translocation to the cell membrane, ras undergoes a posttranslational lipid modification (farnesylation) catalyzed by farnesyltransferase (FTase).

Ras gene mutations resulting in constitutive activation are common in cancer but not gliomas. Nonetheless, activated ras is overexpressed in a large proportion of GBM. It is currently thought that overactive TKR, including EGFR, drive this increased activity.

Given the importance of ras in oncogenesis, pharmaceutic companies have developed FTase inhibitors that competitively inhibit FTase, thereby blocking farnesylation of ras. FTase inhibitors inhibit glioma growth through various mechanisms [140–142]. Furthermore, they are active regardless of ras mutational status [143]. One such agent, tipifarnib, was evaluated in a phase II study of patients who had recurrent high-grade glioma in which 6-month progression-free survival was only 11% among glioblastoma patients. Radiographic response rate was low and significant interaction with enzyme-inducing anticonvulsants was found [144,145]. Lonafarnib (SCH66336), another FTase inhibitor, has antiglioma activity in the preclinical setting [146].

## Angiogenesis, cell migration, and invasion

Neoangiogenesis remains a critical target of cancer therapeutics. This incompletely understood process involves a complex interaction of endothelial cells and the extracellular matrix [147]. In addition, glioma cells have remarkable invasive capabilities and can infiltrate the "normal" surrounding brain [148], which is perhaps their most malignant feature. Several approaches to inhibiting the migration of endothelial and tumor cells are being evaluated, including integrin antagonists (EMD-121,974, cilengitide), metrix metalloprotease inhibitors (marimastat, BB-2516), VEGFR TK inhibitors (sunitinib malate, Sutent), endothelin receptor antagonists (atrasentan, ABT-627), protein kinase C inhibitors (enzastaurin), and thalidomide and its analogs (lenolidamide), among others. Such approaches will be the focus of much research in the future, although little data are available currently.

## Other novel therapies

### TM-601

Novel methods of targeting tumor cells are being explored. TM-601, a synthetic version of the chlorotoxin found in the venom of the scorpion *Leiurus quinquestriatus*, has good blood-brain barrier penetration and selectively binds to glioma cells [149]. TM-601 has been conjugated with radioactive iodine and administered into the surgical cavity by way of an Ommaya or Rickham reservoir. Distribution of radioactivity following a single injection extended beyond the enhancing lesion, as demonstrated on T1-weighted postgadolinium images, and correlated more closely with the T2-hyperintense signal [150]. In addition, 131I-TM-601 localized to, and remained concentrated in and around, the surgical cavity for at least 5 to 7 days [150,151]. Systemic exposure was insignificant. A single injection was well tolerated without significant toxicity [151]. A phase II trial is in progress.

*Immunotherapy, gene therapy, and convection-enhanced delivery*

The use of immunotherapeutic approaches to fight gliomas has received substantial attention over the last 3 decades. Approaches have included adoptive immunotherapy (the passive administration of sensitized immune cells, largely abandoned in recent years), passive immunotherapy (target-specific exogenous antibodies), and active immunotherapy with tumor vaccines. Immunotherapy faces several major challenges within the CNS, including the absence of a lymphatic system, the presence of a blood-brain barrier, the paucity of tumor-specific antigens, and the secretion by gliomas of immunosuppressive factors including transforming growth factor (TGF)-$\beta$2 and interleukin (IL)-10.

A full discussion of immunotherapy is beyond the scope of this article. Several promising strategies are undergoing evaluation in clinical trials. These include passive immunotherapy approaches with radioactive iodine–labeled monoclonal antibodies to tenascin (an extracellular matrix protein) delivered into a tumor resection cavity [91,150]. Active immunotherapy approaches typically use dendritic cells, which are potent antigen-presenting cells that can be loaded with tumor lysates or peptides [85,91,152–154]. Another approach has been to use cells primed to recognize the EGFR vIII variant; of course, this approach may only be useful in the 30% of patients expressing this variant [155,156].

Convection-enhanced delivery is a novel method of delivering an agent that allows for the distribution of substances throughout the interstitial space by way of positive pressure infusion through stereotactically placed catheters. This technique allows the delivery of agents, independent of their size, beyond the blood-brain barrier to a targeted region. Several agents are being evaluated. Perhaps the most extensively studied agent is cintredekin besudotox (IL-13-PE38QQR), an IL-13 cytotoxin composed of human IL-13 (which targets the agent to the IL-13 receptor, which is differentially overexpressed in high-grade gliomas) and truncated pseudomonal exotoxin. Although initial phase I and II data were encouraging, a recent phase III study in which patients who had recurrent glioblastoma were randomized to the cintredekin besudotox or Gliadel wafers failed to show superiority of the study agent. Successful treatment depends on homogenous diffusion of the agent throughout the targeted region. Elevated interstitial pressure characteristic of brain tumors, however, may interfere with this process. Outcome also depends on optimal placement of the catheters, which influences drug delivery and distribution [157]. Other agents being evaluated are TP-38 (TGF-$\alpha$ conjugated to a mutated pseudomonal toxin), TransMID (transferring conjugated to a modified diphtheria toxin), and monoclonal antibodies [158,159].

Gene therapy is another venue of active investigation in high-grade gliomas. Gene therapies use viral vectors administered systemically or intratumorally by neurosurgeons. Two types of viral vectors are used: nonreplicating viruses that deliver transgenes whose expression leads to an anticancer effect, or replicating oncolytic viruses that achieve an anticancer effect through viral replication leading to cellular lysis [160]. Transgenes used in replication-deficient viruses (most commonly retroviruses and adenoviruses) inhibit angiogenesis, stimulate an antitumor immune response, correct genetic defects (ie, introduction of wild-type *p53* gene into *p53*-deficient gliomas), or encode a prodrug activating enzyme (ie, introduce the *HSV-TK* gene, which encodes a protein that converts ganciclovir into its toxic form). Replicating viruses consist of DNA viruses engineered to achieve tumor selectivity (herpes simplex virus) and wild-type attenuated RNA viruses with intrinsic tumor selectivity (ie, reovirus, poliovirus, measles). Gene therapy strategies have been evaluated in several studies that have demonstrated treatment to be safe, although larger studies are necessary to determine its effectiveness [160,161]. Limitations of these approaches include the efficiency of gene transduction into tumor cells, limited spatial distribution of transgenes or vector, and selection of appropriate targets in the setting of heterogeneous tumors.

## Summary

The impact of cytotoxic therapies on the outcome of glioblastoma has been modest thus far. Yet it is clear that subsets of high-grade gliomas exist that are sensitive to treatment, as the association between *MGMT*/AGT tumor status and temozolomide response suggests. Patients deemed resistant to the current standard approach may be selected for alternative therapies, thereby avoiding treatment toxicity from an ineffective treatment. However, commercially available assays to evaluate the *MGMT*/AGT system have not been developed, and the optimal method to evaluate *MGMT*/AGT status has yet to be determined. Several methods, including methylation-specific polymerase chain reaction, expanded segment gene sequencing, mRNA, and protein expression levels, have been used. It is conceivable that future studies will stratify patients by their *MGMT*/AGT status and ultimately select groups of patients for alternative therapies. A paradigm shift has already occurred for codeleted oligodendrogliomas, which are primarily being treated with upfront chemotherapy with deferred radiotherapy. Large collaborative group studies are ongoing to validate and refine this approach.

Mechanisms of resistance to cytotoxic chemotherapy are currently being elucidated. Consequently, protocols combining chemotherapeutics with treatment sensitizers are being explored. Thus far, toxicity has been significant, suggesting that many of the mechanisms are natural defenses in normal tissues. Nonetheless, additional study is warranted and ongoing. Focal therapies (such as convection-enhanced delivery or Gliadel wafers) combined with treatment sensitizers may minimize systemic toxicity.

Alternatively, rescue or protective strategies to minimize or correct systemic toxicity may allow for dose intensification of treatment. Furthermore, alternative treatment sensitizers, such as PARP inhibitors, may not result in significant toxicity. Molecular markers of response are also critical because mechanisms of resistance may differ among different tumors.

An increase in our knowledge of the molecular biology of malignant glioma has led to a dramatic increase in the number of potential therapeutics. The development of targeted therapies will allow for tailored treatment for specific tumors, based on the individual molecular profile. Thus far, however, such therapies have failed to improve outcomes significantly. Disappointing results may stem from the fact that most studies have evaluated monotherapy approaches. Yet it is well recognized that parallel pathways exist that converge and diverge, thereby allowing for bypass of a single molecular blockade. The most extensively studied molecular therapies thus far have been specific in their target. Novel agents that are broader in their targets are emerging. For example, sunitinib malate (Sutent), a multi-TK inhibitor of PDGFR and VEGFR, may be more active than imatinib mesylate, a selective PDGFR inhibitor. Furthermore, the heterogeneity of gliomas is such that all tumors will not respond to identical therapies. Rather, the sensitivity of a specific tumor to an agent may be predicated on specific molecular abnormalities within that tumor. As such, it is critical to identify markers of response to certain therapies. For example, PTEN-deleted glioblastomas and tumors with increased expression of phospho-Akt may be resistant to EGFR inhibitors, thereby negatively influencing the results of studies of these agents. Yet tumor without these abnormalities may still benefit from this approach. Future studies focusing on subsets of high-grade gliomas predicted, based on molecular markers, to be responsive to specific treatments will potentially improve on the discouraging results of the studies reported thus far. Furthermore, rational combination of agents, based on the molecular profile of tumors and their stem cells, may sensitize otherwise resistant tumors. To continue the above example, PTEN-deleted high-grade gliomas resistant to EGFR inhibitors may respond to the addition of mTOR inhibitors. Nonetheless, several obstacles exist to this approach. Adequate tissue for molecular analysis is not available at the time of tumor progression in most cases of recurrent glioblastoma. To date, standardized methods of evaluating molecular abnormalities are still lacking. Furthermore, completion of clinical trials evaluating specific subsets of glioblastoma would require extensive multi-institutional collaboration for timely accrual. Nevertheless, it is critical that the research community continue to focus on identifying tumor markers of response and ultimately refine our treatments in a more rational manner.

The future of novel therapies lies in our understanding of the molecular biology of gliomas and their stem cells. Not only will this drive the development of new agents, it will also lead to tailored therapies for specific tumors. Yet much research is still needed at all levels, from the identification of molecular markers to the development and application of novel therapeutics.

## References

[1] Walker MD, Green SB, Byar DP, et al. Randomized comparisons of radiotherapy and nitrosoureas for the treatment of malignant glioma after surgery. N Engl J Med 1980; 303(23):1323–9.

[2] Green SB, Byar DP, Walker MD, et al. Comparisons of carmustine, procarbazine, and high-dose methylprednisolone as additions to surgery and radiotherapy for the treatment of malignant glioma. Cancer Treat Rep 1983;67(2):121–32.

[3] Fine HA, Dear KB, Loeffler JS, et al. Meta-analysis of radiation therapy with and without adjuvant chemotherapy for malignant gliomas in adults. Cancer 1993;71(8):2585–97.

[4] Stewart LA. Chemotherapy in adult high-grade glioma: a systematic review and meta-analysis of individual patient data from 12 randomised trials. Lancet 2002;359(9311): 1011–8.

[5] Brandes AA, Tosoni A, Amista P, et al. How effective is BCNU in recurrent glioblastoma in the modern era? a phase II trial. Neurology 2004;63(7):1281–4.

[6] Cairncross G, Berkey B, Shaw E, et al. Phase III trial of chemotherapy plus radiotherapy compared with radiotherapy alone for pure and mixed anaplastic oligodendroglioma: Intergroup Radiation Therapy Oncology Group Trial 9402. J Clin Oncol 2006;24(18): 2707–14.

[7] van den Bent MJ, Carpentier AF, Brandes AA, et al. Adjuvant procarbazine, lomustine, and vincristine improves progression-free survival but not overall survival in newly diagnosed anaplastic oligodendrogliomas and oligoastrocytomas: a randomized European Organisation for Research and Treatment of Cancer phase III trial. J Clin Oncol 2006; 24(18):2715–22.

[8] Stupp R, Mason WP, van den Bent MJ, et al. Radiotherapy plus concomitant and adjuvant temozolomide for glioblastoma. N Engl J Med 2005;352(10):987–96.

[9] Colman H, Hess KR, Turner MC, et al. Impact of duration of temozolomide therapy on progression-free survival in recurrent malignant glioma (abstract 218). Neuro Oncol 2002;4(4):368.

[10] Hau P, Koch D, Hundsberger T, et al. Safety and feasibility of long-term temozolomide treatment in patients with high-grade glioma. Neurology 2007;68(9):688–90.

[11] Su YW, Chang MC, Chiang MF, et al. Treatment-related myelodysplastic syndrome after temozolomide for recurrent high-grade glioma. J Neuro oncol 2005;71(3):315–8.

[12] Noronha V, Berliner N, Ballen KK, et al. Treatment-related myelodysplasia/AML in a patient with a history of breast cancer and an oligodendroglioma treated with temozolomide: case study and review of the literature. Neuro oncol 2006;8(3):280–3.

[13] Tolcher AW, Gerson SL, Denis L, et al. Marked inactivation of O6-alkylguanine-DNA alkyltransferase activity with protracted temozolomide schedules. Br J Cancer 2003; 88(7):1004–11.

[14] Kim JT, Kim JS, Ko KW, et al. Metronomic treatment of temozolomide inhibits tumor cell growth through reduction of angiogenesis and augmentation of apoptosis in orthotopic models of gliomas. Oncol Rep 2006;16(1):33–9.

[15] Kong DS, Lee JI, Kim WS, et al. A pilot study of metronomic temozolomide treatment in patients with recurrent temozolomide-refractory glioblastoma. Oncol Rep 2006;16(5): 1117–21.

[16] Brandes AA, Tosoni A, Cavallo G, et al. Temozolomide 3 weeks on and 1 week off as first-line therapy for recurrent glioblastoma: phase II study from Gruppo Italiano Cooperativo di Neuro-Oncologia (GICNO). Br J Cancer 2006;95(9):1155–60.

[17] Tosoni A, Cavallo G, Ermani M, et al. Is protracted low-dose temozolomide feasible in glioma patients? Neurology 2006;66(3):427–9.

[18] Gerber DE, Grossman SA, Zeltzman M, et al. The impact of thrombocytopenia from temozolomide and radiation in newly diagnosed adults with high-grade gliomas. Neuro oncol 2007;9(1):47–52.

[19] Wick W, Steinbach JP, Kuker WM, et al. One week on/one week off: a novel active regimen of temozolomide for recurrent glioblastoma. Neurology 2004;62(11):2113–5.

[20] Friedman HS, McLendon RE, Kerby T, et al. DNA mismatch repair and O6-alkylguanine-DNA alkyltransferase analysis and response to temodal in newly diagnosed malignant glioma. J Clin Oncol 1998;16(12):3851–7.

[21] Belanich M, Pastor M, Randall T, et al. Retrospective study of the correlation between the DNA repair protein alkyltransferase and survival of brain tumor patients treated with carmustine. Cancer Res 1996;56(4):783–8.

[22] Jaeckle KA, Eyre HJ, Townsend JJ, et al. Correlation of tumor O6 methylguanine-DNA methyltransferase levels with survival of malignant astrocytoma patients treated with bischloroethylnitrosourea: a Southwest Oncology Group study. J Clin Oncol 1998;16(10): 3310–5.

[23] Esteller M, Garcia-Foncillas J, Andion E, et al. Inactivation of the DNA-repair gene MGMT and the clinical response of gliomas to alkylating agents. N Engl J Med 2000; 343(19):1350–4.

[24] Gerson SL. Clinical relevance of MGMT in the treatment of cancer. J Clin Oncol 2002; 20(9):2388–99.

[25] Hegi ME, Diserens AC, Gorlia T, et al. MGMT gene silencing and benefit from temozolomide in glioblastoma. N Engl J Med 2005;352(10):997–1003.

[26] Kanzawa T, Bedwell J, Kondo Y, et al. Inhibition of DNA repair for sensitizing resistant glioma cells to temozolomide. J Neurosurg 2003;99(6):1047–52.

[27] Friedman HS, Kokkinakis DM, Pluda J, et al. Phase I trial of O6-benzylguanine for patients undergoing surgery for malignant glioma. J Clin Oncol 1998;16(11): 3570–5.

[28] Friedman HS, Pluda J, Quinn JA, et al. Phase I trial of carmustine plus O6-benzylguanine for patients with recurrent or progressive malignant glioma. J Clin Oncol 2000;18(20): 3522–8.

[29] Quinn JA, Pluda J, Dolan ME, et al. Phase II trial of carmustine plus O(6)-benzylguanine for patients with nitrosourea-resistant recurrent or progressive malignant glioma. J Clin Oncol 2002;20(9):2277–83.

[30] Ryan CW, Dolan ME, Brockstein BB, et al. A phase II trial of O6-benzylguanine and carmustine in patients with advanced soft tissue sarcoma. Cancer Chemother Pharmacol 2006; 58(5):634–9.

[31] Gajewski TF, Sosman J, Gerson SL, et al. Phase II trial of the O6-alkylguanine DNA alkyltransferase inhibitor O6-benzylguanine and 1,3-bis(2-chloroethyl)-1-nitrosourea in advanced melanoma. Clin Cancer Res 2005;11(21):7861–5.

[32] Hansen RJ, Nagasubramanian R, Delaney SM, et al. Role of O6-alkylguanine-DNA alkyltransferase in protecting against 1,3-bis(2-chloroethyl)-1-nitrosourea (BCNU)-induced long-term toxicities. J Pharmacol Exp Ther 2005;315(3):1247–55.

[33] Quinn JA, Desjardins A, Weingart J, et al. Phase I trial of temozolomide plus O6-benzylguanine for patients with recurrent or progressive malignant glioma. J Clin Oncol 2005; 23(28):7178–87.

[34] Blumenthal DT, Rankin C, Stelzer K, et al. SWOG S0001: a phase III study of radiation therapy and O6-Benzylguanine plus BCNU versus BCNU alone for newly diagnosed glioblastoma and gliosarcoma (Abstract TA-404). Neuro Oncol 2006;8(4):438.

[35] Warren KE, Aikin AA, Libucha M, et al. Phase I study of O6-benzylguanine and temozolomide administered daily for 5 days to pediatric patients with solid tumors. J Clin Oncol 2005;23(30):7646–53.

[36] Weingart J, Grossman SA, Carson KA, et al. Phase I trial of polifeprosan 20 with carmustine implant plus continuous infusion of intravenous O6-benzylguanine in adults with

recurrent malignant glioma: new approaches to brain tumor therapy CNS consortium trial. J Clin Oncol 2007;25(4):399–404.

[37] Kreklau EL, Pollok KE, Bailey BJ, et al. Hematopoietic expression of O(6)-methylguanine DNA methyltransferase-P140K allows intensive treatment of human glioma xenografts with combination O(6)-benzylguanine and 1,3-bis-(2-chloroethyl)-1-nitrosourea. Mol Cancer Ther 2003;2(12):1321–9.

[38] Reese JS, Davis BM, Liu L, et al. Simultaneous protection of G156A methylguanine DNA methyltransferase gene-transduced hematopoietic progenitors and sensitization of tumor cells using O6-benzylguanine and temozolomide. Clin Cancer Res 1999;5(1):163–9.

[39] D'Atri S, Tentori L, Lacal PM, et al. Involvement of the mismatch repair system in temozolomide-induced apoptosis. Mol Pharmacol 1998;54(2):334–41.

[40] Cahill DP, Levine KK, Betensky RA, et al. Loss of the mismatch repair protein MSH6 in human glioblastomas is associated with tumor progression during temozolomide treatment. Clin Cancer Res 2007;13(7):2038–45.

[41] Curtin NJ, Wang LZ, Yiakouvaki A, et al. Novel poly(ADP-ribose) polymerase-1 inhibitor, AG14361, restores sensitivity to temozolomide in mismatch repair-deficient cells. Clin Cancer Res 2004;10(3):881–9.

[42] Tentori L, Leonetti C, Scarsella M, et al. Brain distribution and efficacy as chemosensitizer of an oral formulation of PARP-1 inhibitor GPI 15427 in experimental models of CNS tumors. Int J Oncol 2005;26(2):415–22.

[43] Cheng CL, Johnson SP, Keir ST, et al. Poly(ADP-ribose) polymerase-1 inhibition reverses temozolomide resistance in a DNA mismatch repair-deficient malignant glioma xenograft. Mol Cancer Ther 2005;4(9):1364–8.

[44] Friedman HS, Petros WP, Friedman AH, et al. Irinotecan therapy in adults with recurrent or progressive malignant glioma. J Clin Oncol 1999;17(5):1516–25.

[45] Chamberlain MC. Salvage chemotherapy with CPT-11 for recurrent glioblastoma multiforme. J Neurooncol 2002;56(2):183–8.

[46] Raymond E, Fabbro M, Boige V, et al. Multicentre phase II study and pharmacokinetic analysis of irinotecan in chemotherapy-naive patients with glioblastoma. Ann Oncol 2003;14(4):603–14.

[47] Cloughesy TF, Filka E, Kuhn J, et al. Two studies evaluating irinotecan treatment for recurrent malignant glioma using an every-3-week regimen. Cancer 2003;97(9 Suppl): 2381–6.

[48] Buckner JC, Reid JM, Wright K, et al. Irinotecan in the treatment of glioma patients: current and future studies of the North Central Cancer Treatment Group. Cancer 2003; 97(9 Suppl):2352–8.

[49] Prados MD, Lamborn K, Yung WK, et al. A phase 2 trial of irinotecan (CPT-11) in patients with recurrent malignant glioma: a North American Brain Tumor Consortium study. Neuro oncol 2006;8(2):189–93.

[50] Batchelor TT, Gilbert MR, Supko JG, et al. Phase 2 study of weekly irinotecan in adults with recurrent malignant glioma: final report of NABTT 97-11. Neuro oncol 2004;6(1): 21–7.

[51] Prados MD, Yung WK, Jaeckle KA, et al. Phase 1 trial of irinotecan (CPT-11) in patients with recurrent malignant glioma: a North American Brain Tumor Consortium study. Neuro oncol 2004;6(1):44–54.

[52] Gilbert MR, Supko JG, Batchelor T, et al. Phase I clinical and pharmacokinetic study of irinotecan in adults with recurrent malignant glioma. Clin Cancer Res 2003;9(8):2940–9.

[53] Coggins CA, Elion GB, Houghton PJ, et al. Enhancement of irinotecan (CPT-11) activity against central nervous system tumor xenografts by alkylating agents. Cancer Chemother Pharmacol 1998;41(6):485–90.

[54] Storm PB, Renard VM, Moriarity JL, et al. Systemic BCNU enhances the efficacy of local delivery of a topoisomerase I inhibitor against malignant glioma. Cancer Chemother Pharmacol 2004;54(4):361–7.

[55] Patel VJ, Elion GB, Houghton PJ, et al. Schedule-dependent activity of temozolomide plus CPT-11 against a human central nervous system tumor-derived xenograft. Clin Cancer Res 2000;6(10):4154–7.

[56] Pourquier P, Waltman JL, Urasaki Y, et al. Topoisomerase I-mediated cytotoxicity of N-methyl-N'-nitro-N-nitrosoguanidine: trapping of topoisomerase I by the O6-methylguanine. Cancer Res 2001;61(1):53–8.

[57] Quinn JA, Reardon DA, Friedman AH, et al. Phase 1 trial of irinotecan plus BCNU in patients with progressive or recurrent malignant glioma. Neuro oncol 2004;6(2):145–53.

[58] Reardon DA, Quinn JA, Rich JN, et al. Phase 2 trial of BCNU plus irinotecan in adults with malignant glioma. Neuro oncol 2004;6(2):134–44.

[59] Brandes AA, Tosoni A, Basso U, et al. Second-line chemotherapy with irinotecan plus carmustine in glioblastoma recurrent or progressive after first-line temozolomide chemotherapy: a phase II study of the Gruppo Italiano Cooperativo di Neuro-Oncologia (GICNO). J Clin Oncol 2004;22(23):4779–86.

[60] Reardon DA, Quinn JA, Rich JN, et al. Phase I trial of irinotecan plus temozolomide in adults with recurrent malignant glioma. Cancer 2005;104(7):1478–86.

[61] Gruber ML, Buster WP. Temozolomide in combination with irinotecan for treatment of recurrent malignant glioma. Am J Clin Oncol 2004;27(1):33–8.

[62] Cavaliere R, Newton H. Cytotoxic and molecular chemotherapy for high-grade glioma: an emerging strategy for the future. Expert Opin Pharmacother 2006;7(6):749–65.

[63] Knobbe CB, Merlo A, Reifenberger G. PTEN signaling in gliomas. Neuro Oncol 2002;4(3): 196–211.

[64] Raizer JJ. HER1/EGFR tyrosine kinase inhibitors for the treatment of glioblastoma multiforme. J Neurooncol 2005;74(1):77–86.

[65] Halatsch ME, Schmidt U, Behnke-Mursch J, et al. Epidermal growth factor receptor inhibition for the treatment of glioblastoma multiforme and other malignant brain tumours. Cancer Treat Rev 2006;32(2):74–89.

[66] Chinnaiyan P, Huang S, Vallabhaneni G, et al. Mechanisms of enhanced radiation response following epidermal growth factor receptor signaling inhibition by erlotinib (Tarceva). Cancer Res 2005;65(8):3328–35.

[67] Stea B, Falsey R, Kislin K, et al. Time and dose-dependent radiosensitization of the glioblastoma multiforme U251 cells by the EGF receptor tyrosine kinase inhibitor ZD1839 ('Iressa'). Cancer Lett 2003;202(1):43–51.

[68] Carlson BL, Schroeder MA, Mladek AC, et al. Radiosensitization by OSI-774 of serially transplantable human GBM xenografts. Neuro-oncol 2003;5(4):321.

[69] Iwata KK, Provancha K, Gibson N. Inhibition of mutant EGFRvIII transformed cells by tyrosine kinase inhibitor OSI-774 [Abstract 79]. In: Proc Am Soc Clin Oncol 2002. p. 21a.

[70] Hofer S, Frei K, Rutz HP. Gefitinib accumulation in glioblastoma tissue. Cancer Biol Ther 2006;5(5):483–4.

[71] Broniscer A, Panetta JC, O'Shaughnessy M, et al. Plasma and cerebrospinal fluid pharmacokinetics of erlotinib and its active metabolite OSI-420. Clin Cancer Res 2007;13(5): 1511–5.

[72] Rich JN, Reardon DA, Peery T, et al. Phase II trial of gefitinib in recurrent glioblastoma. J Clin Oncol 2004;22(1):133–42.

[73] Uhm JH, Ballman KV, Giannini C, et al. Phase II study of ZD 1839 in patients with newly diagnosed grade 4 astrocytoma [Abstract 1505]. In: Proc Am Soc Clin Oncol 2004. p. 108.

[74] Li B, Yuan M, Kim IA, et al. Mutant epidermal growth factor receptor displays increased signaling through the phosphatidylinositol-3 kinase/AKT pathway and promotes radioresistance in cells of astrocytic origin. Oncogene 2004;23(26):4594–602.

[75] Barker FG 2nd, Simmons ML, Chang SM, et al. EGFR overexpression and radiation response in glioblastoma multiforme. Int J Radiat Oncol Biol Phys 2001;51(2):410–8.

[76] Chakravarti A, Chakladar A, Delaney MA, et al. The epidermal growth factor receptor pathway mediates resistance to sequential administration of radiation and chemotherapy

in primary human glioblastoma cells in a RAS-dependent manner. Cancer Res 2002;62(15): 4307–15.

[77] Lammering G, Valerie K, Lin PS, et al. Radiosensitization of malignant glioma cells through overexpression of dominant-negative epidermal growth factor receptor. Clin Cancer Res 2001;7(3):682–90.

[78] Chakravarti A, Berkley B, Robins HI, et al. An update of the phase II study results from RTOG 0211: a phase I/II study of gefitinib with radiotherapy in newly diagnosed glioblastoma multiforme [Abstract TA-408]. Neuro Oncol 2006;8(4):439.

[79] Peereboom D, Brewer C, Suh J, et al. Phase II trial of erlotinib with temozolomide and concurrent radiation therapy in patients with newly diagnosed glioblastoma multiforme: final results [Abstract TA-441]. Neuro Oncol 2006;8(4):448.

[80] Krishnan S, Brown PD, Ballman KV, et al. Phase I trial of erlotinib with radiation therapy in patients with glioblastoma multiforme: results of North Central Cancer Treatment Group protocol N0177. Int J Radiat Oncol Biol Phys 2006;65(4):1192–9.

[81] Chang SM, Wen P, Cloughesy T, et al. Phase II study of CCI-779 in patients with recurrent glioblastoma multiforme. Invest New Drugs 2005;23(4):357–61.

[82] Galanis E, Buckner JC, Maurer MJ, et al. Phase II trial of temsirolimus (CCI-779) in recurrent glioblastoma multiforme: a North Central Cancer Treatment Group Study. J Clin Oncol 2005;23(23):5294–304.

[83] Halatsch ME, Gehrke EE, Vougioukas VI, et al. Inverse correlation of epidermal growth factor receptor messenger RNA induction and suppression of anchorage-independent growth by OSI-774, an epidermal growth factor receptor tyrosine kinase inhibitor, in glioblastoma multiforme cell lines. J Neurosurg 2004;100(3):523–33.

[84] Marie Y, Carpentier AF, Omuro AM, et al. EGFR tyrosine kinase domain mutations in human gliomas. Neurology 2005;64(8):1444–5.

[85] Mellinghoff IK, Wang MY, Vivanco I, et al. Molecular determinants of the response of glioblastomas to EGFR kinase inhibitors. N Engl J Med 2005;353(19):2012–24.

[86] Haas-Kogan DA, Prados MD, Tihan T, et al. Epidermal growth factor receptor, protein kinase B/Akt, and glioma response to erlotinib. J Natl Cancer Inst 2005;97(12): 880–7.

[87] Lassman AB, Rossi MR, Raizer JJ, et al. Molecular study of malignant gliomas treated with epidermal growth factor receptor inhibitors: tissue analysis from North American Brain Tumor Consortium Trials 01-03 and 00-01. Clin Cancer Res 2005; 11(21):7841–50.

[88] Rao RD, Mladek AC, Lamont JD, et al. Disruption of parallel and converging signaling pathways contributes to the synergistic antitumor effects of simultaneous mTOR and EGFR inhibition in GBM cells. Neoplasia 2005;7(10):921–9.

[89] Doherty L, Gigas DC, Kesari S, et al. Pilot study of the combination of EGFR and mTOR inhibitors in recurrent malignant gliomas. Neurology 2006;67(1):156–8.

[90] Wen P, Chang SM, Kuhn J, et al. Phase I study of erlotinib and temsirolimus for patients with recurrent malignant glioma. Neuro Oncol 2006;8(4):454.

[91] Reardon DA, Quinn JA, Vredenburgh JJ, et al. Phase 1 trial of gefitinib plus sirolimus in adults with recurrent malignant glioma. Clin Cancer Res 2006;12(3 Pt 1):860–8.

[92] Badruddoja M, Das A, Chu RM, et al. Gefitinib and Rapamycin for adult patients with recurrent glioblastoma multiforme. Neuro Oncol 2006;8(4):438.

[93] Nguyen TDL, AB, Lis E, et al. A pilot study to assess the tolerability and efficacy of RAD-001 (Everolimus) with gefitinib in patients with glioblastoma multiforme. Neuro Oncol 2006;8(4):447.

[94] Hellstrom M, Kalen M, Lindahl P, et al. Role of PDGF-B and PDGFR-beta in recruitment of vascular smooth muscle cells and pericytes during embryonic blood vessel formation in the mouse. Development 1999;126(14):3047–55.

[95] Lindahl P, Johansson BR, Leveen P, et al. Pericyte loss and microaneurysm formation in PDGF-B-deficient mice. Science 1997;277(5323):242–5.

[96] Sano H, Ueda Y, Takakura N, et al. Blockade of platelet-derived growth factor receptor-beta pathway induces apoptosis of vascular endothelial cells and disrupts glomerular capillary formation in neonatal mice. Am J Pathol 2002;161(1):135–43.

[97] Bergers G, Song S, Meyer-Morse N, et al. Benefits of targeting both pericytes and endothelial cells in the tumor vasculature with kinase inhibitors. J Clin Invest 2003;111(9): 1287–95.

[98] Plate KH, Breier G, Farrell CL, et al. Platelet-derived growth factor receptor-beta is induced during tumor development and upregulated during tumor progression in endothelial cells in human gliomas. Lab Invest 1992;67(4):529–34.

[99] Holmen SL, Williams BO. Essential role for Ras signaling in glioblastoma maintenance. Cancer Res 2005;65(18):8250–5.

[100] Chakravarti A, Zhai G, Suzuki Y, et al. The prognostic significance of phosphatidylinositol 3-kinase pathway activation in human gliomas. J Clin Oncol 2004;22(10):1926–33.

[101] Hermanson M, Funa K, Hartman M, et al. Platelet-derived growth factor and its receptors in human glioma tissue: expression of messenger RNA and protein suggests the presence of autocrine and paracrine loops. Cancer Res 1992;52(11):3213–9.

[102] Guha A, Dashner K, Black PM, et al. Expression of PDGF and PDGF receptors in human astrocytoma operation specimens supports the existence of an autocrine loop. Int J Cancer 1995;60(2):168–73.

[103] Uhrbom L, Hesselager G, Nister M, et al. Induction of brain tumors in mice using a recombinant platelet-derived growth factor B-chain retrovirus. Cancer Res 1998;58(23): 5275–9.

[104] Dai C, Celestino JC, Okada Y, et al. PDGF autocrine stimulation dedifferentiates cultured astrocytes and induces oligodendrogliomas and oligoastrocytomas from neural progenitors and astrocytes in vivo. Genes Dev 2001;15(15):1913–25.

[105] Clarke ID, Dirks PB. A human brain tumor-derived PDGFR-alpha deletion mutant is transforming. Oncogene 2003;22(5):722–33.

[106] Shih AH, Dai C, Hu X, et al. Dose-dependent effects of platelet-derived growth factor-B on glial tumorigenesis. Cancer Res 2004;64(14):4783–9.

[107] Guo P, Hu B, Gu W, et al. Platelet-derived growth factor-B enhances glioma angiogenesis by stimulating vascular endothelial growth factor expression in tumor endothelia and by promoting pericyte recruitment. Am J Pathol 2003;162(4):1083–93.

[108] Lokker NA, Sullivan CM, Hollenbach SJ, et al. Platelet-derived growth factor (PDGF) autocrine signaling regulates survival and mitogenic pathways in glioblastoma cells: evidence that the novel PDGF-C and PDGF-D ligands may play a role in the development of brain tumors. Cancer Res 2002;62(13):3729–35.

[109] Kilic T, Alberta JA, Zdunek PR, et al. Intracranial inhibition of platelet-derived growth factor-mediated glioblastoma cell growth by an orally active kinase inhibitor of the 2-phenylaminopyrimidine class. Cancer Res 2000;60(18):5143–50.

[110] Fleming TP, Matsui T, Heidaran MA, et al. Demonstration of an activated platelet-derived growth factor autocrine pathway and its role in human tumor cell proliferation in vitro. Oncogene 1992;7(7):1355–9.

[111] Takeuchi H, Kanzawa T, Kondo Y, et al. Inhibition of platelet-derived growth factor signalling induces autophagy in malignant glioma cells. Br J Cancer 2004;90(5):1069–75.

[112] Strawn LM, Mann E, Elliger SS, et al. Inhibition of glioma cell growth by a truncated platelet-derived growth factor-beta receptor. J Biol Chem 1994;269(33):21215–22.

[113] Vassbotn FS, Andersson M, Westermark B, et al. Reversion of autocrine transformation by a dominant negative platelet-derived growth factor mutant. Mol Cell Biol 1993;13(7): 4066–76.

[114] Farhadi MR, Capelle HH, Erber R, et al. Combined inhibition of vascular endothelial growth factor and platelet-derived growth factor signaling: effects on the angiogenesis, microcirculation, and growth of orthotopic malignant gliomas. J Neurosurg 2005;102(2): 363–70.

[115] Erber R, Thurnher A, Katsen AD, et al. Combined inhibition of VEGF and PDGF signaling enforces tumor vessel regression by interfering with pericyte-mediated endothelial cell survival mechanisms. FASEB J 2004;18(2):338–40.

[116] Wang D, Huang HJ, Kazlauskas A, et al. Induction of vascular endothelial growth factor expression in endothelial cells by platelet-derived growth factor through the activation of phosphatidylinositol 3-kinase. Cancer Res 1999;59(7):1464–72.

[117] Roberts WG, Whalen PM, Soderstrom E, et al. Antiangiogenic and antitumor activity of a selective PDGFR tyrosine kinase inhibitor, CP-673,451. Cancer Res 2005;65(3): 957–66.

[118] Dunn IF, Heese O, Black PM. Growth factors in glioma angiogenesis: FGFs, PDGF, EGF, and TGFs. J Neurooncol 2000;50(1–2):121–37.

[119] Plate KH, Breier G, Weich HA, et al. Vascular endothelial growth factor is a potential tumour angiogenesis factor in human gliomas in vivo. Nature 1992;359(6398): 845–8.

[120] Chaudhry IH, O'Donovan DG, Brenchley PE, et al. Vascular endothelial growth factor expression correlates with tumour grade and vascularity in gliomas. Histopathology 2001; 39(4):409–15.

[121] Ke LD, Shi YX, Im SA, et al. The relevance of cell proliferation, vascular endothelial growth factor, and basic fibroblast growth factor production to angiogenesis and tumorigenicity in human glioma cell lines. Clin Cancer Res 2000;6(6):2562–72.

[122] Ikeda E, Achen MG, Breier G, et al. Hypoxia-induced transcriptional activation and increased mRNA stability of vascular endothelial growth factor in C6 glioma cells. J Biol Chem 1995;270(34):19761–6.

[123] Kieser A, Weich HA, Brandner G, et al. Mutant p53 potentiates protein kinase C induction of vascular endothelial growth factor expression. Oncogene 1994;9(3):963–9.

[124] Yu JL, Rak JW, Coomber BL, et al. Effect of p53 status on tumor response to antiangiogenic therapy. Science 2002;295(5559):1526–8.

[125] Jiang BH, Jiang G, Zheng JZ, et al. Phosphatidylinositol 3-kinase signaling controls levels of hypoxia-inducible factor 1. Cell Growth Differ 2001;12(7):363–9.

[126] Pore N, Liu S, Haas-Kogan DA, et al. PTEN mutation and epidermal growth factor receptor activation regulate vascular endothelial growth factor (VEGF) mRNA expression in human glioblastoma cells by transactivating the proximal VEGF promoter. Cancer Res 2003;63(1):236–41.

[127] Kim KJ, Li B, Winer J, et al. Inhibition of vascular endothelial growth factor-induced angiogenesis suppresses tumour growth in vivo. Nature 1993;362(6423):841–4.

[128] Millauer B, Shawver LK, Plate KH, et al. Glioblastoma growth inhibited in vivo by a dominant-negative Flk-1 mutant. Nature 1994;367(6463):576–9.

[129] Millauer B, Longhi MP, Plate KH, et al. Dominant-negative inhibition of Flk-1 suppresses the growth of many tumor types in vivo. Cancer Res 1996;56(7):1615–20.

[130] Saleh M, Stacker SA, Wilks AF. Inhibition of growth of C6 glioma cells in vivo by expression of antisense vascular endothelial growth factor sequence. Cancer Res 1996;56(2): 393–401.

[131] Kunkel P, Ulbricht U, Bohlen P, et al. Inhibition of glioma angiogenesis and growth in vivo by systemic treatment with a monoclonal antibody against vascular endothelial growth factor receptor-2. Cancer Res 2001;61(18):6624–8.

[132] Wen PY, Yung WK, Lamborn KR, et al. Phase I/II study of imatinib mesylate for recurrent malignant gliomas: North American Brain Tumor Consortium Study 99-08. Clin Cancer Res 2006;12(16):4899–907.

[133] Raymond E, Brandes A, Van Oosterom AT, et al. Multicentre phase II study of imatinib mesylate in patients with recurrent glioblastoma: an EORTC: NDDG/BTG Intergroup Study. In: Proc Am Soc Clin Oncol 2004. p. 107.

[134] Dresemann G. Imatinib and hydroxyurea in pretreated progressive glioblastoma multiforme: a patient series. Ann Oncol 2005;16(10):1702–8.

[135] Reardon DA, Egorin MJ, Quinn JA, et al. Phase II study of imatinib mesylate plus hydroxyurea in adults with recurrent glioblastoma multiforme. J Clin Oncol 2005;23(36): 9359–68.

[136] Stark-Vance V. Bevacizumab and CPT-11 in the treatment of relapsed malignant glioma. Neuro-oncol 2005;7(3):369.

[137] Vredenburgh JJ, Desjardins A, Herndon JE 2nd, et al. Phase II trial of bevacizumab and irinotecan in recurrent malignant glioma. Clin Cancer Res 2007;13(4):1253–9.

[138] Bokstein F, Blumenthal DT. Treatment of recurrent high-grade glial tumors with bevacizumab and intrinotecan: preliminary results (Abstract TA-405). Neuro Oncol 2006;8(4): 438.

[139] Batchelor TT, Sorensen AG, di Tomaso E, et al. AZD2171, a pan-VEGF receptor tyrosine kinase inhibitor, normalizes tumor vasculature and alleviates edema in glioblastoma patients. Cancer Cell 2007;11(1):83–95.

[140] Delmas C, End D, Rochaix P, et al. The farnesyltransferase inhibitor R115777 reduces hypoxia and matrix metalloproteinase 2 expression in human glioma xenograft. Clin Cancer Res 2003;9(16 Pt 1):6062–8.

[141] Feldkamp MM, Lau N, Guha A. Growth inhibition of astrocytoma cells by farnesyl transferase inhibitors is mediated by a combination of anti-proliferative, pro-apoptotic and antiangiogenic effects. Oncogene 1999;18(52):7514–26.

[142] Pollack IF, Bredel M, Erff M, et al. Inhibition of Ras and related guanosine triphosphate-dependent proteins as a therapeutic strategy for blocking malignant glioma growth: II–preclinical studies in a nude mouse model. Neurosurgery 1999;45(5):1208–14 [discussion: 1214–5].

[143] Feldkamp MM, Lau N, Roncari L, et al. Isotype-specific Ras-GTP-levels predict the efficacy of farnesyl transferase inhibitors against human astrocytomas regardless of Ras mutational status. Cancer Res 2001;61(11):4425–31.

[144] Cloughesy TF, Wen PY, Robins HI, et al. Phase II trial of tipifarnib in patients with recurrent malignant glioma either receiving or not receiving enzyme-inducing antiepileptic drugs: a North American Brain Tumor Consortium Study. J Clin Oncol 2006;24(22): 3651–6.

[145] Cloughesy TF, Kuhn J, Robins HI, et al. Phase I trial of tipifarnib in patients with recurrent malignant glioma taking enzyme-inducing antiepileptic drugs: a North American Brain Tumor Consortium Study. J Clin Oncol 2005;23(27):6647–56.

[146] Glass TL, Liu TJ, Yung WK. Inhibition of cell growth in human glioblastoma cell lines by farnesyltransferase inhibitor SCH66336. Neuro oncol 2000;2(3):151–8.

[147] Wesseling P, Ruiter DJ, Burger PC. Angiogenesis in brain tumors; pathobiological and clinical aspects. J Neurooncol 1997;32(3):253–65.

[148] Nakada M, Nakada S, Demuth T, et al. Molecular targets of glioma invasion. Cell Mol Life Sci 2007;64(4):458–78.

[149] Lyons SA, O'Neal J, Sontheimer H. Chlorotoxin, a scorpion-derived peptide, specifically binds to gliomas and tumors of neuroectodermal origin. Glia 2002;39(2):162–73.

[150] Hockaday DC, Shen S, Fiveash J, et al. Imaging glioma extent with 131I-TM-601. J Nucl Med 2005;46(4):580–6.

[151] Mamelak AN, Rosenfeld S, Bucholz R, et al. Phase I single-dose study of intracavitary-administered iodine-131-TM-601 in adults with recurrent high-grade glioma. J Clin Oncol 2006;24(22):3644–50.

[152] Reardon DA, Akabani G, Coleman RE, et al. Phase II trial of murine (131)I-labeled anti-tenascin monoclonal antibody 81C6 administered into surgically created resection cavities of patients with newly diagnosed malignant gliomas. J Clin Oncol 2002;20(5):1389–97.

[153] Wheeler CJ, Das A, Liu G, et al. Clinical responsiveness of glioblastoma multiforme to chemotherapy after vaccination. Clin Cancer Res 2004;10(16):5316–26.

[154] Yu JS, Luptrawan A, Black KL, et al. Mahaley Clinical Research Award: chemosensitization of glioma through dendritic cell vaccination. Clin Neurosurg 2006;53:345–51.

[155] Heimberger AB, Crotty LE, Archer GE, et al. Epidermal growth factor receptor VIII peptide vaccination is efficacious against established intracerebral tumors. Clin Cancer Res 2003;9(11):4247–54.

[156] Hussain AE, Blakley BW, Nicolas M, et al. Assessment of the protective effects of amifostine against cisplatin-induced toxicity. J Otolaryngol 2003;32(5):294–7.

[157] Kunwar S, Prados MD, Chang SM, et al. Direct intracerebral delivery of cintredekin besudotox (IL13-PE38QQR) in recurrent malignant glioma: a report by the Cintredekin Besudotox Intraparenchymal Study Group. J Clin Oncol 2007;25(7):837–44.

[158] Hall WA, Rustamzadeh E, Asher AL. Convection-enhanced delivery in clinical trials. Neurosurg Focus 2003;14(2):e2.

[159] Vogelbaum MA. Convection enhanced delivery for the treatment of malignant gliomas: symposium review. J Neuro oncol 2005;73(1):57–69.

[160] Aghi M, Chiocca EA. Gene therapy for glioblastoma. Neurosurg Focus 2006;20(4):E18.

[161] Pulkkanen KJ, Yla-Herttuala S. Gene therapy for malignant glioma: current clinical status. Mol Ther 2005;12(4):585–98.

ELSEVIER
SAUNDERS

NEUROLOGIC
CLINICS

Neurol Clin 25 (2007) 1173–1192

# Brain Metastases

## Teri D. Nguyen, MD, Lisa M. DeAngelis, MD*

*Department of Neurology, Memorial Sloan-Kettering Cancer Center, 1275 York Avenue,
New York, NY 10021, USA*

Brain metastases are a common complication of cancer and can affect 20% to 40% of patients [1]. This often-quoted estimate is derived primarily from large autopsy series describing patients from 3 decades ago, and probably underestimates the true current lifetime prevalence. Advances in oncology have extended survival for cancer patients since that time period, leading to a larger population at risk for this late complication of disease. Brain metastases are 10 times more common than primary brain tumors, and are often approached with the same nihilism. Central nervous system (CNS) dissemination is distinguished from other sites of advanced disease by conferring morbidity from neurologic disability, and the need to interrupt systemic treatment to provide palliation. Untreated, CNS metastases lead to progressive neurologic deterioration and death secondary to increased intracranial pressure in 1 to 2 months [2,3]. Avoiding or delaying this fate requires a working knowledge of supportive and definitive treatments for brain metastases.

Brain metastases share early cellular events with metastases to other organs, such as mutations that facilitate cellular detachment from basement membranes, intravasation, and endothelial adhesion. The systemic circulation distributes intravascular tumor cells to multiple organs in proportion to blood flow, but some cancers tend to metastasize to other organs preferentially. In 1889, the pathologist Stephen Paget first posited tropism of certain histologies for specific sites of dissemination. This "seed and soil" hypothesis applies to brain metastases, where malignancies such as melanoma and small cell lung cancer (SCLC) have a disproportionately high rate of brain metastasis (Table 1) [4–8].

Even within the brain, there is regional selectivity for growth of metastases from different primaries; melanoma is more common in the frontal and temporal lobes, breast carcinoma in the cerebellum and basal ganglia,

---
\* Corresponding author.
*E-mail address:* deangell@mskcc.org (L.M. DeAngelis).

0733-8619/07/$ - see front matter © 2007 Elsevier Inc. All rights reserved.
doi:10.1016/j.ncl.2007.07.011      *neurologic.theclinics.com*

Table 1
Brain metastases by primary tumor

| Primary tumor | Chason et al [4] (N=200) | Hunter and Newcastle [5] (N=393) | Posner and Chernik [6] (N=572) | Nussbaum et al [7] (N=729) | Zimm et al [8] (N=191) |
|---|---|---|---|---|---|
| Lung | 61% | 34% | 18% | 39% | 64% |
| Breast | 16% | 19% | 17% | 17% | 14% |
| Colorectal | 4% | 6% | 2% | — | 3% |
| Melanoma | 5% | 6% | 16% | 11% | 4% |
| Renal | 4% | 4% | 2% | 6% | 2% |
| Thyroid | <1% | 2% | — | — | — |
| Leukemia | — | — | 12% | — | — |
| Lymphoma | — | — | 10% | — | — |
| Unknown | 1% | 4% | — | 5% | 8% |

and non–small cell lung cancer (NSCLC) in the occipital lobes [9]. Clearly, tumor-specific interactions with brain physiology mediate the establishment and proliferation of brain metastases. Only recently has work been done to elucidate such molecular mechanisms. For example, hormone receptor and human epidermal growth factor receptor-2 (HER2)/neu status in breast cancer patients are predictive of brain metastases, and astrocytic contributions to their invasiveness have been described [10,11]. Research in this field is moving toward histology-specific investigations, appropriately recognizing that brain metastases have to be studied as separately as their original tumors.

## Diagnosis

Clinically evident brain metastases present with signs of increased intracranial pressure (headache, nausea, and vomiting), mental status changes, seizures, or focal signs. Focal signs are most frequently reported as hemiparesis, but aphasia and ataxia are common. Leptomeningeal carcinomatosis can present similarly, except that cranial nerve abnormalities are more common. Vertebral body metastases, although not considered CNS disease, can extend into the epidural space and cause spinal cord compression syndromes presenting with back pain, gait impairment, and myelopathy. Bulky, nodular leptomeningeal disease (LMD) can invade the spinal cord and also cause myelopathy. Intraparenchymal spinal metastases are rare.

Usually, new neurologic symptoms prompt evaluation with imaging. In an acute presentation (rapid change in examination within 24 hours), a CT without contrast of the brain is appropriate, to identify quickly life-threatening pathologies such as parenchymal or subarachnoid hemorrhage, acute hydrocephalus, or impending herniation from tumor and edema-related mass effect. In a potentially unstable patient, MRI is an inappropriate study because it can take more than half an hour to complete, leaving the patient unmonitored for an unacceptably long period of time. Some lesions may appear hyperdense on noncontrast CT because of acute intratumoral hemorrhage, or from increased tissue density of the tumor itself. Lesions typically have an impaired blood-brain barrier and are best distinguished using contrast-enhanced CT or MRI, with MRI being significantly more sensitive and the imaging modality of choice [12]. MRI also has the ability to differentiate metastases from other diagnoses such as stroke. Leptomeningeal and posterior fossa disease are better imaged with contrast-enhanced MRI. CT of the brain often produces artifact from the skull that is most apparent in the posterior fossa, making smaller cerebellar lesions difficult to diagnose, even with the administration of contrast (Fig. 1).

In a patient who has widespread systemic tumor, multiple intracranial lesions on MRI usually leave little doubt as to the diagnosis. However, immunosuppressed or septic patients may develop brain abscesses that can have a similar appearance and distribution. Single or solitary brain lesions may be more challenging diagnostically, because primary brain tumors

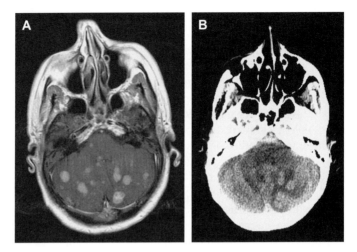

Fig. 1. Superior resolution of MRI for brain metastases. (*A*) Gadolinium-enhanced T1-weighted MRI of brain metastases in the posterior fossa. (*B*) Noncontrast CT of the same patient who has hyperdense lesions and significant beam-hardening artifact.

can occur in patients who have systemic malignancies. About 3% of patients who have high-grade glioma were found to have a systemic malignancy in one retrospective study [13]. Patients may also have a history of more than one active systemic neoplasm. Distinguishing which cancer has metastasized to the brain cannot be accomplished from imaging alone, and may require surgical resection if a pathologic diagnosis is necessary. In one prospective study of surgery for single brain metastasis, 11% of patients had pathology consistent with primary brain tumor, or infectious or inflammatory disease [14].

Suspected LMD requires either radiographic confirmation with contrast-enhanced MRI, or positive cytology from spinal fluid analysis. The sensitivity of both methods is about 75%, but serial lumbar punctures can increase the sensitivity to more than 90% with the third sample [15,16]. Specificity of cytology (100%) is also superior to MRI, where false positives may result from infectious or inflammatory disease. Meningeal enhancement from intracranial hypotension can occur as a result of lumbar puncture. Therefore, neuroimaging should precede cerebrospinal fluid sampling, when possible. Imaging also allows an assessment of safety before lumbar puncture in a patient with potential risk for herniation. Evidence of LMD in the spine or brain should prompt imaging of the remainder of the neuraxis to complete the evaluation.

## Supportive treatments for central nervous system metastases

Management of a patient who has CNS metastases is composed of symptomatic and definitive therapies. The mainstays of symptomatic control are steroids for tumor-related edema, antiepileptic drugs (AEDs) for seizure control, and multidisciplinary interventions aimed at minimizing neurologic disability.

Steroids stabilize the integrity of the tumor vasculature, which has increased permeability relative to the normal blood-brain barrier. Decreasing intracerebral pressure can alleviate symptoms, such as headache, nausea, weakness, and confusion, within hours of steroid administration. Decreasing interstitial pressure can improve the penetration of chemotherapeutic agents that rely on hydrostatic pressure to penetrate brain parenchyma. Dexamethasone is preferred for its low mineralocorticoid activity. The pharmacokinetics of the drug permit twice-daily dosing, which is optimal for patients because the medication can interfere with sleep if dosed too close to bedtime. Some side effects can be beneficial, such as improved appetite in a cachectic patient, increased energy for generalized fatigue, and inherent antiemetic activity. However, convention dictates that high doses used in the acute period (8–24 mg daily) should be tapered to the lowest effective dose as soon as possible to minimize side effects. The rate of taper should be slower once lower doses (4–6 mg/d) are achieved to avoid rebound edema, which especially occurs in patients with extensive edema or who have had longstanding steroid use. Patients starting radiation therapy may need sustained moderate doses at least 2 days before, and during the early stages of treatment, when peritumoral edema can be exacerbated by radiation effects.

The importance of using steroids in managing brain metastases often means accepting the addition of other treatments required to minimize side effects. The risk of *Pneumocystis jiroveci* pneumonia is greatest when a patient has been treated with steroids for 6 weeks or longer. Prophylaxis is achieved with standard regimens using sulfamethoxazole/trimethoprim, pentamidine, or dapsone. Gastrointestinal prophylaxis is warranted for symptomatic dyspepsia or reflux, but is not necessary in the asymptomatic patient. Psychosis or mood lability is best managed with dose reduction, but sometimes short-term neuroleptics are required. Steroid myopathy, which can develop in a matter of weeks in some patients, is reversed only with dose reductions. Enhanced physical activity and a high protein diet may ameliorate this complication. Premorbid hypertension and diabetes mellitus must be monitored carefully and standing medications adjusted appropriately.

In the absence of clinical seizures, prophylactic use of AEDs is not justified. Prophylactic AEDs in patients who have brain metastases do not decrease the rate of first clinical seizure and are associated with higher rates of complications caused by drug interactions [17]. Neurosurgeons occasionally use AEDs in the perioperative period, but these agents can be tapered off postoperatively if there has been no history of a clinical event. Seizures occurring only in the immediate postoperative period may not require long-term therapy if the event can be attributed to temporarily lowered seizure threshold from craniotomy.

About 20% of patients who have brain metastases present with seizures. The AED most commonly started in this population tends to be the enzyme-inducing agent phenytoin. Enzyme-inducing AEDs markedly upregulate the hepatic microsomal system, leading to adverse interactions with other drugs the patient may be taking, including chemotherapy drugs and glucocorticosteroids. Newer AEDs such as leviteracetam and topiramate, which are not metabolized by the hepatic cytochrome P450 systems, are used increasingly and with success in the brain tumor population.

A critical aspect of care for patients who have brain metastases is ensuring access to services for neurologic disability. Paresis, gait impairment, incontinence, and cognitive impairment are common manifestations of CNS disease that require special considerations. Unlike an enlarged or new visceral lesion, progression of disease in the brain or spinal cord can trigger the need for chronic bladder catheterization, physical therapy, 24-hour supervision, or durable medical equipment at home. Without recognition of these needs, patients can leave physician encounters with a treatment plan for their CNS metastases, but without a mechanism for managing their new level of function.

**Occult brain metastases**

Of growing interest and frequency is the acquisition of brain imaging to screen for brain metastases before starting treatment in a patient who has no neurologic symptoms. In some instances, asymptomatic patients are screened to qualify for enrollment in a clinical trial. Most therapeutic trials exclude patients who have CNS involvement because it carries a poor prognosis, and certain investigational agents, such as the new angiogenesis inhibitors, may have a theoretic increased risk of hemorrhage.

The diagnosis of occult brain metastases poses a therapeutic dilemma because little data exist to guide appropriate management. One study by Miller and colleagues [18] retrospectively reviewed 155 brain-screening CT and MRI scans obtained before enrollment in four separate therapeutic clinical trials for breast cancer that required exclusion of CNS disease. Twenty-three patients (14.8%) were reported to have occult CNS metastases, comparable to other studies reporting occult brain metastases in breast cancer patients with a range of 14% to 20% [19–21]. This cohort was compared with a group of symptomatic patients referred for whole-brain radiation therapy (WBRT) during the same time period. The investigators demonstrated that CNS dissemination, whether occult or symptomatic, conferred a worse prognosis, and both groups had similar survival. This result is expected because both groups had the same extent of disease (merely detected at different time points), and most patients were treated with WBRT. This study begs the question as to whether treating occult lesions at diagnosis with WBRT or other definitive treatment modalities is appropriate or necessary. Perhaps deferring treatment until radiographic or clinical progression is equivalent in efficacy would delay radiation toxicity, and allow more flexibility in offering systemic regimens.

## Definitive treatments for central nervous system metastases

The treatment and prognosis of CNS metastases depend on patient characteristics and the location and burden of disease in the CNS and elsewhere. Definitive therapies include radiation therapy, surgery, and chemotherapy. Optimal treatment is determined by age, performance status, extent of systemic disease, and distribution of tumor in the CNS. In 1997, the Radiation Therapy Oncology Group (RTOG) proposed classifying patients who have brain metastases according to prognostic factors identified by a recursive partitioning analysis (RPA) of 1200 patients treated with radiotherapy in several RTOG trials (Fig. 2) [22]. This schema has been validated in subsequent studies, and many publications stratify patients by RPA class.

### Whole-brain radiation therapy

The mainstay of treatment for brain metastases has been WBRT, conventionally given in 10 fractions to a total dose of 30 Gy, and it remains the first-line treatment of choice for treating multifocal, symptomatic brain metastases. Patients who are RPA class III or class II, with poorly controlled systemic disease, are best treated with WBRT for rapid palliation. Bulky, radiographically evident LMD of the brain, causing cranial nerve dysfunction, hydrocephalus, or increased intracranial pressure, is also best addressed with WBRT, which can encompass all sites of disease. The

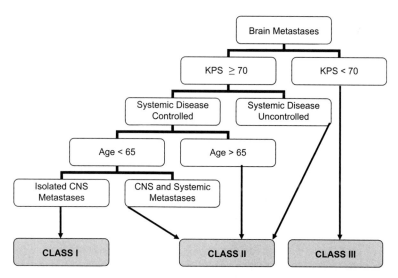

Fig. 2. RTOG recursive partitioning analysis classification of brain metastases. KPS, Karnofsky Performance Status score.

treatment is effective in palliating symptoms for 50% to 60% of patients, and can be completed in 2 weeks, minimizing the delay in systemic therapy that is often being changed in the setting of disease progression [22,23]. WBRT alone gives an overall median survival of 3 to 5 months [24–26]. Survival depends on RPA class (8.3 versus 2.4 months for class I and III, respectively) [27]. Short-term toxicities of WBRT include confusion, headache, fatigue, nausea, scalp erythema, and alopecia. Long-term survivors face an increased risk of dementia and radionecrosis, especially if treated at higher doses of radiation [28]. Despite treatment, approximately one half of patients succumb to CNS progression.

Repeat WBRT can be used for disease progression, usually at lower doses, and has been shown to produce clinical improvement in 27% to 70% of patients. Median survival after reirradiation ranges from 1.8 to 5.5 months, making concerns about the delayed effects of radiation less compelling in these patients [29–33]. Although WBRT remains a useful treatment, some patients benefit from more focused therapy with either surgery or stereotactic radiosurgery (SRS).

## Surgery

A small proportion of patients present with single or oligometastases in surgically accessible locations, and are also well enough to tolerate a craniotomy. Single brain lesions raise the possibility of alternate diagnoses in patients with a history of more than one active malignancy, who are long-term survivors of a prior cancer, or who have lesions that are not radiographically classic for metastases. In these instances, surgical resection provides a tissue diagnosis and offers therapeutic debulking. Often, surgery is required to address acute neurologic symptoms caused by mass effect, especially for large lesions in the posterior fossa, where decompression lowers the risk of obstructive hydrocephalus and rapid decompensation. Some posterior fossa lesions may require extirpation, even if multiple smaller metastases also exist. A landmark randomized prospective trial of surgery for single brain metastasis was reported by Patchell and colleagues [14]. Forty-eight patients who had a Karnofsky Performance Status score greater than 70 and confirmed metastases from solid tumors with intermediate radiosensitivity were evaluated for the added benefit of resection before WBRT. The surgical group had less frequent local recurrence, improved overall survival (40 versus 15 weeks, $P < .01$), and longer functional independence (38 versus 8 weeks, $P < .005$). Age and the presence of widely disseminated disease had a negative impact on overall survival in both groups, but neurologic survival was significantly associated with surgery. The survival benefit observed for this select population was also reported in a similar study by Vecht and colleagues [34], but was not corroborated in a third trial by Mintz and colleagues [35], which had more liberal inclusion criteria. In this last study, 23% of patients who received WBRT alone later required surgical resection, which may have obscured any survival benefit from surgery as part of initial therapy. Patchell and colleagues [36] conducted a second trial, randomizing patients to receive WBRT or not, after complete resection of a single brain metastasis. Radiation significantly decreased the rate of local (10% versus 46%, $P < .001$) and distal recurrence in the brain (14% versus 37%, $P < .01$), and death from neurologic causes (14% versus 44%, $P = .003$). These data support following resection of a single brain metastasis with WBRT, although overall survival and duration of functional independence was not different between the two groups. Although delaying neurologic disability from recurrence is important, certain patients with potential long-term survival may benefit from deferring WBRT to avoid the cognitive sequelae of brain radiation.

## Stereotactic radiosurgery

Unfortunately, many patients present with single or oligometastases situated deeply in the brain, inaccessible to surgical resection. An alternative for these patients is SRS, highly focused radiotherapy delivered in single or several fractions to a discreet area of tissue to a total dose of 14 to 20 Gy. Multiple lesions can be treated at one time. Linear accelerator and gamma knife delivery systems are equivalent. This noninvasive procedure is performed on an outpatient basis with minimal to no recovery time, making it a preferred modality of treatment for patients and their physicians. Because the maximum tolerated dose of radiation is inversely proportional to the size of the lesion, tumors are eligible for treatment if they are less than 3 to 4 cm in diameter. These higher doses, delivered as a singe fraction, increase the risk of radionecrosis (20% versus 5% for WBRT). The risk is highest in patients who receive SRS for recurrent brain tumors after progressing through WBRT, or in those who require WBRT for progression after SRS. Radionecrosis can be difficult to distinguish from true tumor recurrence, even with the use of positron emission tomography imaging or MR spectroscopy. Radionecrosis often requires long-term use of steroids (and development of attendant complications), or resection for pathologic verification and symptom control.

SRS for the initial treatment of brain metastases is used increasingly as a substitute for surgery, even for resectable lesions. Currently, however, no data directly compare the two methods. Retrospective studies suggest these two techniques are comparable. SRS can be used to treat multiple brain metastases, but has been proven to have a survival benefit only in patients who have single metastases when added to WBRT (6.5 months for WBRT + SRS versus 4.9 months for WBRT alone, $P = .0393$) [37]. A recent prospective trial of SRS alone versus WBRT + SRS did not show a survival benefit (8.0 months versus 7.5 months, $P = .42$), confirming observations from prior large retrospective studies. Similar to the data for surgery, WBRT decreased the rate of local and distant recurrence when added to focal therapy with SRS. However, it had no impact on neurologic cause of death or level of function, implying that WBRT can be deferred and used as salvage therapy, delaying the risk of late radionecrosis [38]. Most patients enrolled in these randomized studies had lung cancer, and it is unknown if these results can be extrapolated with equal efficacy to brain metastases from other primaries.

## Chemotherapy

Chemotherapy has been regarded historically as ineffective for brain metastases, with no class I evidence to support any one regimen. By the time brain metastases have developed, tumors have likely acquired resistance to many drugs used to treat the systemic disease. The blood-brain barrier not only provides a physical barrier to most substances, by way of endothelial tight junctions, but is also maintained by active efflux of drugs by p-glycoprotein and multidrug resistance proteins. Although contrast-enhancing metastases have an impaired blood-brain barrier, intracranial pressure dynamics make drug delivery to brain tumor tissue unreliable, and nonenhancing tumor cells are left untreated by most agents.

Chemotherapy is most commonly used for patients once surgical and radiation options have been exhausted; thus, the CNS disease may be highly resistant by the time chemotherapy is even tried. Patients who have recurrent brain disease often have active systemic tumor, and need treatment regimens with activity against all sites of their disease. Table 2 [39–54] lists some recent studies of chemotherapy in cohorts that include patients with recurrent disease who had progressed after receiving surgery or radiation for their brain metastases.

The patient who has newly diagnosed brain metastases may not be symptomatic enough to require urgent treatment with focused interventions or WBRT. This situation is particularly true of patients whose brain metastases were identified by screening neuroimaging. For patients who have nondisabling CNS metastases and active systemic disease, chemotherapy provides an opportunity to treat both compartments, potentially deferring the need for radiation and surgery. These patients are ideal candidates in whom to study chemotherapy regimens with expected activity against the primary tumor. Table 3 [55–68] details recent studies of upfront treatment for brain metastases with chemotherapy alone, and Table 4 [69–78] describes initial use of chemotherapy in combination with WBRT.

Some regimens have demonstrated clear activity against brain metastases from specific histologies. Brain metastases from NSCLC have responded to platinum-based mono- and combination therapy, temozolomide, and tyrosine kinase inhibitors. Brain metastases from breast cancer are more treatment responsive, and have response rates of 30% to 60% to various regimens, particularly those that include cyclophosphamide and methotrexate. Capecitabine and gemcitabine have also shown activity in isolated

Table 2
Chemotherapy alone for brain metastases

| Study | Study size (N) | Histology | Patients who have recurrent BM[a] | Chemotherapy | Response rate (CR + PR) | Median overall survival | TTP/PFS |
|---|---|---|---|---|---|---|---|
| Boogerd et al [39] | 22 | Breast | 32% | CMF CAF | 12/16 (75%) | 6.3 mo | — |
| Rivera et al [40] | 24 | Breast | 42% | temozolomide + capecitabine | 4/14 (18%) | — | 3.0 mo[b] |
| Lassman et al [41] | 23 | Breast (91%) | 83% | methotrexate | 5/23 (22%) | 5.0 mo | — |
| Christodoulou et al [42] | 32 | Breast (47%) NSCLC (38%) | 53% | temozolomide + cisplatin | 10/32 (31%) | 5.5 mo | 2.9 mo[b] |
| Ceresoli et al [43] | 41 | NSCLC | 44% | gefitinib | 4/41 (10%) | 5.0 mo | 3.0 mo[c] |
| Hotta et al [44] | 14 | NSCLC | 43% | gefitinib | 6/14 (43%) | — | 8.8 mo[b] |
| Namba et al [45] | 15 | NSCLC | 60% | gefitinib | 9/15 (60%) | 8.3 mo | — |
| Giorgio et al [46] | 30 | NSCLC | 100% | temozolomide | 3/30 (10%) | 6.0 mo | 3.6 mo[b] |
| Boogerd et al [47] | 13 | NSCLC | 46% | teniposide | 3/13 (23%) | — | — |
| Abrey et al [48] | 41 | NSCLC (54%) Breast (24%) | 100% | temozolomide | 2/34 (6%) all NSCLC | 6.6 mo | 2.0 mo[b] |
| Kaba et al [49] | 115 | NSCLC (42%) Breast (24%) SCLC (8%) Melanoma (8%) | 100% | TPDC-FuHu | 27/97 (28%) | 6.3 mo | 3.0 mo[b] |
| Omuro et al [50] | 21 | NSCLC (48%) Breast (29%) SCLC (14%) | 100% | temozolomide + vinorelbine | 2/18 (11%) | 4.3 mo | — |
| Caraglia et al [51] | 19 | NSCLC (60%) SCLC (40%) | 68% | temozolomide + pegylated liposomal doxorubicin | 7/19 (37%) | 10 mo | 5.5 mo[c] |
| Korfel et al [52] | 30 | SCLC | 100% | topotecan | 10/30 (33%) | 3.6 mo | 3.1 mo[b] |
| Hwu et al [53] | 26 | Melanoma | 100% | temozolomide + thalidomide | 3/15 (20%) | 5.0 mo | — |
| Jacquillat et al [54] | 36 | Melanoma | 14% | fotemustine | 9/36 (25%) | — | — |

*Abbreviations*: BM, brain metastases; CAF, cyclophosphamide, doxorubicin, fluorouracil; CMF, cyclophosphamide, methotrexate, fluorouracil; CR, complete response; PFS, median progression-free survival; PR, partial response; TPDC-FuHu, thioguanine, dibromodulcitol, lomustine, fluorouracil, hydroxyurea; TTP, median time to tumor progression.

[a] Patient has received prior treatment for brain metastases with radiation or surgery.

[b] TTP.

[c] PFS.

Table 3
Upfront chemotherapy alone for newly diagnosed brain metastases

| Study | Study size (N) | Histology | Chemotherapy | Response rate (CR + PR) | Median overall survival | TTP/PFS |
|---|---|---|---|---|---|---|
| Rosner et al [55] | 100 | Breast | CFP<br>CFP-M<br>FP<br>CFP-MV<br>MVP<br>CA | 50/100 (50%) | CR 39.5 mo<br>PR 10.5 mo<br>PD 1.5 mo<br>All 5.5 mo | — |
| Oberhoff et al [56] | 24 | Breast | topotecan | 6/16 (38%) | 6.3 mo | — |
| Franciosi et al [57] | 116 | Breast (52%)<br>NSCLC (40%)<br>Melanoma (8%) | cisplatin + etoposide | 21/56 (38%) Breast<br>13/43 (30%) NSCLC<br>0% Melanoma | 7.8 mo Breast<br>8 mo NSCLC<br>4.3 mo Melanoma | — |
| Agarwala et al [58] | 151 | Melanoma | temozolomide | 9/151 (6%) | 3.2 mo | — |
| Boogerd et al [59] | 13 | Melanoma (with systemic response to temozolomide) | temozolomide | 5/13 (38%) | 5.6 mo | 7.0 mo[a] |
| Fujita et al [60] | 30 | NSCLC | cisplatin + ifosfamide + irinotecan | 14/28 (50%) | 12.5 mo | — |
| Minotti et al [61] | 23 | NSCLC | cisplatin + teniposide | 8/23 (35%) | 5.2 mo | — |
| Bernardo et al [62] | 22 | NSCLC | vinorelbine + gemcitabine + carboplatin | 9/20 (45%) | 8.5 mo | — |
| Colleoni et al [63] | 28 | NSCLC (71%)<br>Breast (21%) | lomustine + carboplatin + vinorelbine + 1-leucovorin + fluorouracil | 9/26 (35%) | 7.4 mo | 3.7 mo[a] |
| Vinolas et al [64] | 14 | NSCLC (57%)<br>Breast (29%) | cisplatin + etoposide | 2/14 (14%) | 6.0 mo | — |

| Study | N | Tumor types | Regimen | Response | Survival | |
|---|---|---|---|---|---|---|
| Lorusso et al [65] | 19 | NSCLC (42%) Breast (32%) SCLC (16%) Colon (12%) | topotecan | 2/19 (10%) all SCLC | | — |
| Tummarello et al [66] | 23 | NSCLC (61%) SCLC (39%) | cisplatin + vinblastine + mitomycin *or* cyclophosphamide + doxorubicin + vincristine | 2/14 (14%) NSCLC 5/9 (55%) SCLC | | — |
| Malacarne et al [67] | 30 | NSCLC (60%) SCLC (40%) | carboplatin + etoposide | 3/18 (17%) NSCLC 7/12 (58%) SCLC | 7.5 mo NSCLC5.8 mo SCLC | — |
| Seute et al [68] | 22 | SCLC | cyclophosphamide + doxorubicin + etoposide | 6/22 (27%) | 8.3 mo | 2.3 mo[b] |

*Abbreviations:* CA, cyclophosphamide, doxorubicin; CFP, cyclophosphamide, fluorouracil, prednisone; CFP-M, cyclophosphamide, fluorouracil, prednisone, methotrexate; CFP-MV, cyclophosphamide, fluorouracil, prednisone, methotrexate, vincristine; CR, complete response; FP, fluorouracil, prednisone; MVP, methotrexate, vincristine, prednisone; PD, progressed disease; PFS, median progression-free survival; PR, partial response; TTP, median time to tumor progression.

[a] TTP.
[b] PFS.

Table 4
Upfront chemotherapy ± whole-brain radiation therapy for newly diagnosed brain metastases

| Study | Study size (N) | Histology | Regimen or regimens | Response rate (CR + PR) | Median OS | TTP/PFS |
|---|---|---|---|---|---|---|
| Kollmannsberger et al [69] | 22 | Germ cell | cisplatin/etoposide/ifosfamide with stem cell transplant (WBRT in 12 pts) | 20/22 (91%) 100% chemo-only patients | 2y OS=81% | 2y PFS=72% |
| Cocconi et al [70] | 22 | Breast | platinum/etoposide (WBRT in 5 pts) | 12/22 (55%) | 14.5 mo | — |
| Verger et al [71] | 82 | NSCLC (53%) Breast (17%) Other (29%) | A: WBRT B: WBRT + temozolomide | A: 13/31 (42%) B: 13/35 (37%) | A: 3.1 mo B: 4.5 mo | — |
| Robinet et al [72] | 174 | NSCLC | A: cisplatin/vinorelbine + WBRT B: WBRT after 2–6 cycles of cisplatin/vinorelbine | A: 23/76 (30%) B: 28/73 (38%) P = .12 | A: 6.0 mo B: 5.3 mo P = .83 | A: 3.3 mo[a] B: 2.8 mo[a] P = .92 |
| Guerrieri et al [73] | 42 | NSCLC | A: WBRT B: WBRT + carboplatin | A: 10% B: 29% P = .24 | A: 4.4 mo B: 3.7 mo P = .64 | — |
| Cortot et al [74] | 50 | NSCLC | temozolomide/cisplatin (≤ 6 cycles) followed by WBRT | 8/50 (16%) | 5.0 mo | 2.3 mo[a] |
| Pronzato et al [75] | 20 | NSCLC | WBRT + carboplatin/teniposide | 3/20 (15%) | 7.0 mo | — |
| Moscetti et al [76] | 156 | NSCLC | A: platinum-based chemo alone (110 pts) B: WBRT followed by platinum-based chemo (46 pts) | A: 30/107 (28%) B: 16/46 (35%) P = .07 | A: 10.0 mo B: 14.0 mo P = .07 | A: 6.0 mo[b] B: 6.0 mo[b] |
| Ushio et al [77] | 88 | NSCLC (75%) SCLC (11%) | A: WBRT aloneB: WBRT + nitrosureasC: WBRT + nitrosureas/tegafur | A: 5/14 (36%) B: 11/16 (69%) C: 14/19 (74%) | A: 6.8 mo B: 7.6 mo C: 7.3 mo | — |
| Postmus et al [78] | 120 | SCLC | A: teniposide B: teniposide + WBRT | A: 22% B: 57% P<.001 | A: 3.2 mo B: 3.5 mo P = .087 | A: 1.7 mo[a] B: 2.9 mo[a] P = .005 |

Abbreviations: CR, complete response; OS, overall survival; PR, partial response; TTP, median time to tumor progression. PFS, median progression-free survival;

a TTP.
b PFS.

patients, whereas temozolomide is not as effective in this population as in NSCLC. SCLC brain metastases have a broader range of active regimens, the most popular combination being cisplatin and etoposide. When germ cell tumors and non-Hodgkin's lymphoma disseminate to the CNS, chemotherapy is usually the first-line treatment. In stark contrast, malignant melanoma and renal cell carcinoma are frequent culprits of CNS spread, with no success stories. Temozolomide, although reducing the risk of developing brain metastases from advanced melanoma, does not produce impressive response rates once intracranial lesions have developed [79].

Researchers are also exploring potential synergy between radiation and compounds that serve as radiation sensitizers. Efaproxiral is a synthetic modifier of hemoglobin that, when given in combination with WBRT, significantly improved response rates for NSCLC (24% versus 13%) and breast cancer (45% versus 18%), but did not affect survival [80]. It is currently being studied in a phase III trial for patients who have brain metastases from breast cancer. Motexafin gadolinium was studied in 401 patients and did not improve overall survival when added to WBRT; however, in a subgroup analysis, patients who had NSCLC had improved neurologic function [81].

## Management of leptomeningeal disease

Radiation and chemotherapy can be used in patients who have LMD occurring either in isolation or concomitantly with parenchymal brain disease. Survival in this population is dismal, so preventing disability and preserving quality of life are paramount. Steroids can be effective in treating headache and pain, but do not improve neurologic disability from LMD the way they do in patients who have brain metastases. Radiation therapy is necessary to treat symptomatic areas. Rarely, a patient who has secondary hydrocephalus can respond quickly to WBRT, abrogating the need for a ventriculoperitoneal shunt. Contrast-enhancing LMD is usually defined as "bulky" disease and is best treated with radiation, whether in the brain or spine. Large fields can lead to severe myelosuppression, especially in heavily pretreated patients. Intrathecal therapy penetrates only the first few millimeters into tumor tissue and is not effective against thick or nodular disease. Furthermore, thick enhancement, in either the spine or the brain, may impair cerebrospinal fluid flow, which cannot circulate properly, increasing the risk of leukoencephalopathy from intrathecal therapy. A nuclear flow study should be performed before treating with intrathecal agents if there is bulky, radiographically evident LMD. An Ommaya reservoir is the most reliable and comfortable mode of drug delivery for patients, who usually require multiple treatments. Prophylaxis with steroids for chemical meningitis is required when using liposomal cytarabine, but is not necessary for most other agents. Aggressive approaches beyond palliative radiation should be reserved for patients who have limited systemic disease and good performance status.

## Summary

Brain metastases are a common complication of cancer and alter patient management more than any other site of distant progression. Single and solitary metastases that are resectable in relatively healthy patients should be removed surgically, with or without subsequent WBRT. Multiple symptomatic metastases should be treated with WBRT. Inoperable single or oligometastases can be treated successfully with SRS. SRS for resectable lesions has not been proven equivalent or superior to surgery and carries the possibility of radionecrosis and incomplete response. SRS carries a lower procedural risk and is more tolerable, but is most effective for small lesions. Chemotherapy plays a role primarily in the population with recurrent brain metastases, and merits further study. Chemotherapy has a special role in the upfront treatment of brain metastases from chemosensitive primary tumors, particularly when found in the asymptomatic patient. Delaying or decreasing neurologic cause of death and disability are important therapeutic goals that should be included in any trial for brain metastases. While better definitive strategies are investigated, physicians must remember to optimize the use of supportive therapies to ameliorate symptoms and maintain quality of life.

## References

[1] Landis SH, Murray T, Bolden S, et al. Cancer statistics, 1999. CA Cancer J Clin 1999;49(1): 8–31, 31.

[2] DiStefano A, Yong Yap Y, Hortobagyi GN, et al. The natural history of breast cancer patients with brain metastases. Cancer 1979;44(5):1913–8.

[3] Markesbery WR, Brooks WH, Gupta GD, et al. Treatment for patients with cerebral metastases. Arch Neurol 1978;35(11):754–6.

[4] Chason JL, Walker FB, Landers JW. Metastatic carcinoma in the central nervous system and dorsal root ganglia. A prospective autopsy study. Cancer 1963;16:781–7.

[5] Hunter KM, Newcastle NB. Metastatic neoplasms of the brain stem. Can Med Assoc J 1968; 98(1):1–7.

[6] Posner JB, Chernik NL. Intracranial metastases from systemic cancer. Adv Neurol 1978;19: 579–92.

[7] Nussbaum ES, Djalilian HR, Cho KH, et al. Brain metastases. Histology, multiplicity, surgery, and survival. Cancer 1996;78(8):1781–8.

[8] Zimm S, Wampler GL, Stablein D, et al. Intracerebral metastases in solid-tumor patients: natural history and results of treatment. Cancer 1981;48(2):384–94.

[9] Graf AH, Buchberger W, Langmayr H, et al. Site preference of metastatic tumours of the brain. Virchows Arch A Pathol Anat Histopathol 1988;412(5):493–8.

[10] Gabos Z, Sinha R, Hanson J, et al. Prognostic significance of human epidermal growth factor receptor positivity for the development of brain metastasis after newly diagnosed breast cancer. J Clin Oncol 2006;24(36):5658–63.

[11] Sierra A, Price JE, Garcia-Ramirez M, et al. Astrocyte-derived cytokines contribute to the metastatic brain specificity of breast cancer cells. Lab Invest 1997;77(4):357–68.

[12] Sze G, Milano E, Johnson C, et al. Detection of brain metastases: comparison of contrast-enhanced MR with unenhanced MR and enhanced CT. AJNR Am J Neuroradiol 1990; 11(4):785–91.

[13] Maluf FC, DeAngelis LM, Raizer JJ, et al. High-grade gliomas in patients with prior systemic malignancies. Cancer 2002;94(12):3219–24.

[14] Patchell RA, Tibbs PA, Walsh JW, et al. A randomized trial of surgery in the treatment of single metastases to the brain. N Engl J Med 1990;322(8):494–500.

[15] Straathof CS, de Bruin HG, Dippel DW, et al. The diagnostic accuracy of magnetic resonance imaging and cerebrospinal fluid cytology in leptomeningeal metastasis. J Neurol 1999;246(9):810–4.

[16] Wasserstrom WR, Glass JP, Posner JB. Diagnosis and treatment of leptomeningeal metastases from solid tumors: experience with 90 patients. Cancer 1982;49(4):759–72.

[17] Glantz MJ, Cole BF, Forsyth PA, et al. Practice parameter: anticonvulsant prophylaxis in patients with newly diagnosed brain tumors. Report of the Quality Standards Subcommittee of the American Academy of Neurology. Neurology 2000;54(10):1886–93.

[18] Miller KD, Weathers T, Haney LG, et al. Occult central nervous system involvement in patients with metastatic breast cancer: prevalence, predictive factors and impact on overall survival. Ann Oncol 2003;14(7):1072–7.

[19] Amer MH. Chemotherapy and pattern of metastases in breast cancer patients. J Surg Oncol 1982;19(2):101–5.

[20] Hagemeister FB Jr, Buzdar AU, Luna MA, et al. Causes of death in breast cancer: a clinicopathologic study. Cancer 1980;46(1):162–7.

[21] Tsukada Y, Fouad A, Pickren JW, et al. Central nervous system metastasis from breast carcinoma. Autopsy study. Cancer 1983;52(12):2349–54.

[22] Gaspar L, Scott C, Rotman M, et al. Recursive partitioning analysis (RPA) of prognostic factors in three Radiation Therapy Oncology Group (RTOG) brain metastases trials. Int J Radiat Oncol Biol Phys 1997;37(4):745–51.

[23] Gaspar LE, Scott C, Murray K, et al. Validation of the RTOG recursive partitioning analysis (RPA) classification for brain metastases. Int J Radiat Oncol Biol Phys 2000;47(4):1001–6.

[24] Borgelt B, Gelber R, Kramer S, et al. The palliation of brain metastases: final results of the first two studies by the Radiation Therapy Oncology Group. Int J Radiat Oncol Biol Phys 1980;6(1):1–9.

[25] Horton J, Baxter DH, Olson KB. The management of metastases to the brain by irradiation and corticosteroids. Am J Roentgenol Radium Ther Nucl Med 1971;111(2):334–6.

[26] Kurtz JM, Gelber R, Brady LW, et al. The palliation of brain metastases in a favorable patient population: a randomized clinical trial by the Radiation Therapy Oncology Group. Int J Radiat Oncol Biol Phys 1981;7(7):891–5.

[27] Pease NJ, Edwards A, Moss LJ. Effectiveness of whole brain radiotherapy in the treatment of brain metastases: a systematic review. Palliat Med 2005;19(4):288–99.

[28] DeAngelis LM, Mandell LR, Thaler HT, et al. The role of postoperative radiotherapy after resection of single brain metastases. Neurosurgery 1989;24(6):798–805.

[29] Cooper JS, Steinfeld AD, Lerch IA. Cerebral metastases: value of reirradiation in selected patients. Radiology 1990;174(3 Pt 1):883–5.

[30] Hazuka MB, Kinzie JJ. Brain metastases: results and effects of re-irradiation. Int J Radiat Oncol Biol Phys 1988;15(2):433–7.

[31] Kurup P, Reddy S, Hendrickson FR. Results of re-irradiation for cerebral metastases. Cancer 1980;46(12):2587–9.

[32] Shehata WM, Hendrickson FR, Hindo WA. Rapid fractionation technique and re-treatment of cerebral metastases by irradiation. Cancer 1974;34(2):257–61.

[33] Wong WW, Schild SE, Sawyer TE, et al. Analysis of outcome in patients reirradiated for brain metastases. Int J Radiat Oncol Biol Phys 1996;34(3):585–90.

[34] Vecht CJ, Haaxma-Reiche H, Noordijk EM, et al. Treatment of single brain metastasis: radiotherapy alone or combined with neurosurgery? Ann Neurol 1993;33(6):583–90.

[35] Mintz AH, Kestle J, Rathbone MP, et al. A randomized trial to assess the efficacy of surgery in addition to radiotherapy in patients with a single cerebral metastasis. Cancer 1996;78(7): 1470–6.

[36] Patchell RA, Tibbs PA, Regine WF, et al. Postoperative radiotherapy in the treatment of single metastases to the brain: a randomized trial. JAMA 1998;280(17):1485–9.

[37] Andrews DW, Scott CB, Sperduto PW, et al. Whole brain radiation therapy with or without stereotactic radiosurgery boost for patients with one to three brain metastases: phase III results of the RTOG 9508 randomised trial. Lancet 2004;363(9422):1665–72.

[38] Aoyama H, Shirato H, Tago M, et al. Stereotactic radiosurgery plus whole-brain radiation therapy vs stereotactic radiosurgery alone for treatment of brain metastases: a randomized controlled trial. JAMA 2006;295(21):2483–91.

[39] Boogerd W, Dalesio O, Bais EM, et al. Response of brain metastases from breast cancer to systemic chemotherapy. Cancer 1992;69(4):972–80.

[40] Rivera E, Meyers C, Groves M, et al. Phase I study of capecitabine in combination with temozolomide in the treatment of patients with brain metastases from breast carcinoma. Cancer 2006;107(6):1348–54.

[41] Lassman AB, Abrey LE, Shah GD, et al. Systemic high-dose intravenous methotrexate for central nervous system metastases. J Neurooncol 2006;78(3):255–60.

[42] Christodoulou C, Bafaloukos D, Linardou H, et al. Temozolomide (TMZ) combined with cisplatin (CDDP) in patients with brain metastases from solid tumors: a Hellenic Cooperative Oncology Group (HeCOG) phase II study. J Neurooncol 2005;71(1):61–5.

[43] Ceresoli GL, Cappuzzo F, Gregorc V, et al. Gefitinib in patients with brain metastases from non-small-cell lung cancer: a prospective trial. Ann Oncol 2004;15(7):1042–7.

[44] Hotta K, Kiura K, Ueoka H, et al. Effect of gefitinib ('Iressa', ZD1839) on brain metastases in patients with advanced non-small-cell lung cancer. Lung Cancer 2004;46(2): 255–61.

[45] Namba Y, Kijima T, Yokota S, et al. Gefitinib in patients with brain metastases from non-small-cell lung cancer: review of 15 clinical cases. Clin Lung Cancer 2004;6(2):123–8.

[46] Giorgio CG, Giuffrida D, Pappalardo A, et al. Oral temozolomide in heavily pre-treated brain metastases from non-small cell lung cancer: phase II study. Lung Cancer 2005;50(2): 247–54.

[47] Boogerd W, van der Sande JJ, van Zandwijk N. Teniposide sometimes effective in brain metastases from non-small cell lung cancer. J Neurooncol 1999;41(3):285–9.

[48] Abrey LE, Olson JD, Raizer JJ, et al. A phase II trial of temozolomide for patients with recurrent or progressive brain metastases. J Neurooncol 2001;53(3):259–65.

[49] Kaba SE, Kyritsis AP, Hess K, et al. TPDC-FuHu chemotherapy for the treatment of recurrent metastatic brain tumors. J Clin Oncol 1997;15(3):1063–70.

[50] Omuro AM, Raizer JJ, Demopoulos A, et al. Vinorelbine combined with a protracted course of temozolomide for recurrent brain metastases: a phase I trial. J Neurooncol 2006;78(3): 277–80.

[51] Caraglia M, Addeo R, Costanzo R, et al. Phase II study of temozolomide plus pegylated liposomal doxorubicin in the treatment of brain metastases from solid tumours. Cancer Chemother Pharmacol 2006;57(1):34–9.

[52] Korfel A, Oehm C, von Pawel J, et al. Response to topotecan of symptomatic brain metastases of small-cell lung cancer also after whole-brain irradiation. A multicentre phase II study. Eur J Cancer 2002;38(13):1724–9.

[53] Hwu WJ, Lis E, Menell JH, et al. Temozolomide plus thalidomide in patients with brain metastases from melanoma: a phase II study. Cancer 2005;103(12):2590–7.

[54] Jacquillat C, Khayat D, Banzet P, et al. Final report of the French multicenter phase II study of the nitrosourea fotemustine in 153 evaluable patients with disseminated malignant melanoma including patients with cerebral metastases. Cancer 1990;66(9):1873–8.

[55] Rosner D, Nemoto T, Lane WW. Chemotherapy induces regression of brain metastases in breast carcinoma. Cancer 1986;58(4):832–9.

[56] Oberhoff C, Kieback DG, Wurstlein R, et al. Topotecan chemotherapy in patients with breast cancer and brain metastases: results of a pilot study. Onkologie 2001;24(3):256–60.

[57] Franciosi V, Cocconi G, Michiara M, et al. Front-line chemotherapy with cisplatin and etoposide for patients with brain metastases from breast carcinoma, nonsmall cell lung carcinoma, or malignant melanoma: a prospective study. Cancer 1999;85(7):1599–605.

[58] Agarwala SS, Kirkwood JM, Gore M, et al. Temozolomide for the treatment of brain metastases associated with metastatic melanoma: a phase II study. J Clin Oncol 2004; 22(11):2101–7.

[59] Boogerd W, de Gast GC, Dalesio O. Temozolomide in advanced malignant melanoma with small brain metastases: can we withhold cranial irradiation? Cancer 2007;109(2): 306–12.

[60] Fujita A, Fukuoka S, Takabatake H, et al. Combination chemotherapy of cisplatin, ifosfamide, and irinotecan with rhG-CSF support in patients with brain metastases from nonsmall cell lung cancer. Oncology 2000;59(4):291–5.

[61] Minotti V, Crino L, Meacci ML, et al. Chemotherapy with cisplatin and teniposide for cerebral metastases in non-small cell lung cancer. Lung Cancer 1998;20(2):93–8.

[62] Bernardo G, Cuzzoni Q, Strada MR, et al. First-line chemotherapy with vinorelbine, gemcitabine, and carboplatin in the treatment of brain metastases from non-small-cell lung cancer: a phase II study. Cancer Invest 2002;20(3):293–302.

[63] Colleoni M, Graiff C, Nelli P, et al. Activity of combination chemotherapy in brain metastases from breast and lung adenocarcinoma. Am J Clin Oncol 1997;20(3):303–7.

[64] Vinolas N, Graus F, Mellado B, et al. Phase II trial of cisplatinum and etoposide in brain metastases of solid tumors. J Neurooncol 1997;35(2):145–8.

[65] Lorusso V, Galetta D, Giotta F, et al. Topotecan in the treatment of brain metastases. A phase II study of GOIM (Gruppo Oncologico dell'Italia Meridionale). Anticancer Res 2006;26(3B):2259–63.

[66] Tummarello D, Lippe P, Bracci R, et al. First line chemotherapy in patients with brain metastases from non-small and small cell lung cancer. Oncol Rep 1998;5(4):897–900.

[67] Malacarne P, Santini A, Maestri A. Response of brain metastases from lung cancer to systemic chemotherapy with carboplatin and etoposide. Oncology 1996;53(3):210–3.

[68] Seute T, Leffers P, Wilmink JT, et al. Response of asymptomatic brain metastases from small-cell lung cancer to systemic first-line chemotherapy. J Clin Oncol 2006;24(13): 2079–83.

[69] Kollmannsberger C, Nichols C, Bamberg M, et al. First-line high-dose chemotherapy +/− radiation therapy in patients with metastatic germ-cell cancer and brain metastases. Ann Oncol 2000;11(5):553–9.

[70] Cocconi G, Lottici R, Bisagni G, et al. Combination therapy with platinum and etoposide of brain metastases from breast carcinoma. Cancer Invest 1990;8(3–4):327–34.

[71] Verger E, Gil M, Yaya R, et al. Temozolomide and concomitant whole brain radiotherapy in patients with brain metastases: a phase II randomized trial. Int J Radiat Oncol Biol Phys 2005;61(1):185–91.

[72] Robinet G, Thomas P, Breton JL, et al. Results of a phase III study of early versus delayed whole brain radiotherapy with concurrent cisplatin and vinorelbine combination in inoperable brain metastasis of non-small-cell lung cancer: Groupe Francais de Pneumo-Cancerologie (GFPC) Protocol 95-1. Ann Oncol 2001;12(1):59–67.

[73] Guerrieri M, Wong K, Ryan G, et al. A randomised phase III study of palliative radiation with concomitant carboplatin for brain metastases from non-small cell carcinoma of the lung. Lung Cancer 2004;46(1):107–11.

[74] Cortot AB, Geriniere L, Robinet G, et al. Phase II trial of temozolomide and cisplatin followed by whole brain radiotherapy in non-small-cell lung cancer patients with brain metastases: a GLOT-GFPC study. Ann Oncol 2006;17(9):1412–7.

[75] Pronzato P, Bruna F, Neri E, et al. Radiotherapy plus carboplatin and teniposide in patients with brain metastases from non small cell lung cancer. Anticancer Res 1995;15(2):517–9.

[76] Moscetti L, Nelli F, Felici A, et al. Up-front chemotherapy and radiation treatment in newly diagnosed nonsmall cell lung cancer with brain metastases: survey by Outcome Research Network for Evaluation of Treatment Results in Oncology. Cancer 2007;109(2):274–81.

[77] Ushio Y, Arita N, Hayakawa T, et al. Chemotherapy of brain metastases from lung carcinoma: a controlled randomized study. Neurosurgery 1991;28(2):201–5.

[78] Postmus PE, Haaxma-Reiche H, Smit EF, et al. Treatment of brain metastases of small-cell lung cancer: comparing teniposide and teniposide with whole-brain radiotherapy–a phase III study of the European Organization for the Research and Treatment of Cancer Lung Cancer Cooperative Group. J Clin Oncol 2000;18(19):3400–8.

[79] Paul MJ, Summers Y, Calvert AH, et al. Effect of temozolomide on central nervous system relapse in patients with advanced melanoma. Melanoma Res 2002;12(2):175–8.

[80] Stea B, Suh JH, Boyd AP, et al. Whole-brain radiotherapy with or without efaproxiral for the treatment of brain metastases: determinants of response and its prognostic value for subsequent survival. Int J Radiat Oncol Biol Phys 2006;64(4):1023–30.

[81] Meyers CA, Smith JA, Bezjak A, et al. Neurocognitive function and progression in patients with brain metastases treated with whole-brain radiation and motexafin gadolinium: results of a randomized phase III trial. J Clin Oncol 2004;22(1):157–65.

NEUROLOGIC
CLINICS

Neurol Clin 25 (2007) 1193–1207

# Primary Central Nervous System Lymphoma

Nimish A. Mohile, MD, Lauren E. Abrey, MD*

*Department of Neurology, Memorial Sloan-Kettering Cancer Center,
1275 York Avenue, New York, NY 10021, USA*

## Cause

Primary central nervous system lymphoma (PCNSL) is uncommon and accounts for approximately 1% to 3% of all central nervous system (CNS) malignancies [1]. Although PCNSL is a subtype of non-Hodgkin's lymphoma (NHL), it is by definition restricted to the CNS. It makes up less than 5% of NHLs. The vast majority of PCNSLs are B-cell lymphomas. The most prevalent histology is diffuse large B-cell lymphoma (DLBCL) and most of these are germinal center in origin [2]. Immunoblastic and lymphoblastic types are also seen but are rare. T-cell variants account for less than 4% of all PCNSL cases in the western world. One large series suggests that their presentation and outcome are similar to B-cell PCNSL, but because of the small numbers, their biologic activity and prognostic factors are not well understood [3]. All histologies observed in PCNSL are identical to their systemic counterparts. For this reason, they are classified as stage IE NHL indicating restriction of disease to a single extranodal site.

The cause and behavior of PCNSL differ based on the affected population. Immunocompromised patients are at particular risk for developing PCNSL and it is typically secondary to HIV, organ transplantation, or congenital immunodeficiency syndromes. PCNSL in this setting arises from Epstein-Barr virus (EBV) infection of B-lymphocytes [1]. Affected B-cells proliferate unchecked by the immune system and tend to form tumors in the immuno-privileged environment of the CNS. In contrast, there is no well-established cause for PCNSL in the immunocompetent patient. EBV and the human herpesviruses have been investigated, but no correlation has been discovered. Exactly how these neoplasms develop and grow in

---

* Corresponding author.
*E-mail address:* abreyl@mskcc.org (L.E. Abrey).

the CNS is a mystery. B-lymphocytes have no known role in normal brain. Initial reports of PCNSL discounted the idea that this disease represented metastatic dissemination from systemic lymphoma. Some recent work suggests that occult systemic disease may be more common than previously recognized and theorizes that quiescent malignant cells may be residing in the body [4].

## Epidemiology

PCNSL has a propensity for elderly populations with a median age at diagnosis of 60 years. Most patients are between the ages of 45 and 70 years but the incidence increases with rising age. Estimates from the Central Brain Tumor Registry of the United States suggest that the overall incidence rate is 0.46 per 100,000 person-years. Males are marginally more affected, and there is no known disproportionate representation by race [5]. There has been considerable speculation over the years that the incidence of PCNSL is increasing. Frequency among immunocompetent populations has probably increased, but much of the epidemiologic data are complicated by increasing trends in the incidence and prevalence of HIV [6]. In fact, the age-adjusted incidence tripled between 1973 to 1984 and 1985 to 1997, underscoring earlier work that demonstrated a similar increase from 1973 to 1984 [7,8]. This finding raised the possibility that PCNSL could become the most common type of brain tumor by the year 2000 [9]. In other studies, incidence rates are reported as stable or decreasing, suggesting that part of the reported increase may have been related to the AIDS epidemic [10,11]. The impact of newer imaging modalities and an increase in organ transplantation must also be considered. None of these factors can sufficiently explain the observed increase in patients older than 60 years. These observations may represent a real rise or they may simply be related to more aggressive clinical evaluation in elderly patients. In either case, this highlights the importance of developing less-toxic treatments for a population that is exceptionally vulnerable to the effects of brain irradiation.

More recent epidemiologic data found that the survival rates in the community have not reflected the advances seen in clinical trials that use methotrexate (MTX)–based regimens. Some of the data from the community may reflect a higher proportion of HIV-associated PCNSL or the possibility that elderly patients in the community may be incorrectly treated. These data underscore the importance of treating this rare disease in tertiary care facilities [12].

## Prognostic factors

Age and performance status are recognized as two of the most important prognostic factors for PCNSL [13]. Some authors contend that the impact of age influences outcome even more than treatment [14]. Prognostic factors identified in the literature for systemic NHL include serum lactate dehydrogenase (LDH), a marker of more aggressive disease, along with age and Karnofsky Performance Score (KPS). There are other factors that are specific to PCNSL. Elevation of cerebrospinal fluid (CSF) protein, for instance, is associated with poorer survival [15]. The location of the tumor and its presence in deeper structures predicts worse outcomes. These five parameters together compose the elements of a prognostic score, confirmed by the International Extranodal Lymphoma Study Group (IELSG), that divides patients into three risk groups [16].

A simpler prognostic model developed at Memorial Sloan-Kettering Cancer Center (MSKCC) is based purely on age and KPS. A comparison of the two prognostic indices is displayed in Table 1. External validation was performed using data obtained from prospective trials of the Radiation Therapy Oncology Group (RTOG) [17]. This model also divides patients into three groups and predicts median survivals of 8.5 years, 3.2 years, and 1.1 years based on age and KPS. This score is simple to use and relies on data that are universally obtained. The identification and assessment of prognostic factors enables separation of PCNSL patients into specific risk groups that can help to define appropriate therapies and predict survival. These parameters are useful when interpreting results of clinical trials which, because of the low incidence of PCNSL, are rarely randomized.

## Clinical features

Patients typically present with symptoms that are suggestive of focal neurologic dysfunction that depend on the location of the tumor. Patients

Table 1
Description of International Extranodal Lymphoma Study Group and Memorial Sloan-Kettering Cancer Center prognostic scores for primary central nervous system lymphoma

| IELSG | MSKCC |
|---|---|
| Poor prognostic factors | |
|   Age >60 | Age >50 |
|   ECOG performance status >1 | Karnofsky performance status <70 |
|   Elevated serum LDH | |
|   Elevated CSF protein | |
|   Location of tumor in deep structures | |
| Risk groups | |
|   Group 1: 0 or 1 poor prognostic feature | Class 1 (Age <50) |
|   Group 2: 2 or 3 poor prognostic features | Class 2 (Age ≥50, KPS ≥70) |
|   Group 3: 4 or 5 poor prognostic features | Class 3 (Age ≥50, KPS <70) |
| 2-Year survival | Median survival |
|   Group 1: 80% ± 8% |   Class 1: 8.5 y |
|   Group 2: 48% ± 7% |   Class 2: 3.2 y |
|   Group 3: 15% ± 7% |   Class 3: 1.1 y |

often develop cognitive, behavioral, and personality changes related to the common location of PCNSL in the corpus callosum and deep frontal lobes. Signs of increased intracranial pressure, most commonly manifested by headaches or hydrocephalus, are also common. Cortical structures are infrequently involved and seizures are uncommon. Patients often present with acute onset of weakness, aphasia, or sensory disturbances that can be confused with manifestations of cerebral ischemia. The presentation of PCNSL is therefore nonspecific; important clues to the cause of symptoms are not clear until neuroimaging is obtained. Gadolinium-enhanced MRI of the brain tends to demonstrate a supratentorial mass that is commonly deep or periventricular in location. The most common locations are the cerebral hemispheres, basal ganglia, and corpus callosum (Fig. 1) [18]. PCNSL is usually hypointense on T1 images and hypo- to isointense on T2 images. Contrast enhancement is diffuse and relatively homogeneous. These tumors often appear cloud-like with indistinct borders. Occasionally, PCNSL is multifocal or heterogeneous and can be confused with metastases or astrocytic tumors; tissue is ultimately required for definitive diagnosis.

Patients who complain of blurry or clouded vision or floaters may have ocular lymphoma. Slit-lamp testing must be done to specifically look for evidence of lymphoma; otherwise, patients can be misdiagnosed with uveitis. Leptomeningeal involvement at presentation tends to be asymptomatic, but some patients may present with cranial neuropathies, back or limb pain, or radiculopathy. A detailed history seeking evidence of bladder incontinence, peripheral sensory loss, or other nonspecific pain should be obtained to evaluate signs and symptoms of CSF dissemination.

## Diagnostic workup

The purpose of the diagnostic workup is twofold: to obtain tissue for a definitive pathologic diagnosis of lymphoma and to evaluate the extent of

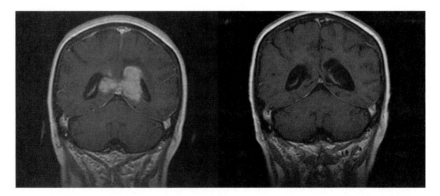

Fig. 1. Patient who has PCNSL with a lesion in the splenium of the corpus callosum. Image on left demonstrates homogeneous contrast enhancement before treatment. Image on right is consistent with a complete response after five cycles of an HD-MTX–based chemotherapy regimen.

CNS and systemic disease. Brain biopsy, lumbar puncture for CSF cytology, or vitrectomy can be done to establish tissue diagnosis. Evaluation of CSF with flow cytometry can be helpful in identifying malignant B-cells. After diagnosis is confirmed, the nervous system and the body need to be staged (Table 2) [19]. Evaluation of the CSF, if not done for diagnosis, is necessary to investigate for leptomeningeal involvement. Tumor markers, such as LDH, β-glucuronidase, and β2-microglobulin are often measured but their prognostic and diagnostic value is uncertain. CSF protein, however, is used for prognostic purposes as already discussed. Ophthalmologic examination with a slit lamp is performed to rule out ocular lymphoma even in asymptomatic patients. Gadolinium-enhanced MRI of the brain serves as an important pretreatment baseline. Gadolinium-enhanced MRI of the spine is not part of routine staging, but should be done in patients with suspicion of spinal cord or leptomeningeal spread. Body staging is important and is necessary to rule out systemic NHL. Approximately 3% to 5% of PCNSLs are found to have systemic foci at diagnosis [13,20,21]. Staging is done with computed tomography (CT) of the chest, abdomen, and pelvis, along with bone marrow biopsy. [18]Flouro-deoxyglucose positron emission tomography can be useful to identify foci of systemic disease, but this has not yet been prospectively evaluated [22]; HIV testing must be done in all patients. A diagnosis of PCNSL in the setting of HIV has significantly different implications for treatment and prognosis. A complete diagnostic workup is comprehensive and time-consuming for all patients. In patients who have poor performance status or neurologic disability, we often recommend an in-patient admission to complete all of the tests. In addition, a 24-hour urine

Table 2
Recommended staging of primary central nervous system lymphoma

| Staging for extent of central nervous system involvement | Staging for extent of systemic involvement |
| --- | --- |
| MRI brain with gadolinium | CT of chest/abdomen/pelvis |
| Ophthalmology evaluation with slit-lamp exam | Bone marrow biopsy |
| Lumbar puncture for: CSF protein | HIV testing |
| Cytology, including flow cytometry | |
| Optional exams | Optional exams |
| Lumbar puncture for: | [18]FDG PET body |
| β-glucuronidase | Testicular ultrasound |
| β-2 microglobulin | Serum LDH |
| LDH isozyme 5 | |
| MRI total spine with gadolinium (if clinically indicated) | |

*Abbreviation:* [18]FDG PET, [18]flouro-deoxyglucose positron emission tomography.
*Data from* Abrey LE, Batchelor TT, Ferreri AJM, et al. Report of an international workshop to standardize baseline evaluation and response criteria for primary CNS lymphoma. J Clin Oncol 2005;23(22):5034–43.

collection in preparation for potential treatment with high-dose MTX (HD-MTX) can be obtained.

**Primary central nervous system lymphoma therapy**

*Corticosteroids*

Corticosteroids in the patient who has PCNSL are known to lead to significant tumor regression often associated with clinical improvement [23]. Corticosteroids induce apoptosis in lymphoma cells, contributing to cytotoxic effects rather than reduction in cerebral edema [24]. Neuroimaging response can be dramatic, sometimes demonstrating complete remission of contrast-enhancing abnormalities. Most responses are temporary, although durable remissions have been reported. Prolonged exposure to steroid medications can result in resistance to their cytotoxic actions. Steroids should be avoided in suspected but undiagnosed PCNSL because they can impact biopsy results and delay definitive diagnosis. When symptoms, especially those from increased intracranial pressure, are severe or life threatening, steroids need to be administered to relieve symptoms and prevent herniation. It is important, as with steroid use in almost all conditions, to try to maintain patients on the minimum dose for as short a period as possible in an effort to avoid the many associated long-term toxicities.

*Surgery*

There is no known survival benefit to debulking surgery other than in patients who have masses large enough to cause herniation. When PCNSL is not strongly suspected in the differential diagnosis and craniotomy for debulking is performed, a frozen section consistent with PCNSL should lead the surgeon to terminate further resection. In symptomatic patients, tumor sensitivity to steroids, chemotherapy, and radiotherapy preclude the necessity for maximal resection. The primary role for surgery, therefore, is to obtain an appropriate and adequate sample of tissue with stereotactic needle biopsy. This biopsy is the optimal procedure for evaluating a malignancy that often lies in or adjacent to deep structures of the brain.

*Radiotherapy*

Radiotherapy is a fundamental part of PCNSL therapy considering the known radiosensitivity of systemic NHL. Based purely on CT and MR imaging, one would presume that PCNSL is a well-circumscribed disease that could be treated with focal radiotherapy. Autopsy studies have confirmed otherwise and demonstrate that MRI appreciably underestimates the extent of tumor involvement and that PCNSL is, in fact, a diffuse infiltrative neoplasm [25]. Consistent with these findings, patients who received focal radiotherapy had significant recurrence of disease within and outside of the radiation field [26]. Whole brain radiation therapy (WBRT) has been a standard component of therapy for a long time, but the optimal dose has never been definitively established. The ideal dose is somewhere in the range of 40 to 50 Gy based on several studies [13,27,28]. Patients receiving less than 40 Gy had shorter survival, whereas those receiving more than 50 Gy suffered from greater toxicity [13,27,29]. The addition of a boost, as studied prospectively by the RTOG, demonstrated no benefit [28]. In this study, 41 patients received a 20-Gy boost in addition to a 40-Gy dose. Median survival was only 12.2 months from time of diagnosis, which compared poorly to contemporary studies that reported a survival range from 1 to 2 years. Current recommendations are essentially a compromise of the studied regimens: 45 Gy (WBRT) with no boost. Some authors advocate deferring radiotherapy (RT) in patients older than 60 years of age with the intent of restricting neurotoxicity without compromising survival [30,31]. Ongoing protocols are examining the options of either deferring radiotherapy or using lower doses in patients who are older or who have achieved a complete response to initial chemotherapy [29,32].

## Combined-modality therapy

The chemosensitivity of PCNSL is exceptional. Not surprisingly, the addition of chemotherapy to standard radiotherapy has had an appreciable impact on tumor response and patient survival. This impact was first noted with the use of doxorubicin-based chemotherapy regimens devised for systemic NHL. Early reports resulted in radiographic responses but they were not durable. The use of cyclophosphamide, doxorubicin, vincristine, and prednisone (CHOP) demonstrated no benefit over radiotherapy alone and radiographic responses were brief [33–35]. The initial response to therapy can result in blood–brain barrier reconstitution and may prevent these drugs from adequately penetrating the brain. When low-dose MTX and bleomycin were added to the regimen (MACOP-B), the results were no different [36]. The basis of MTX use in PCNSL stems from observations of its activity in patients who had systemic lymphoma and CNS metastases [37]. MTX has limited ability to cross the blood–brain barrier. Its efficacy in PCNSL is from use at higher doses ($1-8$ g/m$^2$) when MTX is physically forced across the blood–brain barrier and achieves effective levels in the brain and CSF. Single-agent and combination regimens have both been studied and the latter have demonstrated superior response and survival rates.

The administration of HD-MTX requires detailed clinical evaluation and close clinical follow-up. In this setting, it is safe and tolerated in patients who have adequate renal function (creatinine clearance greater than 60 mL/min or 100 mL/min for patients receiving MTX 8 g/m$^2$). It should be administered with ample hydration and urine pH should be measured frequently and alkalinized if too low. Oral leucovorin is given beginning

24 hours after administration and continues for 1 to 2 days after MTX is cleared. In our institution, administration of HD-MTX is done on an inpatient basis to ensure patient safety. Daily MTX levels are followed until the drug is adequately cleared. Interesting retrospective studies suggest that prolonged clearance and higher MTX area under the curve is associated with better outcome, but this has not been corroborated [38].

In the early 1990s, DeAngelis and colleagues [20] reported a decrease in the rate of leptomeningeal relapse in patients treated with chemotherapy. These data suggested that RT alone is probably insufficient to treat disease involving the subarachnoid space. It is not clear if the decrement in CSF relapse was attributable to better penetration of the blood–brain barrier by high doses of MTX and cytarabine (ara-C) or to intra-CSF delivery of chemotherapy. HD-MTX and HD ara-C result in CSF levels of chemotherapy; however, their levels are neither consistent nor sustained [39]. Introduction of drug directly into the subarachnoid space results in therapeutic levels for 48 hours. Shorter infusions are associated with better CNS penetration and more thorough clearing of malignant cells from CSF [40]. Although retrospective data suggest that delivery into the CSF offers no added benefit to HD-MTX regimens, this has not been evaluated prospectively [41]. We treat patients who have malignant cells in their CSF with 12 mg MTX infused directly into the ventricular space by way of an Ommaya reservoir at the end of each cycle. We prefer intra-Ommaya (IO) administration because data suggest that intrathecal (IT) administration is inconsistent [42]. Additionally, IT treatments can be burdensome and require repeated intervention with lumbar puncture.

Combined-modality regimens prolong survival compared with radiotherapy alone and are the mainstay of treatment of PCNSL. They consist of HD-MTX–based combination chemotherapy, radiotherapy, and treatment of leptomeningeal disease [20]. These regimens result in impressive survival benefit with median overall survival ranging from 25 to 60 months [43]. Common MTX-based combination regimens along with their median survivals are listed in Table 3 [30,44–49]. MTX is typically infused over several hours to optimize CSF penetration and is given either weekly or every 2 weeks. HD-MTX–based regimens are given in multiple cycles with the goal of inducing a radiographic complete response. This regimen is followed by WBRT, the dose of which is determined by the extent of radiographic response and patient age. Some regimens include consolidation treatment, typically with cytarabine, and this can be given before or after WBRT. Comparing treatments can be difficult because there is variation not only in the chemotherapy regimen but also in patient age, performance status, IT treatment, radiation dose, and salvage therapies. The prognostic indices described by Abrey and colleagues [17] and Ferreri and colleagues [16] earlier in this article may be of benefit in sorting out this survival data.

The use of maintenance MTX has been studied in 31 patients who were treated with 8 $g/m^2$ for up to eight cycles until they had a complete response

Table 3
Median survival in months for high-dose methotrexate–based combined-modality regimens

| Ref | N | Combination chemotherapy regimen | | | WBRT dose (cGY) | Consolidation chemotherapy | Median survival (mo) |
|---|---|---|---|---|---|---|---|
| Abrey et al [30] | 52 | IV | MTX | 3.5 g/m$^2$ | 4500 (12 elderly patients deferred RT) | IV Ara-C 3 g/m$^2$/d × 2 | 60 |
| | | PO | PCB | 100 mg/m$^2$ | | | |
| | | IV | VCR | 1.4 g/m$^2$ | | | |
| | | IO | MTX | 12 mg | | | |
| De Angelis et al [45] | 102 | IV | MTX | 2.5 g/m$^2$ | 3600 to 4500 | IV Ara-C 3 g/m$^2$/d × 2 | 36.9 |
| | | PO | PCB | 100 mg/m$^2$ | | | |
| | | IV | VCR | 1.4 g/m$^2$ | | | |
| | | IO | MTX | 12 mg | | | |
| Omuro et al [47] | 17 | IV | MTX | 1 g/m$^2$ | 4140 + 1440 boost | None | 32 |
| | | IV | TTP | 30 mg/m$^2$ | | | |
| | | PO | PCB | 75 mg/m$^2$ | | | |
| | | IT | MTX | 12 mg × 5 | | | |
| Ferreri et al [46] | 41 | IV | MTX | 3.5 g/m$^2$ | 3000 in patients with CR; 3600 in patients with PR; 4500 in all others | None | 15 |
| | | IV | Ara-C | 2 g/m$^2$ × 2 | | | |
| | | IV | Ida | 15 mg/m$^2$ | | | |
| | | IV | TTP | 35 mg/m$^2$ | | | |
| Poortmans et al [48] | 52 | IV | MTX | 3 g/m$^2$ | 3000 + 1000 boost | None | 46 |
| | | PO | Pred | 60 mg/m$^2$ | | | |
| | | IV | Ten | 100 mg/m$^2$ | | | |
| | | IV | BCNU | 100 mg/m$^2$ | | | |
| | | IT | MTX | 15 mg × 4 | | | |
| | | IT | Ara-C | 40 mg × 4 | | | |
| Bessell et al [49] | 77 | IV | BCNU | 100 mg/m$^2$ | 4500 | None | 38 |
| | | IV | VCR | 1.4 mg/m$^2$ | | | |
| | | IV | MTX | 1.5 g/m$^2$ | | | |
| | | IV | Ara-C | 3 g/m$^2$ | | | |

*Abbreviations:* Ara-C, cytarabine; BCNU, carmustine; cGy, centigray; CR, complete remission; Ida, idarubicin; IV, intravenous; N, number of patients in study; PCB, procarbazine; PO, by mouth; PR, partial remission; Pred, prednisone; Ref, references; Ten, teniposide; TTP, thiotepa; VCR, vincristine.

[50]. Following this, they received monthly maintenance at a lower dose (3.5 g/m$^2$). Median overall survival was more than 2.5 years, but the median time to progression was just over 1 year. A follow-up study by the New Approaches to Brain Tumor Therapy group using single-agent MTX resulted in a median progression-free survival of 12.8 months [51].

*Chemotherapy dose intensification*

Much of the focus of current research is on optimizing chemotherapy and allowing patients to defer radiotherapy and its sequelae. A common experimental approach is to deliver myeloablative doses of chemotherapy followed by autologous stem cell rescue (ASCR). This strategy has proved to be successful in the treatment of systemic NHL [52]. The aim of such regimens is to attain cure with cytotoxic therapies alone, allowing patients to avoid radiation-induced long-term neurotoxicity.

Abrey and colleagues [53] treated 28 patients with an induction regimen (MTX 3.5 g/m$^2$ and ara-C 3 g/m$^2$ each for 2 days) followed by a conditioning regimen that included carmustine, etoposide, cytarabine, and melphalan. Only 57% of patients attained a complete response with the induction regimen. For those who were transplanted, median time to progression was 9.3 months. A similar ongoing effort by the same group now includes a more potent conditioning regimen. Cheng and colleagues [54] also used an HD-MTX–based regimen for induction followed by thiotepa, busulfan, and cyclophosphamide. In their small series of patients who had poor prognoses, six of seven achieved a complete response, which was maintained in five patients at last follow-up. Their results suggest that this may be an option in patients who have poor prognostic factors. A German group reported the use of HD chemotherapy and ASCR in conjunction with a hyperfractionated course of WBRT [55]. Their regimen consisted of three cycles of MTX (8 g/m$^2$), a 2-day course of ara-C (3 g/m$^2$), and thiotepa (40 mg/m$^2$). Patients received carmustine and thiotepa before transplant; the WBRT dose was 45 Gy for patients who had a complete response and 50 Gy for patients who had a partial response. Fifteen patients of 30 had a complete response with induction therapy and an additional 6 achieved a complete response after WBRT. Neurotoxicity was rare, but follow-up was short.

Other approaches aimed at intensifying dose or delivery of chemotherapy have been tried. Intra-arterial (IA) MTX in conjunction with blood–brain barrier disruption has been studied by Neuwelt and colleagues [56]. Response rates are impressive and comparable to intravenous (IV) HD-MTX. Although the regimen is associated with less long-term neurotoxicity, acute toxicities are significant and IA therapy requires general anesthesia.

*Salvage therapy*

Although response rates to combined modality therapy are high, most patients eventually relapse. At relapse, patients need to be re-staged for extent of CNS, leptomeningeal, and systemic disease; results of a re-staging workup often dictate further therapies. For those who have deferred radiotherapy, it is an important salvage option and is palliative. Clinical trials evaluating the efficacy of various single agents and combination regimens have yielded reasonable response rates [57–61]. Prior HD-MTX responders may find benefit with a second course of MTX-based treatment. Patients may be at a higher risk for neurotoxicity, however. Soussain and colleagues [61] examined a regimen in which patients who were successfully salvaged with cytarabine and etoposide were consolidated with thiotepa, busulfan, and cyclophosphamide followed by ASCR. Sixteen of 22 patients had a complete response after stem cell transplant and the authors predicted a 3-year survival of 63.7%. Temodar (150 mg/m$^2$) for 5 days in a 28-day cycle yielded a response in one fourth of patients [60]. The addition of Rituximab (750 mg/m$^2$ weekly) to temozolomide (100 to 200 mg/m$^2$, 7 days on, 7 days off) resulted in a 53% response rate when studied in 15 patients [62]. On the whole, response rates with salvage regimens tend to be less durable than those seen with upfront treatment.

*Acute and chronic toxicity*

Therapy is generally well tolerated by patients, particularly in the acute setting. All therapies are associated with some side effects, however. During radiotherapy, patients can suffer from significant fatigue. Increasing cerebral edema during this period can result in worsening neurologic deficits. IV MTX can cause a transient encephalopathy several days after treatment characterized by mental status changes, lethargy, and somnolence. IO MTX can lead to an arachnoiditis and is worse in patients concurrently receiving radiotherapy. The high doses of cytarabine given for consolidation are associated with a rarely seen cerebellar syndrome.

In the long term, however, treatment is not without consequences. Most significant is the delayed neurotoxicity seen as a result of the combination of MTX and radiotherapy [63]. Patients often develop symptoms before clinicians expect them and as early as weeks to months after treatment [64]. This syndrome is characterized primarily by cognitive symptoms. Executive dysfunction, behavioral changes, ataxia, and urinary incontinence are reported and tend to be progressive [43]. Clinical deterioration is more pronounced in the elderly and can be devastating. Leukoencephalopathy can be dramatic when viewed on MRI FLAIR imaging. A handful of patients find temporary benefit from ventriculoperitoneal shunting [65]; other treatments are purely palliative. The recognition of this syndrome and its impact on quality of life has been an important step in our understanding of PCNSL therapy. It is a dominant theme in the approach of clinicians and researchers in devising new and less-toxic combination therapies.

**Summary**

PCNSL is an unusual form of NHL that is restricted to the CNS. Although it presents with focal neurologic symptoms, it is characterized pathologically by diffuse infiltration of the brain. PCNSL is sensitive to corticosteroids, radiotherapy, and chemotherapy. HD-MTX–based regimens form the cornerstone of multimodality therapy and have significantly improved response rates and survival. Prolonged survival can be associated with devastating neurotoxicity to which the elderly are particularly susceptible. The development of newer regimens should aim to minimize such toxicity while maintaining the survival benefit of combined modality treatment.

# References

[1] DeAngelis LM, Gutin PH, Leibel SA, et al. Intracranial tumors. Diagnosis and treatment. 1st edition. London: Martin Dunitz; 2002.

[2] Ferreri AJM, Abrey LE, Blay J-Y, et al. Summary statement on primary central nervous system lymphomas from the Eighth International Conference on Malignant Lymphoma, Lugano, Switzerland, June 12 to 15, 2002. J Clin Oncol 2003;21(12):2407–14.

[3] Shenkier TN, Blay J-Y, O'Neill BP, et al. Primary CNS lymphoma of T-cell origin: a descriptive analysis from the international primary CNS lymphoma collaborative group. J Clin Oncol 2005;23(10):2233–9.

[4] Jahnke K, Hummel M, Korfel A, et al. Detection of subclinical systemic disease in primary CNS lymphoma by polymerase chain reaction of the rearranged immunoglobulin heavy-chain genes. J Clin Oncol 2006;24(29):4754–7.

[5] Schabet M. Epidemiology of primary CNS lymphoma. J Neurooncol 1999;43(3):199–201.

[6] Coté TR, Manns A, Hardy CR, et al. Epidemiology of brain lymphoma among people with or without acquired immunodeficiency syndrome. AIDS/Cancer Study Group. J Natl Cancer Inst 1996;88(10):675–9.

[7] Eby NL, Grufferman S, Flannelly CM, et al. Increasing incidence of primary brain lymphoma in the US. Cancer 1988;62(11):2461–5.

[8] Olson JE, Janney CA, Rao RD, et al. The continuing increase in the incidence of primary central nervous system non-Hodgkin lymphoma: a surveillance, epidemiology, and end results analysis. Cancer 2002;95(7):1504–10.

[9] Corn BW, Marcus SM, Topham A, et al. Will primary central nervous system lymphoma be the most frequent brain tumor diagnosed in the year 2000? Cancer 1997;79(12):2409–13.

[10] Hao D, DiFrancesco LM, Brasher PM, et al. Is primary CNS lymphoma really becoming more common? A population-based study of incidence, clinicopathological features and outcomes in Alberta from 1975 to 1996. Ann Oncol 1999;10(1):65–70.

[11] Kadan-Lottick NS, Skluzacek MC, Gurney JG. Decreasing incidence rates of primary central nervous system lymphoma. Cancer 2002;95(1):193–202.

[12] Panageas KS, Elkin EB, DeAngelis LM, et al. Trends in survival from primary central nervous system lymphoma, 1975–1999: a population-based analysis. Cancer 2005;104(11):2466–72.

[13] Pollack IF, Lunsford LD, Flickinger JC, et al. Prognostic factors in the diagnosis and treatment of primary central nervous system lymphoma. Cancer 1989;63(5):939–47.

[14] Corry J, Smith JG, Wirth A, et al. Primary central nervous system lymphoma: age and performance status are more important than treatment modality. Int J Radiat Oncol Biol Phys 1998;41(3):615–20.

[15] Blay JY, Lasset C, Carrie C, et al. Multivariate analysis of prognostic factors in patients with non HIV-related primary cerebral lymphoma. A proposal for a prognostic scoring. Br J Cancer 1993;67(5):1136–41.

[16] Ferreri AJM, Blay J-Y, Reni M, et al. Prognostic scoring system for primary CNS lymphomas: the International Extranodal Lymphoma Study Group experience. J Clin Oncol 2003; 21(2):266–72.

[17] Abrey LE, Ben-Porat L, Panageas KS, et al. Primary central nervous system lymphoma: the Memorial Sloan-Kettering Cancer Center prognostic model. J Clin Oncol 2006;24(36): 5711–5.

[18] Küker W, Nägele T, Korfel A, et al. Primary central nervous system lymphomas (PCNSL): MRI features at presentation in 100 patients. J Neurooncol 2005;72(2):169–77.

[19] Abrey LE, Batchelor TT, Ferreri AJM, et al. Report of an international workshop to standardize baseline evaluation and response criteria for primary CNS lymphoma. J Clin Oncol 2005;23(22):5034–43.

[20] DeAngelis LM, Yahalom J, Thaler HT, et al. Combined modality therapy for primary CNS lymphoma. J Clin Oncol 1992;10(4):635–43.

[21] O'Neill BP, Dinapoli RP, Kurtin PJ, et al. Occult systemic non-Hodgkin's lymphoma (NHL) in patients initially diagnosed as primary central nervous system lymphoma (PCNSL): how much staging is enough? J Neurooncol 1995;25(1):67–71.

[22] Mohile N, DeAngelis L, Abrey L. The role of cranial and body 18 fluoro-deoxyglucose positron emission tomography in primary CNS lymphoma. Proceedings of the American Society of Clinical Oncology 2006;24:665.

[23] Todd FD, Miller CA, Yates AJ, et al. Steroid-induced remission in primary malignant lymphoma of the central nervous system. Surg Neurol 1986;26(1):79–84.

[24] Weller M. Glucocorticoid treatment of primary CNS lymphoma. J Neurooncol 1999;43(3): 237–9.

[25] Lai R, Rosenblum MK, DeAngelis LM. Primary CNS lymphoma: a whole-brain disease? Neurology 2002;59(10):1557–62.

[26] Shibamoto Y, Hayabuchi N, Hiratsuka J-I, et al. Is whole-brain irradiation necessary for primary central nervous system lymphoma? Patterns of recurrence after partial-brain irradiation. Cancer 2003;97(1):128–33.

[27] Blay JY, Conroy T, Chevreau C, et al. High-dose methotrexate for the treatment of primary cerebral lymphomas: analysis of survival and late neurologic toxicity in a retrospective series. J Clin Oncol 1998;16(3):864–71.

[28] Nelson DF, Martz KL, Bonner H, et al. Non-Hodgkin's lymphoma of the brain: can high dose, large volume radiation therapy improve survival? Report on a prospective trial by the Radiation Therapy Oncology Group (RTOG): RTOG 8315. Int J Radiat Oncol Biol Phys 1992;23(1):9–17.

[29] Bessell EM, López-Guillermo A, Villá S, et al. Importance of radiotherapy in the outcome of patients with primary CNS lymphoma: an analysis of the CHOD/BVAM regimen followed by two different radiotherapy treatments. J Clin Oncol 2002;20(1):231–6.

[30] Abrey LE, Yahalom J, DeAngelis LM. Treatment for primary CNS lymphoma: the next step. J Clin Oncol 2000;18(17):3144–50.

[31] Gavrilovic IT, Hormigo A, Yahalom J, et al. Long-term follow-up of high-dose methotrexate-based therapy with and without whole brain irradiation for newly diagnosed primary CNS lymphoma. J Clin Oncol 2006;24(28):4570–4.

[32] Yahalom J, Abrey LE. Reduced-dose whole grain radiotherapy (WBRT) following complete response to immuno-chemotherapy in patients with primary CNS lymphoma (PCNSL). ASTRO Abstract 2006;66(6):584.

[33] Lachance DH, Brizel DM, Gockerman JP, et al. Cyclophosphamide, doxorubicin, vincristine, and prednisone for primary central nervous system lymphoma: short-duration response and multifocal intracerebral recurrence preceding radiotherapy. Neurology 1994;44(9): 1721–7.

[34] Schultz C, Scott C, Sherman W, et al. Preirradiation chemotherapy with cyclophosphamide, doxorubicin, vincristine, and dexamethasone for primary CNS lymphomas: initial report of radiation therapy oncology group protocol 88-06. J Clin Oncol 1996;14(2): 556–64.

[35] Shibamoto Y, Tsutsui K, Dodo Y, et al. Improved survival rate in primary intracranial lymphoma treated by high-dose radiation and systemic vincristine-doxorubicin-cyclophosphamide-prednisolone chemotherapy. Cancer 1990;65(9):1907–12.

[36] Brada M, Dearnaley D, Horwich A, et al. Management of primary cerebral lymphoma with initial chemotherapy: preliminary results and comparison with patients treated with radiotherapy alone. Int J Radiat Oncol Biol Phys 1990;18(4):787–92.

[37] Skarin AT, Zuckerman KS, Pitman SW, et al. High-dose methotrexate with folinic acid in the treatment of advanced non-Hodgkin lymphoma including CNS involvement. Blood 1977;50(6):1039–47.

[38] Ferreri AJM, Guerra E, Regazzi M, et al. Area under the curve of methotrexate and creatinine clearance are outcome-determining factors in primary CNS lymphomas. Br J Cancer 2004;90(2):353–8.

[39] Slevin ML, Piall EM, Aherne GW, et al. Effect of dose and schedule on pharmacokinetics of high-dose cytosine arabinoside in plasma and cerebrospinal fluid. J Clin Oncol 1983;1(9): 546–51.

[40] Hiraga S, Arita N, Ohnishi T, et al. Rapid infusion of high-dose methotrexate resulting in enhanced penetration into cerebrospinal fluid and intensified tumor response in primary central nervous system lymphomas. J Neurosurg 1999;91(2):221–30.

[41] Khan RB, Shi W, Thaler HT, et al. Is intrathecal methotrexate necessary in the treatment of primary CNS lymphoma? J Neurooncol 2002;58(2):175–8.

[42] Shapiro WR, Young DF, Mehta BM. Methotrexate: distribution in cerebrospinal fluid after intravenous, ventricular and lumbar injections. N Engl J Med 1975;293(4):161–6.

[43] Omuro AMP, Ben-Porat LS, Panageas KS, et al. Delayed neurotoxicity in primary central nervous system lymphoma. Arch Neurol 2005;62(10):1595–600.

[44] Cheng AL, Yeh KH, Uen WC, et al. Systemic chemotherapy alone for patients with non-acquired immunodeficiency syndrome-related central nervous system lymphoma: a pilot study of the BOMES protocol. Cancer 1998;82(10):1946–51.

[45] DeAngelis LM, Seiferheld W, Schold SC, et al. Combination chemotherapy and radiotherapy for primary central nervous system lymphoma: Radiation Therapy Oncology Group Study 93-10. J Clin Oncol 2002;20(24):4643–8.

[46] Ferreri AJM, Dell'Oro S, Foppoli M, et al. MATILDE regimen followed by radiotherapy is an active strategy against primary CNS lymphomas. Neurology 2006;66(9):1435–8.

[47] Omuro AMP, DeAngelis LM, Yahalom J, et al. Chemoradiotherapy for primary CNS lymphoma: an intent-to-treat analysis with complete follow-up. Neurology 2005;64(1): 69–74.

[48] Poortmans PMP, Kluin-Nelemans HC, Haaxma-Reiche H, et al. High-dose methotrexate-based chemotherapy followed by consolidating radiotherapy in non-AIDS-related primary central nervous system lymphoma: European Organization for Research and Treatment of Cancer Lymphoma Group Phase II Trial 20962. J Clin Oncol 2003;21(24): 4483–8.

[49] Bessell EM, Graus FF, Lopez-Guillermo A, et al. Primary non-Hodgkin's lymphoma of the CNS treated with CHOD/BVAM or BVAM chemotherapy before radiotherapy: long-term survival and prognostic factors. Int J Radiat Oncol Biol Phys 2004;59(2):501–8.

[50] Guha-Thakurta N, Damek D, Pollack C, et al. Intravenous methotrexate as initial treatment for primary central nervous system lymphoma: response to therapy and quality of life of patients. J Neurooncol 1999;43(3):259–68.

[51] Batchelor T, Carson K, O'Neill A, et al. Treatment of primary CNS lymphoma with methotrexate and deferred radiotherapy: a report of NABTT 96-07. J Clin Oncol 2003;21(6): 1044–9.

[52] Milpied N, Deconinck E, Gaillard F, et al. Initial treatment of aggressive lymphoma with high-dose chemotherapy and autologous stem-cell support. N Engl J Med 2004;350(13): 1287–95.

[53] Abrey LE, Moskowitz CH, Mason WP, et al. Intensive methotrexate and cytarabine followed by high-dose chemotherapy with autologous stem-cell rescue in patients with newly diagnosed primary CNS lymphoma: an intent-to-treat analysis. J Clin Oncol 2003;21(22): 4151–6.

[54] Cheng T, Forsyth P, Chaudhry A, et al. High-dose thiotepa, busulfan, cyclophosphamide and ASCT without whole-brain radiotherapy for poor prognosis primary CNS lymphoma. Bone Marrow Transplant 2003;31(8):679–85.

[55] Illerhaus G, Marks R, Ihorst G, et al. High-dose chemotherapy with autologous stem-cell transplantation and hyperfractionated radiotherapy as first-line treatment of primary CNS lymphoma. J Clin Oncol 2006;24(24):3865–70.

[56] Neuwelt EA, Goldman DL, Dahlborg SA, et al. Primary CNS lymphoma treated with osmotic blood-brain barrier disruption: prolonged survival and preservation of cognitive function. J Clin Oncol 1991;9(9):1580–90.

[57] Arellano-Rodrigo E, López-Guillermo A, Bessell EM, et al. Salvage treatment with etoposide (VP-16), ifosfamide and cytarabine (Ara-C) for patients with recurrent primary central nervous system lymphoma. Eur J Haematol 2003;70(4):219–24.

[58] Herrlinger U, Brugger W, Bamberg M, et al. PCV salvage chemotherapy for recurrent primary CNS lymphoma. Neurology 2000;54(8):1707–8.

[59] Pels H, Schulz H, Schlegel U, et al. Treatment of CNS lymphoma with the anti-CD20 antibody rituximab: experience with two cases and review of the literature. Onkologie 2003;26(4):351–4.

[60] Reni M, Mason W, Zaja F, et al. Salvage chemotherapy with temozolomide in primary CNS lymphomas: preliminary results of a phase II trial. Eur J Cancer 2004;40(11):1682–8.

[61] Soussain C, Suzan F, Hoang-Xuan K, et al. Results of intensive chemotherapy followed by hematopoietic stem-cell rescue in 22 patients with refractory or recurrent primary CNS lymphoma or intraocular lymphoma. J Clin Oncol 2001;19(3):742–9.

[62] Enting RH, Demopoulos A, DeAngelis LM, et al. Salvage therapy for primary CNS lymphoma with a combination of rituximab and temozolomide. Neurology 2004;63(5): 901–3.

[63] Correa D, DeAngelis LM, Shi W, et al. Cognitive functions in survivors of primary central nervous system lymphoma. Neurology 2004;62(4):548–55.

[64] Lai R, Abrey LE, Rosenblum MK, et al. Treatment-induced leukoencephalopathy in primary CNS lymphoma: a clinical and autopsy study. Neurology 2004;62(3):451–6.

[65] Thiessen B, DeAngelis LM. Hydrocephalus in radiation leukoencephalopathy: results of ventriculoperitoneal shunting. Arch Neurol 1998;55(5):705–10.

ELSEVIER
SAUNDERS

NEUROLOGIC
CLINICS

Neurol Clin 25 (2007) 1209–1230

# Current Concepts in Management of Meningiomas and Schwannomas

Ashok R. Asthagiri, MD[a],*,
Gregory A. Helm, MD, PhD[b],
Jason P. Sheehan, MD, PhD[b]

[a]National Institutes of Health/NINDS, Bethesda, MD, USA
[b]Department of Neurological Surgery, University of Virginia Health Sciences Center,
P.O. Box 800212, Charlottesville, VA 22908-0212, USA

Intracranial schwannomas and tumors of the meninges have been reported since the eighteenth century [1,2]. These extra-axial lesions lent themselves to clinical detection by presenting overt and focal changes in appearance and function of the harboring patient. The earliest diagnosis of meningiomas during life occurred by causing hyperostotic changes to the overlying skull. The first presumptive case of a vestibular schwannoma can be dated back to autopsy findings by Sandifort in 1777 in which he documented a small body adherent to the right auditory nerve, as related by Cushing [3]. Since their initial discovery, these often-benign lesions have shared a parallel metamorphosis in their management. The goal of this article is to provide a review of the current literature surrounding the mainstays of therapy for these lesions.

Meningiomas and schwannomas are the two most common extra-axial intracranial tumors in adults. Meningiomas account for approximately 25% to 30.1% of all intracranial tumors diagnosed in the United States [4–7]. Data collected from the Central Brain Tumor Registry between 1998 and 2002 reflect trends in meningioma demographics that have shown only modest changes since 1990. These trends include a female age-specific incidence of 6.01 per 100,000 person-years compared with a male age-specific incidence of 2.75 per 100,000 person-years. Although the classic description associates these tumors with middle-aged women, it may be misguiding because the median age at diagnosis for these tumors is 64 years

---

* Corresponding author.
 *E-mail address:* asthagiria@ninds.nih.gov (A.R. Asthagiri).

0733-8619/07/$ - see front matter © 2007 Elsevier Inc. All rights reserved.
doi:10.1016/j.ncl.2007.07.009       *neurologic.theclinics.com*

and the age-specific incidence increases with each consecutive 10-year age cohort [7,8].

Intracranial nerve sheath tumors compose 8% to 10% of all intracranial tumors [7,9,10]. Schwannomas, which compose the vast majority of these lesions, are the second most common extra-axial intracranial tumor. The male-to-female age-specific incidence ratio (1.01:1) is far less skewed than for meningiomas. These lesions also show a defined peak in incidence during the fifth and sixth decades of life [7].

## Pathogenesis

### Meningiomas

Tumorigenesis of meningiomas is presumed to be multifactorial and likely the result of exogenous and endogenous factors. Among the earliest theories regarding their etiology was a causal relationship with head trauma, as first suggested by Cushing [11] in 1922 and then more assertively published in 1938 [12]. Although this suggestion has been supported with isolated reports and case-control studies, it has been refuted by others [13–17]. The seemingly conflicting data leave us without definitive proof of a causal relationship between head injury and subsequent development of intracranial meningiomas [18]. The best-proven external factor with a pathogenic role is radiation. Numerous reports have shown meningiomas to occur in treatment fields associated with low doses of radiation. This concept gained wide acceptance after Modan and colleagues [19] reported a fourfold increase in the incidence of meningiomas among children treated with the Kienbock-Adamson protocol for tinea capitis, a low-dose radiation treatment protocol targeting the scalp that has since been replaced by pharmaceutic alternatives. Higher doses of radiation have been associated with a decrease in the temporal delay to discovery of meningiomas [20,21]. Less convincing supporting data exist for other exogenous factors including viral infection.

Endogenous factors involved in tumorigenesis include molecular alterations found in meningiomas and the ambiguous role of endogenous hormones in tumor development. Meningiomas were among the first solid tumors evaluated by cytogenetics. They were found to have a chromosomal aberration on the long arm of chromosome 22 in 50% to 72% of cases, which involved the tumor suppressor NF2 gene loci in up to 60% of sporadic meningiomas [22–25]. The presence of the NF2 gene product, schwannomin/merlin, in 26% of one series, confirms the lack of universal deletion and underscores the notion that non-NF2 mechanisms are also important [26,27]. Of interest, the absence in reduction of NF2 protein levels may be as high as 72% in some histologic subtypes of meningiomas [28]. Other chromosomal aberrations and genetic abnormalities, including the loss of other tumor suppressor genes (DAL-1, CDKN2A), oncogene activation, and telomerase reactivation, are being implicated in the tumorigenesis of meningiomas and the progression toward malignant behavior with accrual of these changes [26].

An almost 2:1 female preponderance of meningiomas reported in the literature and a strong association with breast cancer led to initial interest in the role of sex hormones in the development and progression of meningiomas. Investigation has revealed that tumors expressing progesterone receptors behave in a more benign clinical fashion and are less likely to recur. Tumors expressing estrogen receptor or lacking progesterone receptor expression display more frequent genotypic alterations and karyotype abnormalities consistent with more aggressive meningiomas [29,30]. Although the use of steroid hormone receptor antagonists as targets of therapy was initially successful in mice experiments and promising to a limited potential in humans, it now seems less promising after no benefit was seen in a double-blinded, placebo-controlled phase III study [30,31].

## Schwannomas

Schwannomas are slow-growing peripheral nerve sheath tumors that arise distal to the oligodendroglial–Schwann cell myelination transition. Our understanding of these lesions' pathogenesis has been forwarded by the evaluation of the molecular and genetic changes found in neurofibromatosis 2 (NF2). The *NF2* gene was localized to chromosome 22q12 through genetic linkage analysis [32]. Subsequent genetic and physical mapping led to the discovery of the *NF2* gene by two independent groups in 1993 [33,34]. This region of DNA encodes a 595–amino acid protein product termed "merlin" (for *m*oesin-*e*zrin-*r*adixin-like protein) or schwannomin, and it functions as a tumor suppressor. Mutations of the *NF2* gene have been found not only in schwannomas associated with NF2 but also in sporadic cases [35–37]. Extensive screening of vestibular schwannomas, however, has not yielded a universal detection of mutations of the *NF2* gene locus, suggesting that additional mechanisms for inactivation of the tumor suppressor may exist [38].

## Clinical presentation

### Meningiomas

Meningiomas are among the most diverse of all intracranial lesions, presenting with a vast assortment of symptoms, diagnostic imaging results, and histology. The duplicitous nature of these lesions and their ability to mimic diagnostic identifying features of other intracranial pathology have garnered respectful monikers such as the "great masquerader." Meningiomas originate from arachnoid (meningothelial) cap cells, which in general are associated with regions containing the trilamellar meninges. Lesions occurring in obscure locations such as the ventricular system can thus be explained by the presence of these cap cells within the tela choroidea. The most common locations of meningiomas, in descending order of frequency, are convexity

(19%–34%), parasagittal (18%–25%), sphenoid and middle cranial fossa (17%–25%), frontal base (10%) and posterior fossa (9%–15%), cerebellar convexity (5%), cerebellopontine angle (2%–4%), intraventricular (1%–5%), and clivus (<1%) [20,39–41].

Meningiomas present in one of four ways, determined by size and location of the tumor [42,43]. With the advent of CT/MRI diagnostic capabilities, meningiomas are being discovered more frequently in an incidental fashion. Indeed, meningiomas represent the most common incidentally detected intracranial neoplasm, accounting for one third of such tumors [39,44]. Ten percent of patients present in this manner, typically asymptomatic with slow or no tumor growth; however, one study of 40 patients revealed tumor growth in 33% and found 10% of patients became symptomatic [44,45]. The second group, accounting for upwards of 50% of patients, may present due to disruption of cortical electrophysiology and present with seizures. Meningiomas may also cause general symptoms of raised intracranial pressure, directly through tumor size and indirectly through associated hemorrhage, edema, obstructive hydrocephalus, and dural venous sinus obstruction. Finally, these tumors may cause neurologic deficits because of neural compression. The clinical presentation in these patients is determined by tumor location and size. Typical clinical presentations have been extensively described in the literature, the most common of which are outlined in Table 1.

*Schwannomas*

These typically benign tumors may be encountered incidentally but more commonly present to clinical attention secondary to neurologic dysfunction from local mass effect. Some tumors may display a more profound global neurologic effect when cerebrospinal fluid dynamics are altered. Intracranial schwannomas, like their spinal counterparts, show a predilection for involvement of the sensory division of nerves. In order of decreasing frequency, schwannomas arise most commonly from the vestibular component of the eighth nerve (>90%), sensory division of the trigeminal nerve (0.8%–8%), facial nerve (1.9%), nerves of the jugular foramen (2.9%–4%), hypoglossal nerve, extraocular nerves, and the olfactory nerve [46–50]. Because of their intimate relationship with regional cranial nerves, brainstem, and cerebellum, schwannomas may become symptomatic even as relatively small tumors. Conversely, their slow growth rates may mask the insidious progression of neurologic deficits, allow neural elements to deform without a direct loss of function, or both. Typical clinical presentations of intracranial schwannomas are reviewed in Table 2.

**Treatment**

In the interests of brevity, the microsurgical and radiosurgical treatment results for meningiomas and vestibular schwannomas are discussed the

Table 1
Meningioma location and associated typical clinical presentations

| Meningioma | Location | Clinical presentation |
|---|---|---|
| Parasagittal and falcine | Anterior one third | Headache and mental status changes |
| | Middle one third | Jacksonian seizures and progressive hemiparesis |
| | Posterior one third | Headache, visual symptoms, seizures, or mental status changes |
| Spenoid wing | Lateral/pterional | Similar to convexity tumors |
| | Middle one third (alar) | Hemiparesis/dysphasia |
| | Medial (clinoidal) | Visual acuity/field disturbance due to optic nerve compression, proptosis, cranial nerve dysfunction (III, IV, V, VI) |
| Olfactory groove | | Foster Kennedy syndrome (anosmia, ipsilateral optic atrophy with contralateral papilledema), frontal lobe syndromes/mental status changes, urinary incontinence, seizure |
| Tuberculum sella/suprasellar | | Visual acuity/field disturbance, anosmia, hydrocephalus, endocrinologic syndromes |
| Cavernous sinus | | Cranial nerve deficits (III, IV, V, VI) |
| Cerebellopontine angle | | Hearing loss, facial pain/numbness/weakness/spasm, headaches, cerebellar signs |
| Foramen magnum | | Unilateral cervical pain, extremity motor and sensory loss (clockwise involvement), cold and clumsy hands with intrinsic hand atrophy |
| Petroclival | | Hearing loss, vertigo, tinnitus, facial pain, cranial nerve deficits (V, VI, VII, VII) |

following sections. These approaches and the associated results can be generally translated to other more rare tumors such as facial or trigeminal schwannomas.

## Microsurgical management

> There is today nothing in the whole realm of surgery more gratifying than the successful removal of a meningioma with subsequent perfect functional recovery... —Harvey Cushing [11]

Surgical resection of acoustic neuromas and meningiomas has been the mainstay of treatment. Several compelling arguments favor surgery: (1) seemingly difficult tumors can sometimes be removed safely; (2) surgery secures a tissue diagnosis—occasionally, a tumor thought to be a meningioma on imaging is determined to be a different lesion; and (3) most meningiomas and acoustic neuromas are benign tumors, and a "cure" can be achieved by

Table 2
Intracranial schwannomas: typical clinical presentation

| Schwannoma | Clinical presentation |
|---|---|
| Vestibular | Unilateral sensory hearing loss, tinnitus, disequilibrium |
| Trigeminal | Trigeminal nerve dysfunction (numbness, pain), headache, diplopia, hearing loss/tinnitus |
| Facial | Hearing loss, facial paralysis (may be acute), facial pain, hemifacial spasm, tinnitus, vertigo |
| Jugular foramen | Cranial nerve palsies (IX, X, XI) |
| Accessory nerve | Chronic neck and shoulder pain, muscle spasms |
| Hypoglossal | Headache, cranial nerve dysfunction (IX, X, XI), limb weakness |

complete resection. Advanced microsurgical and skull-based techniques have led to reduced morbidity and more thorough resections of meningiomas and acoustic neuromas. Despite these advances, gross total resections cannot always be accomplished without placing the patient at significant risk of morbidity and mortality. The goal of surgery should always be to preserve the quality of the patient's life, even if it means leaving residual tumor.

*Microsurgery results*

*Meningiomas*

The measures used to review operative results in meningioma surgery include radiographic parameters (including recurrence rates) and clinical-based outcomes of morbidity and mortality. In 1957, Simpson [51] retrospectively reviewed the postoperative course of 265 patients who had meningiomas, 55 of whom experienced recurrences (21%). A recurrence rate of 9% was seen in patients who had a grade I excision, a recurrence rate of 19% was seen for grade II excisions, 29% for grade III, and 44% for grade IV (Table 3). The extent of surgical resection is the most important factor in the prevention of recurrence.

Although complete resection is generically the fundamental goal in surgery for these benign lesions, deliberate incomplete resection is often

Table 3
Simpson's classification of the extent of resection of intracranial meningiomas

| Grade | Extent of resection | Recurrence rate |
|---|---|---|
| I | Gross total resection of tumor, dural attachments, and abnormal bone | 9% |
| II | Gross total resection of tumor, coagulation of dural attachments | 19% |
| III | Gross total resection of tumor without resection or coagulation of dural attachments or its extradural extensions | 29% |
| IV | Partial resection of tumor | 44% |
| V | Simple decompression | |

*From* Simpson D. The recurrence of intracranial meningiomas after surgical treatment. J Neurol Neurosurg Psychiatry 1957;20(1):22–39; with permission.

undertaken to minimize associated morbidity. This practice is especially true with regard to petroclival, clinoidal, and tentorial-based tumors to reduce related cranial nerve morbidity, and in posterior parasagittal lesions with incomplete obstruction of the superior sagittal sinus to preserve its patency. Inherent to this, recurrence rates of these tumors are higher; the highest recurrence rates (>20%) are found in patients who have sphenoid wing meningiomas, followed by those who have parasagittal meningiomas (8%–24%) and suprasellar meningiomas (5%–10%) [41]. These findings show that the site of tumor origin and its operative accessibility may limit the potential for complete resection and thus serve as a secondary factor influencing recurrence rate [52,53]. Other factors that correlate with an increased recurrence rate include histopathologic findings of increased mitosis, focal necrosis, nuclear pleomorphism, prominent nucleoli, syncytial tumors, and the presence of brain invasion [54–56]. These findings (except brain invasion) have been incorporated into the World Health Organization classification of meningiomas and denote changes toward malignancy.

The surgical morbidity and mortality associated with resection of these lesions has dramatically decreased since initial undertakings at the turn of the twentieth century. This decrease has been a result of improved diagnostic imaging, introduction of microsurgical techniques and image guidance, and better perioperative critical/medical care. Even in the best hands, however, mortality rates remain at 1% to 14% [57–62]. Factors that increase mortality include poor preoperative clinical condition, compressive symptoms from tumor, old age, incomplete tumor removal, pulmonary embolism, and intracranial hemorrhage [58].

Morbidity associated with meningioma surgery has been cataloged and critically reviewed and should be clustered into two broad categories. The low-risk group includes tumors that provide an easy corridor for access and that are spatially removed from cranial nerves, brainstem, and vital cerebrovascular anatomy. Examples of such tumors include cerebral and cerebellar convexity tumors, lateral- and middle-third sphenoid wing meningiomas, and anterior-third parasagittal and falcine meningiomas. In most cases, convexity meningiomas are amenable to complete resection and improved operative mortality rates [63,64]. Neurologic sequelae associated with these resections typically manifest secondary to compromise of adjacent cerebrovascular structures, immediate postoperative edema, and epilepsy [57]. In one study, convexity meningioma recurrence-free rates at 5, 10, and 15 years were 93%, 80%, and 68%, respectively [65]. Several investigators have reported low mortality rates (0%–3%) and morbidity manifesting as permanent neurologic deficit in 10% of patients [66–68]. Similarly, relatively low rates of postoperative-increased morbidity can be found with anterior-third parasagittal and falcine meningiomas.

The high-risk group of meningiomas includes tumors of the skull base, tentorial-based tumors, foramen magnum meningiomas, and parasagittal lesions associated with the middle third of the superior sagittal sinus. Basal tumors are often intimately associated with cranial nerves and proximal cerebral vessels, thereby making the approach to these lesions a formidable challenge. With resection of skull-base tumors, permanent neurologic deficit ascribed to cranial nerve dysfunction has been reported in a wide range (18%–86%) [69]. The highest of these complication rates is typically associated with petroclival or cavernous sinus meningiomas, especially in cases in which a complete resection is performed [70–72]. Subtotal resection for decompression, even with tumors of the cavernous sinus, can be performed safely, although recurrence rates are naturally higher.

## Schwannomas (vestibular)

The first reported surgical removal of a vestibular schwannoma was performed by Sir Charles Ballance [73] in 1894. Although alive and well over a decade later, the patient suffered ipsilateral facial paralysis and numbness, two neurologic sequelae that were not uncommon during initial undertakings for removal of these tumors. During this time period, Dandy [74] reported the operative mortality to be 67% to 84%. Through improved surgical methodology and technique, Cushing was able to markedly decrease the mortality rates associated with operative management of these lesions, thereby ushering neurosurgeons and neuro-otologists into the modern era of surgery for acoustic neuromas. Since that time, the introduction of the operating microscope, more sensitive diagnostic imaging, and intraoperative facial and cochlear monitoring has steadily reduced the morbidity and mortality associated with resection of these lesions. In a meta-analysis of 16 studies including 5005 patients undergoing microsurgery for sporadic unilateral vestibular schwannomas, it was reported that tumor resection was complete in 96% of cases, with a mortality rate of 0.63%. The most common non-neurologic complication was cerebrospinal fluid leak, which occurred in 6.0% of patients [75].

With an expectant small mortality and major morbidity rate, the more common end points for evaluation of a successful surgery have turned to preservation of facial nerve function and auditory function. In 1985, House and Brackmann [76] developed what has become the most widely accepted measurement of facial nerve function (Table 4). Detailed evaluation of individual large series shows that preservation of facial nerve function is inversely proportional to tumor size. Indeed, when evaluating facial nerve preservation after resection of intracanalicular lesions alone, multiple studies have reported 100% postoperative grade I House-Brackmann function [77–81]. Resection of small tumors (<2.0 cm), medium-sized tumors (2.0–3.9 cm), and large tumors (>4.0 cm) was respectively associated with a 95% to 97%, a 61% to 73%, and a 28% to 57% preservation of grade I to II House-Brackmann function [82–84]. In reviewing the relative rates of facial nerve dysfunction, the suboccipital and translabyrinthine approaches afford comparable and excellent results compared with the middle

Table 4
House-Brackmann scale for assessment of facial nerve function

| Grade | Function | Gross | Motion |
|---|---|---|---|
| I | Normal facial function | | |
| II | Mild dysfunction | • Slight weakness noticeable on close inspection<br>• May have slight synkinesis<br>• At rest, normal symmetry and tone | • Forehead: moderate-to-good function<br>• Eye: complete closure with minimal effort<br>• Mouth: slight asymmetry |
| III | Moderate dysfunction | • Obvious but not disfiguring difference between the two sides<br>• Noticeable but not severe synkinesis, contracture, or hemifacial spasm<br>• At rest, normal symmetry and tone | • Forehead: slight-to-moderate movement<br>• Eye: complete closure with effort<br>• Mouth: slightly weak with maximum effort |
| IV | Moderately severe dysfunction | • Obvious weakness and/or disfiguring asymmetry<br>• At rest, normal symmetry and tone | • Forehead: none<br>• Eye: incomplete closure<br>• Mouth: asymmetric with maximum effort |
| V | Severe dysfunction | • Only barely perceptible motion<br>• At rest, asymmetry | • Forehead: none<br>• Eye: incomplete closure<br>• Mouth: slight movement |
| VI | Total paralysis | • No movement | • No movement |

*From* House JW, Brackmann DE. Facial nerve grading system. Otolaryngol Head Neck Surg 1985;93(2):146–7; with permission.

fossa approach in which increased manipulation of the superiorly located facial nerve in the internal auditory canal may account for a higher risk to facial nerve function [84–86].

Similarly, the importance of preservation of serviceable ipsilateral hearing has become paramount. The translabyrinthine approach, through its destruction of the otic capsule, is not compatible with hearing preservation [85]. Resection of purely intracanalicular tumors is associated with a 57% to 82% preservation of ipsilateral serviceable auditory function [77,79]. Risk to serviceable auditory function is directly related to tumor size. In 1988, Gardner and Robertson [87] compiled results of multiple operative series and found hearing preservation in 131 of 394 patients, athough only 5 of these patients had tumors larger than 3 cm. Subsequent studies have reported retention of functional ipsilateral hearing in 29% to 60% of cases, primarily with tumors less than 3 cm, and a precipitous decline in hearing preservation rates in cases with larger tumors [78,79,88,89]. The objective criteria for the designation of serviceable hearing vary between these studies and may account for the disparity in rates of hearing preservation.

**Radiosurgical management**

Radiosurgery may be used for patients who have recurrent or residual tumors or as a primary treatment in patients unwilling or unable to undergo surgery and who possess a lesion with the typical imaging characteristics of an acoustic neuroma or meningioma. Radiosurgery for meningiomas is usually performed with the gamma knife. Occasionally, modified linear accelarators or proton beam can be used. Patients who have atypical findings on MRI or CT should undergo surgery to obtain a histologic diagnosis. This practice is critical because when gamma knife radiosurgery (GKRS) is used to treat tumors on imaging characteristics alone, the risk of an incorrect diagnosis may be as high as 2% [90].

Location plays a pivotal role in the selection of the appropriate treatment modality. Convexity meningiomas are usually treated with open surgery because they are amenable to complete resection. Acoustic neuromas, skull-base (including cavernous sinus and petroclival) and parasagittal meningiomas, on the other hand, are ideal lesions for radiosurgery due to their anatomy and associated surgical morbidity and mortality.

Residual tumor attached to still-patent vascular or neural structures can be targeted using radiosurgery, allowing less radical microsurgical resection and a lower incidence of morbidity. For radiosurgery, a distance of at least 3 to 4 mm between the tumor and the optic apparatus is ideal. With thin-cut stereotactic planning MRI and shielding, radiosurgery can be used to treat lesions within 2 mm of the optic apparatus. The authors tend to favor early treatment of acoustic neuromas or skull-base meningiomas rather than a "watch and wait" approach because of the favorable benefit-to-risk profile of GKRS.

*Radiosurgery results*

*Meningiomas*
*Neuroimaging outcomes.* The authors have treated more than 300 meningiomas at the University of Virginia since 1989. The most recent evaluation of the authors' material included 206 patients who had meningiomas treated with GKRS, with a follow-up of 1 to 6 years. This evaluation included 142 patients treated for residual disease and 64 patients treated with GKRS primarily. Tumor volume ranged from 1 to 32 cm$^3$. These patients received an average of 38 Gy maximum dose (range, 20–60 Gy) and an average margin dose of 14 Gy (range, 10–20 Gy). Radiographic follow-up was available for 151 patients. Of the evaluated patients, 94 (63%) showed a tumor volume decrease of at least 15% and 40 (26%) showed no change in size, corresponding to an 89% tumor control rate. Tumor growth was noted in 17 patients (11%). The authors now have long-term follow-up (10–21 years) of 31 meningiomas treated with GKRS. Two thirds of these tumors have shrunk significantly or remained stable. Among these tumors are those

in which only the vascular supply for the tumor (ie, the nutritive vessel) was targeted. Such targeting has resulted in significant tumor shrinkage and lasting effect, even in the long-term.

The results of other centers are similar (Table 5) [90–101]. The University of Pittsburgh group recently reported long-term results in 85 patients whose meningiomas were treated with GKRS. With a median follow-up of 10 years, they reported that 53% of the tumors decreased in size and 40% were stable in size, corresponding to a 93% tumor control rate [102]. Kreil and colleagues [103], with a median follow-up of 7.9 years, similarly reported on 200 patients treated with GKRS for meningiomas and found that 56.5% of meningiomas demonstrated a decreased volume and 42.5% showed stable tumor volumes. Pollock and colleagues [104] compared the efficacy of GKRS with that of microsurgery for the treatment of meningiomas that had an average diameter less than 35 mm. They concluded that progression-free survival after radiosurgery is equivalent to that after resection of a Simpson grade 1 tumor and was superior to that after Simpson grade 2, 3, or 4 resections, confirming the efficacy of GKRS, especially in tumors in which gross total resection is difficult to achieve due to anatomic constraints.

*Atypical and malignant meningioma outcomes.* Atypical and malignant meningiomas usually demonstrate recurrence and aggressive growth regardless of the treatment modality (ie, extirpation, radiosurgery, or radiation therapy). Although GKRS appears to work very well for typical meningiomas,

Table 5
Outcome of radiosurgery for meningiomas

| Author (year) [Reference] | N | Follow-up (mo) | Size Decrease (%) | Stable (%) | Increase (%) | Complications (%) | Improved (%) |
|---|---|---|---|---|---|---|---|
| Kondziolka et al (1991) [97] | 50 | 12–36 | 54 | 38 | 2 | 6 | — |
| Pendl et al (1997) [98] | 97 | 48 | 39 | 56 | 5 | 5 | — |
| Liscak et al (1999) [94] | 67 | 2–60 | 52 | 48 | 0 | 4 | 36 |
| Roche et al (2000) [93] | 80 | 12–79 | 31 | 64 | 5 | 4 | 26 |
| Lee et al (2002) [99] | 159 | 2–145 | 34 | 60 | 6 | 7 | 29 |
| Nicolato et al (2002) [91] | 122 | >12 | 61 | 36 | 3 | 3 | — |
| Roche et al (2003) [92] | 32 | 28–188 | 12 | 88 | — | 6 | 41 |
| Kondziolka (2003) [102] | 85 | 120 | 53 | 40 | 7 | 6 | — |
| Flickinger et al (2003) [90] | 219 | 2–164 | — | — | 3 | 5 | — |
| Liscak et al (2004) [100] | 176 | 36 | 73 | 25 | 2 | 15.5 | 63 |
| Kreil et al (2005) [103] | 200 | 60–144 | 57 | 42 | 2 | 3 | 42 |
| Malik et al (2005) [106] | 277 | 39 | — | — | 12 | 3–7 | — |
| Pollock (2005) [101] | 49 | 58 | 59 | 41 | — | 24 | 53 |
| Steiner & Sheehan[a] | 151 | 6–252 | 63 | 26 | 11 | 0 | 8 |

*Abbreviation:* —, n/a.
[a] Unpublished data from the author's series.

the results for atypical and malignant meningiomas are less favorable. In a study from the University of Pittsburgh, Harris and colleagues [105] reported 5-year progression-free survival rates of 83% and 72% for atypical and malignant meningiomas, respectively. Malik and colleagues [106] reported less favorable results, reporting 5-year actuarial control rates of 49% in atypical meningiomas and 0% in malignant meningiomas. Ojemann and colleagues' [107] results were similar to those of Malik and colleagues [106]; they reported a 5-year progression-free survival rate of 26% in patients who had malignant meningiomas treated with GKRS, although outcomes were better in smaller tumors and in young patients. Survival rates, as opposed to control rates, have also been reported for patients after GKRS of atypical and malignant meningiomas. Five-year overall survival rates vary between 59% and 76% in patients who have atypical meningiomas and between 0% and 59% in patients who have malignant meningiomas [105,107,108].

*Radiation-induced meningioma outcomes.* It is well known that fractionated radiation therapy can induce meningiomas. The incidence of radiation-induced tumors following fractionated radiation therapy is 1.9% in 20 years. Some centers (including the authors') have had limited yet favorable early experience with radiosurgical treatment of radiation-induced tumors. For example, the Mayo Clinic group recently reported a 100% 5-year local tumor control rate for 16 patients who had radiation-induced tumors [109]. The median follow-up from the Mayo Clinic report was only 40.2 months. Although it is too early to know whether such an approach is prudent, the concept of treating radiation-induced meningiomas with radiosurgery may have some interesting implications regarding the pathogenesis of intracranial tumors.

*Clinical outcomes following radiosurgery.* Many patients who present for management of meningiomas, especially skull-base lesions, present with neurologic deficits such as cranial nerve dysfunction. It is therefore important not only to evaluate outcomes with respect to tumor control but also clinical outcomes. GKRS is regularly reported to be associated with improved cranial nerve function after treatment of skull-base meningiomas. Pollock and Stafford [110], for example, reported that 12 of 38 patients who presented with cranial neuropathies associated with cavernous sinus meningiomas had improvement in cranial nerve function on follow-up. Roche and colleagues [93] also reported on clinical outcomes in patients who had cavernous sinus meningiomas treated with GKRS. They reported that 23 of 54 patients who had oculomotor palsies improved or completely recovered and that 7 of 13 patients who had trigeminal neuralgia improved or completely recovered. Roche and colleagues [92] reported similar success in GKRS-treated petroclival meningiomas: 13 of 32 patients treated with GKRS for petroclival meningiomas had clinical improvement in cranial nerve dysfunction. Kreil and colleagues [103] reported that 96% of patients who had skull-base meningiomas treated with GKRS had improved or stable neurologic status, with improvement noted in a broad range of areas including vision and other cranial nerve functions, hemiparesis, ataxia, vertigo, seizures, and exophthalmus.

### Vestibular schwannomas

*Neuroimaging outcomes.* At the University of Virginia's Lars Leksell Gamma Knife center, the authors and colleagues have treated 400 patients who had vestibular schwannomas. One hundred fifty-three of these patients who had greater than 12 months' follow-up have been reported [111]. Radiosurgery was the primary treatment for 96 patients and the adjuvant treatment (following microsurgery) in 57 patients. The volume of the treated tumors ranged from 0.02 to 18.3 cm$^3$.

Of the patients treated primarily with GKRS, 81% (78 patients) experienced a decrease in tumor size (Fig. 1), 12% had no change, and 6% had an increase in size. Among the 78 patients who had decreased tumor size, the decrease was greater than 50% in 20 patients. It is the authors' policy to not consider decreases in volume of less than 15% as significant. Radiologic follow-up for these patients ranged from 1 to 10 years.

Of the 57 patients treated with GKRS after microsurgery, 65% obtained a decrease in tumor size, 25% had no change, and 10% had an increase in tumor size. Among the 37 patients who had a decrease in the size of their tumors, the decrease was greater than 50% in 12 patients. The outcome in terms of postradiosurgical volume reduction in patients who had prior microsurgery is worse compared with the outcome in those who were treated primarily with radiosurgery. This difference is likely a result of the increased difficulty with accurate targeting in those who underwent prior microsurgery. Of note, although the authors' experience with treating large vestibular schwannomas is small (n = 19), they have observed a 95% tumor control rate in these patients following radiosurgery. Other centers report similar rates (89%–100%) of tumor control (ie, no change or a decrease in the size of the tumor) in patients (Table 6) [111–118].

The Karolinska group included evaluation of radiographic changes other than size [116]. The most common change was loss of central enhancement within the tumor on contrasted MRI or CT studies. This loss of central enhancement occurred in 70% of patients and was typically observed within 6 to 12 months of treatment. These changes, however, were reversible. Another change that was observed and that the authors have often seen is a transient increase in the size of the tumor during the first 6 months after radiosurgery. This change is commonly seen in tumors that then regress to their original size or smaller.

*Clinical outcomes following radiosurgery.* In the vestibular schwannoma patients treated at the University of Virginia, five had transient changes in

**A**

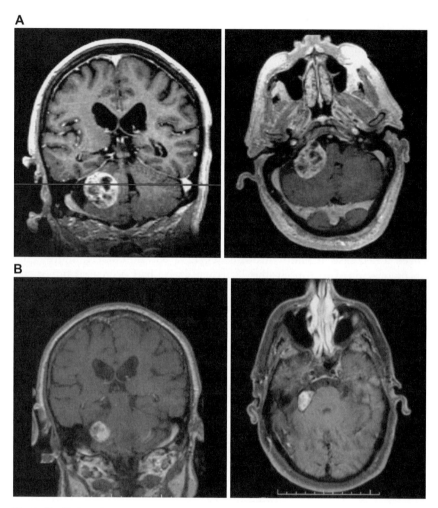

**B**

Fig. 1. Vestibular schwannomas. Of the patients treated primarily with GKRS, a decrease in tumor size was seen in 81% (78 patients). (*A*) Pretreatment T1WI with contrast. (*B*) Post-treatment T1WI with contrast (12 months post-treatment).

trigeminal sensation and three had facial paresis. One of the patients who had facial weakness was operated on shortly after radiosurgery and was lost to follow-up. Another patient recovered completely in 6 weeks, and the third has nearly completely recovered at 10 months. Of the patients who had useful hearing before GKRS, 58% retained their hearing following radiosurgery, 42% experienced some degree of deterioration, and 31% lost useful hearing. Most hearing changes were observed at the 2-year checkup, and additional auditory changes were observed as late as 8 years post radiosurgery.

Table 6
Outcome of radiosurgery for vestibular schwannomas

| Author (year) [Reference] | No. of patients who had follow-up imaging studies | Mean follow-up (mo) | Tumor increased (%) | Tumor unchanged or decreased (%) |
|---|---|---|---|---|
| Noren et al (1993) [116] | 209 | minimum of 12 | 16 | 84 |
| Flickinger et al (1993) [111] | 134 | 24 | 11 | 89 |
| Foote et al (1995) [117] | 35 | 16 | 0 | 100 |
| Kwon et al (1998) [112] | 63 | 52 | 5 | 95 |
| Prasad et al (2000) [118] | 153 | 51 | 7 | 93 |
| Flickinger et al (2001) [113] | 190 | 30 | 3 | 97 |
| Bertalanffy et al (2001) [114] | 40 | 36 | 9 | 91 |
| Iwai et al (2003) [115] | 51 | 60 | 4 | 96 |

Previously published prevalence of cranial neuropathies at other centers were 17% at Karolinska and 29% at Pittsburgh for facial paresis, which in most cases was transient or mild. The trigeminal nerve was affected in a variety of ways in 33% at Pittsburgh, most commonly a mild hypoesthesia. Recent complication rates at these institutions are comparable to those at the authors' center. The authors have not seen an instance of cerebellar edema or hydrocephalus requiring spinal fluid diversion following GKRS for vestibular schwannomas, but these complications have been reported elsewhere [111,116].

## Summary

The initial management of a patient presenting with radiographic evidence of a typically benign extra-axial neoplasm is a complex and evolving process. As we approach an era in which the molecular processes underlying neoplastic transformation and proliferation become more clearly delineated, new chemotherapeutic agents targeting these processes will broaden our armamentarium with which we can target these tumors. Exciting frontiers, such as treatment of meningiomas with cyclo-oxygenase-2 inhibitors, should be embraced with cautious optimism. Enthusiasm generated by successful in vitro and nonprimate experiments in the treatment of meningiomas with antihormonal therapy and hydrosurea has met significant obstacles in the transition to efficacy in human clinical trials. We are hopeful that in the near future we may be enlightened with a chemobiologic treatment advance that is comparable to the contributions brought to meningioma and schwannoma management by radiosurgery over the past several decades.

Patients presenting with asymptomatic, small meningiomas may be best managed conservatively with a trial of expectant management and close surveillance with sequential MRI. In the treatment of these lesions, conservative management may be undertaken with a period of observation for

3 to 12 months before any definitive treatment decision is made [119]. Meningiomas presenting in symptomatic patients due to mass effect should generally be resected completely, especially in the subset of patients harboring tumors that are relatively low risk for surgical complication. Meningioma surgery in the elderly (>65 years old) has been performed with rates of morbidity and mortality similar to a control group of younger patients matched for tumor size and location [120]. Thus, age should not be a deterrent for microsurgical treatment. A decision regarding invasive surgical management versus radiosurgery can be influenced by preinterventional clinical performance status of the patient. When the mass effect of high-risk types of tumors extends beyond local cranial nerve dysfunction, surgical debulking becomes an absolute prequel to adjuvant radiosurgical methods, even when a complete resection is not practical. The greatest amount of controversy exists in treatment of small (<3 cm) skull-base lesions presenting due to focal neurologic signs and symptoms solely from cranial nerve dysfunction. Radiosurgery advocates, in support of primary radiosurgical intervention, note the efficacy of radiosurgical methods in controlling tumor growth and emphasize the high rates of immediate postoperative morbidity associated with attempted surgical resection of these lesions. Supporters of complete surgical resection stress the importance of cure being the ultimate goal, as opposed to control of the disease. They also question the legitimacy of long-term control of tumor growth with radiosurgery, citing the lack of long-term follow-up. A third approach involves the combination of these therapeutic modalities. The benefits from immediate surgical decompression of the cranial nerves with tumor debulking as a pretreatment adjunct to radiosurgical therapy for residual tumor is suggested as a synergistic, rather than mutually exclusive, way to approach the management of these difficult skull-base lesions [121].

The management of small and medium-sized vestibular schwannomas emphasizes the fundamental questions that are brought about in the management of skull-base meningiomas. These lesions arise in the cerebellopontine angle where, even at a small size, they may cause profound effects on cranial nerve function. Surgical management of these lesions allows a cure (recurrence-free) in 92% to 100% of patients undergoing a complete resection, with a small rate of major morbidity and mortality [120–126]. The effectiveness of primary radiosurgical management in the control of tumor growth is indisputable in most patients. Even a tumor with marginal mass effect that extends beyond local cranial nerve involvement may be managed exclusively with radiosurgery. This management is possible because of the large subset of treated tumors that decreases in tumor volume after treatment (see Fig. 1). Monitoring trends in management over the last 2 decades has shown a precipitous decrease in the number of patients undergoing operative intervention, commensurate with a proportional increase in the number of patients treated with radiosurgical methods. The reasons for this are multifactorial, the least of which may be any true indication that radiosurgery is a better alternative than microsurgery for treatment of these lesions. The once-patriarchal patient–physician interaction has been replaced with one of informed patient decision making. Patients are gaining a skeptical understanding of treatment paradigms through use of the Internet and health care advertising, and the wave of enthusiasm for minimally invasive surgery and noninvasive therapeutic modalities is swelling. This, in conjunction with third-party payors helping formulate health care delivery strategies and protocols has placed the management of vestibular schwannomas at the whim of supply and demand economics, rather than a true shift toward superior outcomes. As with any new therapy that comes to the attention of the medical community, this initial crest in interest will subside and an equilibrium will be reached that emphasizes the unique benefits of microsurgery and radiosurgery in the management of these lesions and of their respective definitive niches. At this juncture, providing patients ready accessibility to treatment modalities and education regarding the objectives, risks, and success rates of each will help clarify which management strategy is most suitable for patients on an individual basis.

# References

[1] al-Rodhan NR, Laws ER Jr. Meningioma: a historical study of the tumor and its surgical management. Neurosurgery 1990;26(5):832–46 [discussion: 846–7].

[2] House W, Luetje C. Acoustic tumors. Baltimore (MD): University Park Press; 1979.

[3] Cushing H. Tumors of the nervus acusticus and the syndrome of the cerebellopontine angle. Philadelphia: Saunders; 1917.

[4] Bondy M, Ligon BL. Epidemiology and etiology of intracranial meningiomas: a review. J Neurooncol 1996;29(3):197–205.

[5] Surawicz TS, McCarthy BJ, Kupelian V, et al. Descriptive epidemiology of primary brain and CNS tumors: results from the Central Brain Tumor Registry of the United States, 1990–1994. Neuro oncol 1999;1(1):14–25.

[6] Claus EB, Bondy ML, Schildkraut JM, et al. Epidemiology of intracranial meningioma. Neurosurgery 2005;57(6):1088–95 [discussion: 1088–95].

[7] Central Brain Tumor Registry of the United States. Primary brain tumors in the United States statistical report (1998–2002 years data collected) 2005–2006.

[8] Central Brain Tumor Registry of the United States. Primary brain tumors in the United States statistical report (1990–1994 years data collected) 1999.

[9] Flickinger JC, Lunsford LD, Coffey RJ, et al. Radiosurgery of acoustic neurinomas. Cancer 1991;67(2):345–53.

[10] Harner SG, Laws ER Jr. Clinical findings in patients with acoustic neurinoma. Mayo Clin Proc 1983;58(11):721–8.

[11] Cushing H. The meningiomas (dural endotheliomas): their source, and favoured seats of origin. Brain 1922;45:282–316.

[12] Cushing H, Eisenhardt LC. Meningiomas: their classification, regional behavior, life history and surgical end results. Springfield (IL): Thomas; 1938.

[13] Inskip PD, Mellemkjaer L, Gridley G, et al. Incidence of intracranial tumors following hospitalization for head injuries (Denmark). Cancer Causes Control 1998;9(1):109–16.

[14] Kotzen RM, Swanson RM, Milhorat TH, et al. Post-traumatic meningioma: case report and historical perspective. J Neurol Neurosurg Psychiatry 1999;66(6):796–8.

[15] Preston-Martin S. Descriptive epidemiology of primary tumors of the brain, cranial nerves and cranial meninges in Los Angeles County. Neuroepidemiology 1989;8(6):283–95.

[16] Phillips LE, Koepsell TD, van Belle G, et al. History of head trauma and risk of intracranial meningioma: population-based case-control study. Neurology 2002;58(12):1849–52.

[17] Annegers JF, Laws ER Jr, Kurland LT, et al. Head trauma and subsequent brain tumors. Neurosurgery 1979;4(3):203–6.

[18] Wilkins RH, Rengachary SS. Neurosurgery. 2nd edition. New York: McGraw-Hill Health Professions Division; 1996.

[19] Modan B, Baidatz D, Mart H, et al. Radiation-induced head and neck tumours. Lancet 1974;1(7852):277–9.

[20] Al-Mefty O. Meningiomas. New York: Raven Press; 1991.

[21] Mack EE, Wilson CB. Meningiomas induced by high-dose cranial irradiation. J Neurosurg 1993;79(1):28–31.

[22] Dumanski JP, Rouleau GA, Nordenskjold M, et al. Molecular genetic analysis of chromosome 22 in 81 cases of meningioma. Cancer Res 1990;50(18):5863–7.

[23] Zankl H, Zang KD. Cytological and cytogenetical studies on brain tumors. 4. Identification of the missing G chromosome in human meningiomas as no. 22 by fluorescence technique. Humangenetik 1972;14(2):167–9.

[24] Mark J, Levan G, Mitelman F. Identification by fluorescence of the G chromosome lost in human meningomas. Hereditas 1972;71(1):163–8.

[25] Zang KD. Cytological and cytogenetical studies on human meningioma. Cancer Genet Cytogenet 1982;6(3):249–74.

[26] Drummond KJ, Zhu JJ, Black PM. Meningiomas: updating basic science, management, and outcome. Neurologist 2004;10(3):113–30.

[27] Perry A, Cai DX, Scheithauer BW, et al. Merlin, DAL-1, and progesterone receptor expression in clinicopathologic subsets of meningioma: a correlative immunohistochemical study of 175 cases. J Neuropathol Exp Neurol 2000;59(10):872–9.

[28] Evans JJ, Jeun SS, Lee JH, et al. Molecular alterations in the neurofibromatosis type 2 gene and its protein rarely occurring in meningothelial meningiomas. J Neurosurg 2001;94(1): 111–7.

[29] Pravdenkova S, Al-Mefty O, Sawyer J, et al. Progesterone and estrogen receptors: opposing prognostic indicators in meningiomas. J Neurosurg 2006;105(2):163–73.

[30] Grunberg SM, Rankin C, Townsend J, et al. Phase III double-blind randomized placebo-controlled study of mifepristone (RU) for the treatment of unresectable meningioma. Presented at the American Society of Clinical Oncology. San Francisco (CA), May 12–15, 2001.

[31] Grunberg SM, Weiss MH, Spitz IM, et al. Treatment of unresectable meningiomas with the antiprogesterone agent mifepristone. J Neurosurg 1991;74(6):861–6.

[32] Rouleau GA, Wertelecki W, Haines JL, et al. Genetic linkage of bilateral acoustic neurofibromatosis to a DNA marker on chromosome 22. Nature 1987;329(6136):246–8.

[33] Trofatter JA, MacCollin MM, Rutter JL, et al. A novel moesin-, ezrin-, radixin-like gene is a candidate for the neurofibromatosis 2 tumor suppressor. Cell 1993;75(4):791–800.

[34] Rouleau GA, Merel P, Lutchman M, et al. Alteration in a new gene encoding a putative membrane-organizing protein causes neuro-fibromatosis type 2. Nature 1993;363(6429): 515–21.

[35] Irving RM, Moffat DA, Hardy DG, et al. Somatic NF2 gene mutations in familial and non-familial vestibular schwannoma. Hum Mol Genet 1994;3(2):347–50.

[36] Welling DB, Guida M, Goll F, et al. Mutational spectrum in the neurofibromatosis type 2 gene in sporadic and familial schwannomas. Hum Genet 1996;98(2):189–93.

[37] Jacoby LB, MacCollin M, Louis DN, et al. Exon scanning for mutation of the NF2 gene in schwannomas. Hum Mol Genet 1994;3(3):413–9.

[38] Zucman-Rossi J, Legoix P, Der Sarkissian H, et al. NF2 gene in neurofibromatosis type 2 patients. Hum Mol Genet 1998;7(13):2095–101.

[39] Buetow MP, Buetow PC, Smirniotopoulos JG. Typical, atypical, and misleading features in meningioma. Radiographics 1991;11(6):1087–106.

[40] Schmidek HH. Meningiomas and their surgical management. Philadelphia: Saunders; 1991.

[41] Kaye AH, Laws ER. Brain tumors: an encyclopedic approach. 2nd edition. Edinburgh (UK): Churchill Livingstone; 2001.

[42] Black P. Meningiomas. In: Bernstein M, Berger MS, editors. Neuro-oncology: the essentials. New York: Thieme Medical Publishers; 2000. p. xv, 508.

[43] Fick J, Wilson CB, Fuller G. Intracranial extra-axial tumors: meningiomas. In: Levin VA, editor. Cancer in the nervous system. New York: Churchill Livingstone; 1996. p. 384–90.

[44] Niiro M, Yatsushiro K, Nakamura K, et al. Natural history of elderly patients with asymptomatic meningiomas. J Neurol Neurosurg Psychiatry 2000;68(1):25–8.

[45] Go RS, Taylor BV, Kimmel DW. The natural history of asymptomatic meningiomas in Olmsted County, Minnesota. Neurology 1998;51(6):1718–20.

[46] Pollack IF, Sekhar LN, Jannetta PJ, et al. Neurilemomas of the trigeminal nerve. J Neurosurg 1989;70(5):737–45.

[47] Tan LC, Bordi L, Symon L, et al. Jugular foramen neuromas: a review of 14 cases. Surg Neurol 1990;34(4):205–11.

[48] Samii M, Babu RP, Tatagiba M, et al. Surgical treatment of jugular foramen schwannomas. J Neurosurg 1995;82(6):924–32.

[49] Symon L, Cheesman AD, Kawauchi M, et al. Neuromas of the facial nerve: a report of 12 cases. Br J Neurosurg 1993;7(1):13–22.

[50] McCormick PC, Bello JA, Post KD. Trigeminal schwannoma. Surgical series of 14 cases with review of the literature. J Neurosurg 1988;69(6):850–60.

[51] Simpson D. The recurrence of intracranial meningiomas after surgical treatment. J Neurol Neurosurg Psychiatry 1957;20(1):22–39.

[52] Melamed S, Sahar A, Beller AJ. The recurrence of intracranial meningiomas. Neurochirurgia (Stuttg) 1979;22(2):47–51.

[53] Adegbite AB, Khan MI, Paine KW, et al. The recurrence of intracranial meningiomas after surgical treatment. J Neurosurg 1983;58(1):51–6.

[54] Boker DK, Meurer H, Gullotta F. Recurring intracranial meningiomas. Evaluation of some factors predisposing for tumor recurrence. J Neurosurg Sci 1985;29(1):11–7.

[55] de la Monte SM, Flickinger J, Linggood RM. Histopathologic features predicting recurrence of meningiomas following subtotal resection. Am J Surg Pathol 1986;10(12):836–43.

[56] Marks SM, Whitwell HL, Lye RH. Recurrence of meningiomas after operation. Surg Neurol 1986;25(5):436–40.

[57] Black PM, Loeffler JS. Cancer of the nervous system. 2nd edition. Philadelphia: Lippincott Williams & Wilkins; 2005.

[58] Jaaskelainen J. Seemingly complete removal of histologically benign intracranial meningioma: late recurrence rate and factors predicting recurrence in 657 patients. A multivariate analysis. Surg Neurol 1986;26(5):461–9.

[59] Jan M, Bazeze V, Saudeau D, et al. [Outcome of intracranial meningioma in adults. Retrospective study of a medicosurgical series of 161 meningiomas]. Neurochirurgie 1986;32(2): 129–34 [in French].

[60] Ojemann RG. Skull-base surgery: a perspective. J Neurosurg 1992;76(4):569–70.

[61] Pertuiset B, Farah S, Clayes L, et al. Operability of intracranial meningiomas. Personal series of 353 cases. Acta Neurochir (Wien) 1985;76(1–2):2–11.

[62] Kallio M, Sankila R, Hakulinen T, et al. Factors affecting operative and excess long-term mortality in 935 patients with intracranial meningioma. Neurosurgery 1992;31(1):2–12.

[63] Manelfe C, Lasjaunias P, Ruscalleda J. Preoperative embolization of intracranial meningiomas. AJNR Am J Neuroradiol 1986;7(5):963–72.

[64] Olivecrona H. The meningiomas. In: Olivecrona H, Tonnis W, editors. Handbuch der neurochirugie. Berlin: Springer-Verlag; 1967. p. 1–191.

[65] Morimura T, Takeuchi J, Maeda Y, et al. Preoperative embolization of meningiomas: its efficacy and histopathological findings. Noshuyo Byori 1994;11(2):123–9.

[66] Bonnal J, Thibaut A, Brotchi J, et al. Invading meningiomas of the sphenoid ridge. J Neurosurg 1980;53(5):587–99.

[67] Ojemann RG. Meningiomas of the basal parapituitary region: technical considerations. Clin Neurosurg 1980;27:233–62.

[68] Jaaskelainen J, Ohman J, Kotilainen P, et al. In: Black P, Kaye AH, editors. Operative neurosurgery. Sphenoidal wing meningiomas—outer and middle, vol. 1. London: Harcourt; 2000. p. 587–604.

[69] DeMonte F, Smith HK, al-Mefty O. Outcome of aggressive removal of cavernous sinus meningiomas. J Neurosurg 1994;81(2):245–51.

[70] Al-Mefty O, Smith RR. Surgery of tumors invading the cavernous sinus. Surg Neurol 1988; 30(5):370–81.

[71] Maruyama K, Shin M, Kurita H, et al. Proposed treatment strategy for cavernous sinus meningiomas: a prospective study. Neurosurgery 2004;55(5):1068–75.

[72] Zentner J, Meyer B, Vieweg U, et al. Petroclival meningiomas: is radical resection always the best option? J Neurol Neurosurg Psychiatry 1997;62(4):341–5.

[73] Ballance CA. Some points in the surgery of the brain and its membranes. London: Macmillan; 1907.

[74] Dandy WE. An operation for the total removal of cerebellopontine (acoustic) tumors. Surg Gynecol Obstet 1925;41:129–48.

[75] Yamakami I, Uchino Y, Kobayashi E, et al. Conservative management, gamma-knife radiosurgery, and microsurgery for acoustic neurinomas: a systematic review of outcome and risk of three therapeutic options. Neurol Res 2003;25(7):682–90.

[76] House JW, Brackmann DE. Facial nerve grading system. Otolaryngol Head Neck Surg 1985;93(2):146–7.

[77] Haines SJ, Levine SC. Intracanalicular acoustic neuroma: early surgery for preservation of hearing. J Neurosurg 1993;79(4):515–20.

[78] Nadol JB Jr, Chiong CM, Ojemann RG, et al. Preservation of hearing and facial nerve function in resection of acoustic neuroma. Laryngoscope 1992;102(10):1153–8.

[79] Samii M, Matthies C, Tatagiba M. Intracanalicular acoustic neurinomas. Neurosurgery 1991;29(2):189–98 [discussion: 198–9].

[80] Morrison AW, King TT. Experiences with a translabyrinthine-transtentorial approach to the cerebellopontine angle. Technical note. J Neurosurg 1973;38(3):382–90.

[81] DiTullio MV Jr, Malkasian D, Rand RW. A critical comparison of neurosurgical and otolaryngological approaches to acoustic neuromas. J Neurosurg 1978;48(1):1–12.

[82] Ojemann RG. Management of acoustic neuromas (vestibular schwannomas). [Honored guest presentation]. Clin Neurosurg 1993;40:498–535.

[83] Ebersold MJ, Harner SG, Beatty CW, et al. Current results of the retrosigmoid approach to acoustic neurinoma. J Neurosurg 1992;76(6):901–9.

[84] Sekhar LN, Gormley WB, Wright DC. The best treatment for vestibular schwannoma (acoustic neuroma): microsurgery or radiosurgery? Am J Otol 1996;17(4):676–82 [discussion: 683–9].

[85] Whittaker CK, Luetje CM. Vestibular schwannomas. J Neurosurg 1992;76(6): 897–900.

[86] Shelton C, Brackmann DE, House WF, et al. Middle fossa acoustic tumor surgery: results in 106 cases. Laryngoscope 1989;99(4):405–8.

[87] Gardner G, Robertson JH. Hearing preservation in unilateral acoustic neuroma surgery. Ann Otol Rhinol Laryngol 1988;97(1):55–66.

[88] Baldwin DL, King TT, Morrison AW. Hearing conservation in acoustic neuroma surgery via the posterior fossa. J Laryngol Otol 1990;104(6):463–7.

[89] Fischer G, Fischer C, Remond J. Hearing preservation in acoustic neurinoma surgery. J Neurosurg 1992;76(6):910–7.

[90] Flickinger JC, Kondziolka D, Maitz AH, et al. Gamma knife radiosurgery of imaging-diagnosed intracranial meningioma. Int J Radiat Oncol Biol Phys 2003;56(3):801–6.

[91] Nicolato A, Foroni R, Alessandrini F, et al. Radiosurgical treatment of cavernous sinus meningiomas: experience with 122 treated patients. Neurosurgery 2002;51(5):1153–9 [discussion: 1159–61].

[92] Roche PH, Pellet W, Fuentes S, et al. Gamma knife radiosurgical management of petroclival meningiomas results and indications. Acta Neurochir (Wien) 2003;145(10):883–8 [discussion: 888].

[93] Roche PH, Regis J, Dufour H, et al. Gamma knife radiosurgery in the management of cavernous sinus meningiomas. J Neurosurg 2000;93(Suppl 3):68–73.

[94] Liscak R, Simonova G, Vymazal J, et al. Gamma knife radiosurgery of meningiomas in the cavernous sinus region. Acta Neurochir (Wien) 1999;141(5):473–80.

[95] Kondziolka D, Lunsford LD, Coffey RJ, et al. Stereotactic radiosurgery of meningiomas. J Neurosurg 1991;74(4):552–9.

[96] Steiner L, Lindquist C, Steiner M. Meningiomas and gamma knife surgery. In: Al-Mefty O, editor. Meningiomas. New York: Raven Press; 1991. p. 263–72.

[97] Kondziolka D, Lunsford LD, Coffey RJ, et al. Gamma knife radiosurgery of meningiomas. Stereotact Funct Neurosurg 1991;57(1–2):11–21.

[98] Pendl G, Schrottner O, Eustacchio S, et al. Stereotactic radiosurgery of skull base meningiomas. Minim Invasive Neurosurg 1997;40(3):87–90.

[99] Lee JY, Niranjan A, McInerney J, et al. Stereotactic radiosurgery providing long-term tumor control of cavernous sinus meningiomas. J Neurosurg 2002;97(1):65–72.

[100] Liscak R, Kollova A, Vladyka V, et al. Gamma knife radiosurgery of skull base meningiomas. Acta Neurochir Suppl 2004;91:65–74.

[101] Pollock BE. Stereotactic radiosurgery for intracranial meningiomas: indications and results. Neurosurg Focus 2003;14(5):1–7.

[102] Kondziolka D, Nathoo N, Flickinger JC, et al. Long-term results after radiosurgery for benign intracranial tumors. Neurosurgery 2003;53(4):815–21 [discussion: 821–2].

[103] Kreil W, Luggin J, Fuchs I, et al. Long term experience of gamma knife radiosurgery for benign skull base meningiomas. J Neurol Neurosurg Psychiatry 2005;76(10):1425–30.

[104] Pollock BE, Stafford SL, Utter A, et al. Stereotactic radiosurgery provides equivalent tumor control to Simpson Grade 1 resection for patients with small- to medium-size meningiomas. Int J Radiat Oncol Biol Phys 2003;55(4):1000–5.

[105] Harris AE, Lee JY, Omalu B, et al. The effect of radiosurgery during management of aggressive meningiomas. Surg Neurol 2003;60(4):298–305 [discussion: 305].

[106] Malik I, Rowe JG, Walton L, et al. The use of stereotactic radiosurgery in the management of meningiomas. Br J Neurosurg 2005;19(1):13–20.

[107] Ojemann SG, Sneed PK, Larson DA, et al. Radiosurgery for malignant meningioma: results in 22 patients. J Neurosurg 2000;93(Suppl 3):62–7.

[108] Stafford SL, Pollock BE, Foote RL, et al. Meningioma radiosurgery: tumor control, outcomes, and complications among 190 consecutive patients. Neurosurgery 2001;49(5):1029–37 [discussion: 1037–8].

[109] Jensen AW, Brown PD, Pollock BE, et al. Gamma knife radiosurgery of radiation-induced intracranial tumors: local control, outcomes, and complications. Int J Radiat Oncol Biol Phys 2005;62(1):32–7.

[110] Pollock BE, Stafford SL. Results of stereotactic radiosurgery for patients with imaging defined cavernous sinus meningiomas. Int J Radiat Oncol Biol Phys 2005;62(5):1427–31.

[111] Flickinger JC, Lunsford LD, Linskey ME, et al. Gamma knife radiosurgery for acoustic tumors: multivariate analysis of four year results. Radiother Oncol 1993;27(2):91–8.

[112] Kwon Y, Kim JH, Lee DJ, et al. Gamma knife treatment of acoustic neurinoma. Stereotact Funct Neurosurg 1998;70(Suppl 1):57–64.

[113] Flickinger JC, Kondziolka D, Niranjan A, et al. Results of acoustic neuroma radiosurgery: an analysis of 5 years' experience using current methods. J Neurosurg 2001;94(1):1–6.

[114] Bertalanffy A, Dietrich W, Aichholzer M, et al. Gamma knife radiosurgery of acoustic neurinomas. Acta Neurochir (Wien) 2001;143(7):689–95.

[115] Iwai Y, Yamanaka K, Shiotani M, et al. Radiosurgery for acoustic neuromas: results of low-dose treatment. Neurosurgery 2003;53(2):282–7 [discussion: 287–8].

[116] Noren G, Greitz D, Hirsch A, et al. Gamma knife surgery in acoustic tumours. Acta Neurochir Suppl (Wien) 1993;58:104–7.

[117] Foote RL, Coffey RJ, Swanson JW, et al. Stereotactic radiosurgery using the gamma knife for acoustic neuromas. Int J Radiat Oncol Biol Phys 1995;32(4):1153–60.

[118] Prasad D, Steiner M, Steiner L. Gamma surgery for vestibular schwannoma. J Neurosurg 2000;92(5):745–59.

[119] Black PM. Meningiomas. Neurosurgery 1993;32(4):643–57.

[120] Black P, Kathiresan S, Chung W. Meningioma surgery in the elderly: a case-control study assessing morbidity and mortality. Acta Neurochir (Wien) 1998;140(10):1013–6 [discussion: 1016–7].

[121] Couldwell WT, Kan P, Liu JK, et al. Decompression of cavernous sinus meningioma for preservation and improvement of cranial nerve function. Technical note. J Neurosurg 2006;105(1):148–52.

[122] Pollock BE, Lunsford LD, Noren G. Vestibular schwannoma management in the next century: a radiosurgical perspective. Neurosurgery 1998;43(3):475–81 [discussion: 481–3].

[123] Gormley WB, Sekhar LN, Wright DC, et al. Acoustic neuromas: results of current surgical management. Neurosurgery 1997;41(1):50–8 [discussion: 58–60].

[124] Samii M, Matthies C. Management of 1000 vestibular schwannomas (acoustic neuromas): surgical management and results with an emphasis on complications and how to avoid them. Neurosurgery 1997;40(1):11–21 [discussion: 21–3].

[125] Sampath P, Holliday MJ, Brem H, et al. Facial nerve injury in acoustic neuroma (vestibular schwannoma) surgery: etiology and prevention. J Neurosurg 1997;87(1):60–6.

[126] Wiegand DA, Ojemann RG, Fickel V. Surgical treatment of acoustic neuroma (vestibular schwannoma) in the United States: report from the Acoustic Neuroma Registry. Laryngoscope 1996;106(1 Pt 1):58–66.

ELSEVIER
SAUNDERS

NEUROLOGIC
CLINICS

Neurol Clin 25 (2007) 1231–1249

# Benign Brain Tumors: Sellar/Parasellar Tumors

Jay Jagannathan, MD[a], Adam S. Kanter, MD[b],
Jason P. Sheehan, MD, PhD[a], John A. Jane, Jr, MD[a],*,
Edward R. Laws, Jr, MD, FACS[c]

[a]Department of Neurosurgery, University of Virginia Health System, PO Box 800212,
Charlottesville, VA 22908-0711, USA
[b]Department of Neurosurgery, University of California, San Francisco, CA 94143, USA
[c]Department of Neurosurgery, Stanford University, Palo Alto, CA 94304, USA

Sellar and parasellar tumors include a diverse group of lesions (Table 1). More than 90% of purely intrasellar tumors are pituitary adenomas, although dysembryogenic lesions of the midline (eg, Rathke's cleft cysts and craniopharyngiomas) also occur. Suprasellar tumors include craniopharyngiomas, meningiomas, germinomas, dermoid/epidermoid cysts, lipomas, teratomas, and hamartomas. Over the past 30 years, significant advances in microneurosurgery, neuroimaging, and molecular biology have changed the evaluation and management of these parasellar tumors. This article focuses on current concepts in the understanding and treatment of these diverse pathologic entities.

## Epidemiology

Pituitary adenomas are the most common cause of pituitary disease in adults (10%–15% of all primary brain tumors), with a low incidence in childhood that increases during adolescence [1,2]. Although the incidence varies according to age, gender, and ethnic group, approximately 1 in 10,000 people are diagnosed annually with a pituitary adenoma [3]. Autopsy series indicate that asymptomatic pituitary tumors may exist in up to 25% of the population (Table 2) [2,4]. The majority of these tumors are less than 5 mm in size and do not require medical or surgical intervention. Women are reported to present more frequently than men; this perhaps

* Corresponding author.
*E-mail address:* johnjanejr@virginia.edu (J.A. Jane).

Table 1
Differential diagnosis of sellar and parasellar tumors

Pituitary adenomas
Craniopharyngioma
Rathke's cleft cyst
Arachnoid cyst
Germinoma
Optic nerve glioma
Meningioma
Chordoma/chondrsarcoma
Hamartoma
Hemangioblastoma
Eosinophilic granuloma
Glioma
Hypophysitis

may reflect the relative contribution of prolactinomas and corticotropin-secreting tumors.

Among the varying classes of adenomas, prolactinomas and nonfunctioning adenomas have the highest incidence and account for nearly two thirds of all pituitary tumors, with a peak incidence in women between the ages of 20 to 50 years. Prolactin (PRL)-secreting adenomas account for 40% to 60% of functioning adenomas and are the most common subtype of pituitary tumor diagnosed in adolescents [5–7].

Growth hormone (GH)-secreting adenomas represent approximately 30% of all hormonally active tumors (see Table 2), nearly three quarters of which are macroadenomas. The incidence of acromegaly is 1 in 25,000 with three to four new cases per million people diagnosed each year [2,8]. Most acromegalics present in their third to fifth decades of life after years of symptom development. Acromegaly is associated with an increased incidence of cardiovascular, respiratory, cerebrovascular, and malignant disease, although mortality risk may be different between the sexes [9].

Corticotropin adenomas account for 15% to 25% of all functioning adenomas and are the most common pituitary tumors diagnosed in prepubertal children (see Table 2). The majority of corticotropoin adenomas are microadenomas [10]. Approximately 15 to 20 individuals per million have Cushing's disease (CD) [2,11]. CD is more common in women and tends to present in the third and fourth decades. There is a high incidence of

Table 2
Relative incidence of sellar and parasellar tumors

|                                              | Surgical series (%) | Autopsy series (%) |
| -------------------------------------------- | ------------------- | ------------------ |
| Nonfunctioning (null cell and gonadotrophs)  | 35                  | 34                 |
| Corticotropin staining                       | 12                  | 8                  |
| GH staining                                  | 17                  | 17                 |
| PRL staining                                 | 30                  | 25                 |
| Miscellaneous                                | 11                  | 16                 |

hypertension, diabetes mellitus, and vascular disease–related mortality in patients who have CD [11,12].

Craniopharyngiomas account for 2.5% to 4% of all brain tumors and account for the overwhelming majority (approximately 90%) of pituitary-region neoplasms in children. Two peak incidences are observed, the first from ages 5 to 15 years and the second during the fifth decade of life. No gender predilection exists. Most craniopharyngiomas occur in the intrasellar and suprasellar regions (approximately 70%), with solely intra- or suprasellar locations occurring less frequently (approximately 30%) [2].

Less common than pituitary adenomas are dysembryogenic midline lesions, such as Rathke's cleft cysts. Suprasellar masses, such as germinomas, dermoid/epidermoid tumors, lipomas, meningiomas, and teratomas, are rare but can come to attention by causing mass effect and endocrine dysfunction (see Table 1) [3].

## Clinical presentation and diagnostic evaluation

Although increasing numbers of patients present incidentally, most patients present with signs or symptoms related to tumor type, size, and patient age. Nonfunctioning adenomas, craniopharyngiomas, and Rathke's cleft cysts can produce hypopituitarism and galactorrhea from disturbance of the pituitary stalk and loss of tonic inhibition of PRL (ie, stalk effect). Visual changes, including diminished acuity or field deficits (classically a bitemporal hemianopsia), may result from tumor compression of the optic apparatus (Fig. 1). Increased intracranial pressure may evoke headache, nausea, vomiting, and papilledema. Memory problems and behavioral changes also are observed [3]. Diminished growth velocity or short stature is a common feature in many children harboring pituitary adenomas; this may be accompanied by delayed puberty or hypogonadism.

All patients suspected of harboring a tumor in the sellar region should undergo a complete neurologic, ophthalmologic, endocrinologic, and radiologic work-up. If imaging reveals chiasmal compression, patients should

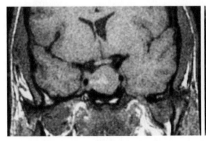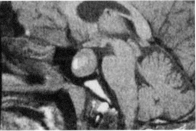

Fig. 1. Preoperative coronal (*left panel*) and sagittal (*right panel*) T1-weighted MRIs with contrast demonstrating a clinically nonfunctioning pituitary adenoma in a patient who presented with headaches. The patient had normal visual field testing.

undergo formal visual field and acuity testing and a dilated fundoscopic examination. Each facet of the hypothalamic-pituitary–end organ axis should be assessed. Mild elevations in serum PRL commonly are the result of stalk effect, whereas levels greater than 200 ng/mL suggest a PRL-secreting adenoma. Thyroid function is evaluated by measuring free thryoxine and thyroid-stimulating hormone. Adrenal function is assessed by a morning serum cortisol assay. In cases of suspected CD, a 24-hour urine-free cortisol (UFC) and a dexamethasone suppression test is performed. Serum GH and insulin-like growth factor I (IGF-1) levels are measured. An oral glucose tolerance test (OGTT) is performed with GH measurements in cases of suspected growth hormone–secreting tumors. In children, a radiograph may be obtained to assess bone age in relation to chronologic age. Radiologic evaluation is achieved with MRI of the sellar region. CT may be useful to assess degree of sinus aeration, particularly in younger patients, who often have incompletely pneumatized sinuses [2,10].

## Hormonally inactive sellar and parasellar tumors

Neurologic disturbances, such as headache and visual field defects, and endocrine deficiencies are the common presenting symptoms of nonfunctioning pituitary adenomas, craniopharyngiomas, meningiomas, and Rathke's cleft cysts. These tumors often stretch the diaphragma sellae and cause headache [1]. Large tumors can obstruct the foramen of Monro, resulting in hydrocephalus, necessitating a cerebrospinal fluid (CSF) diversion procedure. Pituitary adenomas and less common sellar tumors, such as meningiomas involving the optic apparatus and cavernous sinus, may result in cranial nerve palsies, cavernous sinus syndromes, and visual disturbances (Fig. 2).

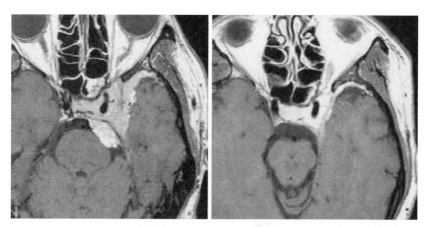

Fig. 2. Preoperative (*left*) and postoperative (*right*) T1-weighted contrasted axial MRI of a 55-year-old woman who presented with worsening diplopia and left-sided facial numbness. Pathology was a parasellar meningioma. The patient had complete resolution of symptoms after craniotomy and resection.

Craniopharyngiomas and nonfunctioning pituitary adenomas commonly present with endocrine dysfunction [1,3]. Nonfunctioning macroadenomas manifest with reduced GH secretion in up to 75% of cases. Follicle-stimulating hormone/luteinizing hormone deficiency (40% of patients) and corticotropin and thyrotropin deficiency (25% of patients) also commonly are seen [1]. Nonfunctioning adenomas can compress the pituitary stalk, but hyperprolactinemia secondary to pituitary stalk compression is present only in approximately 1 in 5 patients because of underlying hypopituitarism. Diabetes insipidus is relatively uncommon, occurring in 9% to 17% of patients, with a tendency to be more common in patients who have Rathke's cleft cysts [13].

## Hormonally active pituitary adenomas: Cushing's disease

The clinical manifestations of CD are a consequence of hypercortisolemia. The clinical presentation remains highly variable, with signs and symptoms ranging from subtle to obvious. Physical manifestations of CD include facial plethora; atrophic striae in the abdomen, legs, and arms; muscle weakness; hypertension; and osteoporosis. Bone mineral density and metabolism in children and adults who have CD reveal marked osteopenia [14]. Recent reports indicate that a long period of time ($>2$ years) is necessary to restore bone mass after a cure from CD, so other therapeutic approaches often are implemented to limit bone loss and accelerate bone recovery in these patients [15].

Children who have CD may have impaired carbohydrate tolerance (although diabetes mellitus is uncommon). Unfortunately, diagnosis often is delayed as growth retardation may be the only perceptible symptom for several years [15]. Excessive adrenal androgens may cause acne and excessive hair growth. Hypercortisolism may cause pubertal delay in adolescent patients. Young patients who have CD may present with neuropsychiatric symptoms that differ from those of adult patients. Frequently, they tend to be obsessive and are high performers in school [2].

The differential diagnosis of CD includes adrenal tumors, ectopic corticotropin production (rare in the pediatric population), and ectopic corticotropin releasing hormone (CRH)-producing tumors. In a child or adolescent who has suspected CD, the diagnosis may be problematic not only because these tumors often are not evident on MRI but also because pseudo-Cushing's states can be difficult to distinguish definitively from true CD. Pseudo-Cushing's syndrome results in a hypercortisolemic state and may include physical features indistinguishable from those of CD. It results from an underlying disease process, such as depression or obesity, although the precise mechanism remains unclear. It seems to be mediated centrally and may involve excessive hypothalamic secretion of CRH. This condition resolves, however, with treatment of the underlying disease. Hence, the initial examination of patients suspected of having CD should screen for disorders that result in pseudo-Cushing's syndrome [15].

Screening for hypercortisolemia involves a 24-hour UFC or low-dose dexamethasone suppression test (LDDST) (Fig. 3). UFC values greater than 220 to 330 nmol/24 hours (80–120 ng/24 hours) are sensitive but relatively nonspecific for a diagnosis of Cushing's syndrome [11]. Failure to suppress morning (0800) serum cortisol levels to 100 to 200 nmol/L (3.6–7.2 ng/dL) the morning after a midnight dose of 0.5 to 2.0 mg of dexamethasone also indicates Cushing's syndrome [11]. Suppression to less than 50 nmol/L or 1.8 ng/dL is highly specific for the exclusion of Cushing's syndrome. When doubt remains as to the possibility of pseudo-Cushing's, a combined CRH-LDDST may be used. As described, patients are administered 0.5 mg of dexamethasone every 6 hours for 24 hours followed by a 1-ng/kg intravenous dose of CRH. In patients who have Cushing's syndrome, CRH should overcome the suppressive effects of dexamethasone, and serum cortisol level at 15 minutes should be greater than 1.4 ng/dL.

Once the presence of Cushing's syndrome is established, the source of cortisol excess must be determined. Although low corticotropin levels (<5 pg/mL) exclude CD, higher levels require further testing to distinguish a pituitary from an ectopic source of corticotropin secretion. No single test provides absolute distinction, but the combined results of several tests generally provide a preponderance of evidence. These tests include the high-dose dexamethasone suppression test (HDDST), dynamic testing with metyrapone (750 mg every 4 hours for 6 doses) or CRH (1 ng/kg intravenously), and inferior petrosal sinus sampling [16].

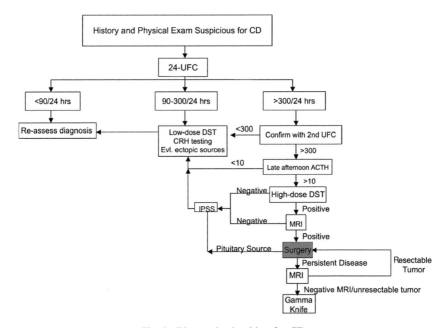

Fig. 3. Diagnostic algorithm for CD.

The HDDST compares steroid levels (either serum cortisol, 24-hour urinary 17-hydroxycorticosteriods [OHCS], or 24-hour UFC) before and the morning after either 2 mg of dexamethsone every 6 hours for 48 hours or a single evening (2300) 8-mg dexamethasone dose. Patients who have pituitary-dependent corticotropin secretion should suppress serum cortisol greater than 50%, UFC greater than 90%, and 17-OHCS greater than 64% to 69% [15]. Fig. 3 shows a complete diagnostic evaluation for CD.

*Hormonally active pituitary adenomas: growth hormone–secreting adenomas*

In adults, chronic GH hypersecretion causes acromegaly. Hallmarks of acromegaly include hyperostosis and hypertrophy of soft tissues. In children and adolescents who have open epiphyseal plates, GH hypersecretion leads to gigantism. The two disorders may be considered along a spectrum of GH excess, with manifestations determined by the age of disease onset. The clinical overlap between gigantism and acromegaly with approximately 10% of acromegalics exhibiting tall stature and the majority of giants eventually demonstrating features of acromegaly supportsthis hypothesis [8].

Physical examination often is sufficient to strongly suggest a diagnosis of acromegaly. Biochemical confirmation is imperative, however, and can be obtained by simple blood tests. The pulsatile nature of GH-secretion makes random serum GH levels limited in diagnostic value, but serum IGF-1 levels and GH levels following a standard glucose load (OGTT) may be used to diagnose acromegaly and monitor for remission and recurrence (Fig. 4) [9]. Fasting patients have serum GH levels drawn at −30, 0, 30, 60, 90, and 120 minutes around the time of oral glucose. Failure to suppress GH levels to less than 1 ng/L (<2 mU/L) confirms the diagnosis [9].

Occasionally, the presence of different GH isoforms in patients who have gigantism/acromegaly may represent a diagnostic problem, as traditional assaying techniques do not distinguish the different isoforms. A greater sensitivity of the GH assay may facilitate the distinction between symptomatic and normal subjects, as shown by the use of a chemiluminescence GH assay. This also may help in demonstrating the persistence of GH hypersecretion after surgery or during medical therapy [9,17].

*Hormonally active pituitary adenomas: prolactin-secreting adenomas*

The clinical manifestations of PRL-secreting adenomas vary depending on the age and gender of the patient. Prepubertal children generally present with a combination of headache, visual disturbance, growth failure, and primary amenorrhea [18]. Women present more commonly with amenorrhea and galactorrhea [6]. Although men may experience galactorrhea, more often they present secondary to tumor mass effect and report headache, visual disturbance, diminished libido, and loss of vitality [19].

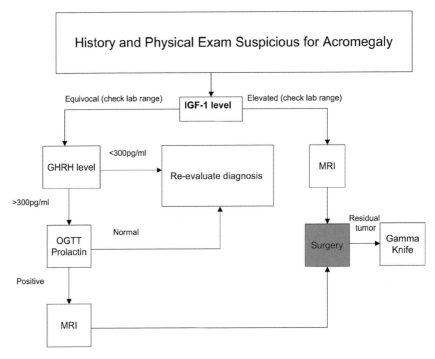

Fig. 4. Diagnostic algorithm for acromegaly.

The biochemical diagnosis of prolactinoma typically is straightforward yet confounding factors exist. Certain drugs (eg, dopamine [DA] antagonists and estrogens), renal and liver failure, hypothyroidism, and the stalk effect can produce moderate elevations in basal PRL levels. Patients who have macroadenomas and moderate elevations in PRL levels should undergo repeated serum PRL testing with serial dilutions. Nevertheless, serum PRL levels greater than 200 ng/mL typically are consistent with a PRL-secreting adenoma [20]. Another pitfall is the serum PRL "hook effect" that may lead to a misdiagnosis of a macroprolactinoma as a nonfunctioning adenoma in the absence of serial dilutions [1,20]. In the hook effect, a large quantity of antigen (PRL) in an immunoassay system impairs antigen-antibody binding, resulting in a falsely low quantity of antigen determined by the assay. The hook effect may occur in any situation when extremely high PRL levels are encountered.

## Treatment of sellar and parasellar tumors

### Hormonally inactive tumors

Surgical decompression remains the treatment of choice for symptomatic craniopharyngiomas, Rathke's cleft cysts, and nonfunctioning pituitary adenomas (Figs. 5 and 6). With the exception of craniopharyngiomas, the most common surgical approach to these tumors is a transsphenoidal procedure to debulk the lesion and decompress parasellar and suprasellar structures (see Figs. 5 and 6) [21]. Transsphenoidal surgery yields low morbidity and mortality rates and leads to improvement in visual symptoms in 87% to 90% of cases (Table 3) [3,21]. For suprasellar tumors that are difficult to resect transsphenoidally, a variety of transcranial approaches (pterional, subfrontal, anterior interhemispheric, and transcallosal) allows adequate visualization and decompression of the optic nerves and chiasm. Variations of the pterional craniotomy are proposed to include resection of the orbital rim and zygoma so as to provide a more basal view and, therefore, better access to the superior aspects of some suprasellar tumors.

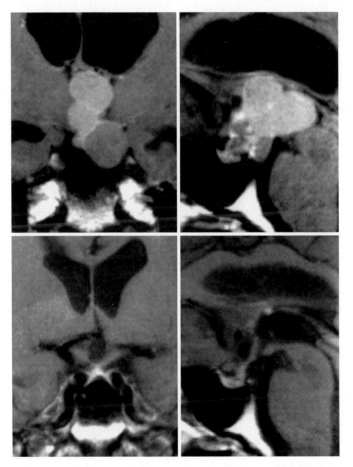

Fig. 5. Preoperative coronal (*top left*) and sagittal (*top right*) and postoperative coronal (*bottom left*) and sagittal (*bottom right*) contrasted MRI of a 5-year-old boy who presented with panhypopituitarism and visual loss. The patient regained vision after transsphenoidal extirpation of the craniopharyngioma.

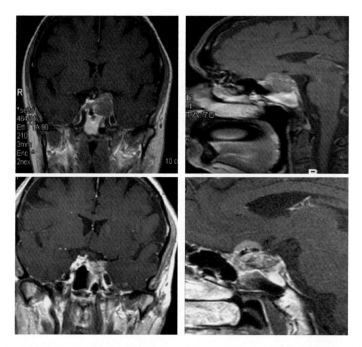

Fig. 6. Preoperative coronal (*top left*) and sagittal (*top right*) and postoperative coronal (*bottom left*) and sagittal (*bottom right*) MRI of a 45-year-old woman who presented with visual loss and a large clinically nonfunctioning pituitary adenoma. The patient regained normal vision and is recurrence free at most recent follow-up (2 years).

After surgery, new endocrine deficits are reported in up to 40% of patients [22]. Recent results indicate, however, that 97% of patients who have microadenomas and 95% of patients who have macroadenomas maintain normal preoperative pituitary function postoperatively [1]. Immediate postoperative polyuria may occur in up to 30% of patients but the majority of cases resolve within the first week after surgery. Delayed hyponatremia, occurring most often 7 to 10 days after surgery, is evident in 1% to 9%

Table 3
Surgical outcomes for pituitary adenomas by pathology with 10-years' follow-up

| Histology | N = | Postoperative remission (%) | Visual recovery[a] | Recurrence (10 years) (%) |
|---|---|---|---|---|
| Nonfunctioning (null cell and honadotrophs) | 1073 | 96 | 91 | 10 |
| Corticotropin secreting | 445 | 86 | 92 | 13 |
| GH secreting | 537 | 73 | 88 | 8 |
| Craniopharyngioma | 226 | 86 | 90 | 12 |
| Miscellaneous pathology | 946 | 92 | 92 | 6 |

[a] When applicable.

*Data from* Jane JA Jr, Laws ER Jr. The surgical management of pituitary adenomas in a series of 3,093 patients. J Am Coll Surg 2001;193:651–9.

of patients [1,23]. Worsening of preoperative visual function is seen in 1% to 4% of patients. Anatomic complications include nasal septal perforations (7%) and fat graft hematomas (rare). Postoperative CSF leaks and meningitis occur in 0.5% to 3.9% of cases [3,22,24].

Recurrences develop over time and as many as 16% of patients who have pituitary adenoma may experience recurrent tumor growth within 10 years after surgical intervention [24–26]. Only 6% of patients experience recurrence requiring repeat surgery [25,26]. Completeness of resection, as is evidenced by postoperative MRI, often can predict recurrence. Up to one third of patients who have residual tumor experience recurrent growth, whereas fewer than 3% of patients after a complete resection experience recurrent disease at a mean follow-up of 3.3 years [27]. For tumors with incomplete resection, adjuvant radiosurgery and medical and radiation therapy may be considered (see discussion later of aduvant treatment). Neither medical therapy nor radiation therapy is recommended as a primary treatment modality, as the long-term effects remain poorly studied.

The recent development of the endoscopic transsphenoidal approach to the pituitary region, which has similar indications to conventional transsphenoidal microsurgery, offers potential advantages over traditional surgical approaches because of its minimal invasiveness and panoramic visualization (Fig. 7). This procedure obviates sublabial incisions or transseptal submucosal dissection and may result in less trauma to the nose. The wider operating field of vision and angled views potentially increase the likelihood of a more thorough and safer tumor removal and preservation of normal gland. Endoscopic modalities also may result in shorter

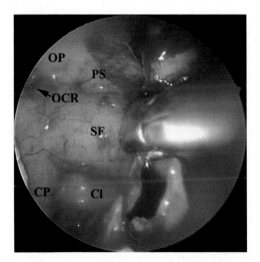

Fig. 7. Intraoperative photograph of endoscopic transsphenoidal surgery demonstrating a panoramic view of the sellar floor (SF). Cl, clivus; CP, carotid protuberance; OCR, opticocarotid recess; OP, optic protuberance; PS, planum sphenoidale.

hospitalizations and more rapid patient recovery, although this is controversial [28–30]. Negatives of the endoscopic approach include a larger sellar opening, which makes it difficult to repair the skull base in the event of a CSF leak. Furthermore, little information exists on the use of the endoscope for the treatment of secretory pituitary adenomas, such as those in CD, where MRI often is normal.

*Prolactin-secreting adenomas*

In the absence of complications necessitating immediate surgery, such as apoplexy, hydrocephalus, or a CSF leak, pharmacotherapy with DA agonists is considered the first-line treatment approach for PRL-secreting adenomas. DA agonists (bromocriptine and cabergoline) effectively normalize PRL levels in as many as 89% of patients [31]. These medications decrease tumor volume by at least 50% in more than two thirds of patients within the first several months of therapy, resulting in visual field improvements in all but 10% of patients. Quinagolide and cabergoline, both selective DA receptor subtype-2 selective agonists, also are effective in reducing PRL secretion and tumor size in adult patients who have prolactinomas, even in those who have a previous poor responsive or intolerance to bromocriptine. Cabergoline in particular has received attention for its tolerability and high compliance rates [28]. Cabergoline has a longer half-life than bromocriptine, and its convenient weekly administration makes it an excellent therapeutic alternative [32,33].

For women who wish to maintain fertile, bromocriptine has been used in several thousand women during pregnancy [33]. There seems to be no increased incidence of birth defects in the more than 2000 children born to women taking bromocriptine. A more limited experience exists in women taking cabergoline during pregnancy but the data suggest no increased risk above baseline in babies exposed during gestation [34].

Although medical therapy can be highly effective, some patients are intolerant of the medications and some tumors are resistant to pharmacotherapy. In patients who are refractory to medical therapy, transsphenoidal surgery can obtain remission in 85% of patients with microprolactinomas (see Table 3). Not unexpectedly, results with macroprolactinomas routinely are less successful, with experienced centers reporting remission rates of approximately 50%, which may reflect a contribution of tumor size or more aggressive biologic behavior [5,25,26,35,36].

*Cushing's disease*

Transsphenoidal resection is the treatment of choice for corticotropin-secreting adenomas. Surgical excision is successful in the majority of patients, with initial remission rates of 70% to 98% and long-term remission of 50% to 98% in most studies (see Table 3) [1,10,37]. The success rate decreases when the patients are followed more than 5 years postoperatively, and patients should be followed carefully for recurrences [10,38]. Surgical morbidity is low when an experienced neurosurgical team performs the procedure [36,39]. Adrenal insufficiency often follows surgery, and patients may require steroid replacement therapy for 6 to 12 months postoperatively until their own hypothalamic-pituitary axis regains function. After normalization of cortisol levels, children may experience resumption of normal growth or even catch-up growth [10].

The optimal treatment modality in patients who have recurrence after transsphenoidal adenomectomy remains controversial; choices include repeat transsphenoidal surgery, radiosurgical treatment, and adrenalectomy [1,27,40]. Radiotherapy with or without concomitant mitotane treatment may be used in patients who have macroadenomas [41], although caution must be exercised, as the long-term risk of side effects, such as radiation necrosis and new neoplasms, remains unknown [42–44]. Although surgery has the potential to cause hypopituitarism or diabetes insipidus, hypothalamic-pituitary dysfunction is a frequent complication of radiation therapy [35]. For recurrent or residual pituitary adenomas, stereotactic radiosurgery with either the Gamma Knife or a modified linear accelerator minimizes the toxic effects of radiation to the brain while still controlling tumor growth and normalizing horomonal overproduction. Bilateral adrenalectomy is the ultimate therapeutic option in case of failure of surgery and radiosurgery.

### Growth hormone–secreting adenomas

The objectives when treating GH-secreting adenomas include resolution of mass effect, restoration of normal basal and stimulated GH secretion, and preservation of normal pituitary function. Although medical therapy steadily is improving, transsphendoidal surgery remains the first-line therapy for treating this disease. Surgery achieves biochemical remission (normal IGF-1 levels and nadir GH < 1 ng/L during OGTT) in approximately 85% of patients who have microadenomas and in 50% of those who have macroadenomas (see Table 3). Transsphenoidal surgery is effective in pediatric patients who have gigantism as it is in adults who have acromegaly [2,45]. Once in remission, up to 8% of patients recur within 10 years, of whom 48% again achieve remission with repeat transsphenoidal surgery [46,47]. Current nonsurgical options for treating acromegaly include stereotactic radiosugery and pharmacologic suppression of GH levels by means of DA agonists, somatostatin analogs, or the GH receptor blocker, pegvisomant [8,9].

Recent reports highlight impressive advancements in the pharmacologic treatment of GH adenomas. Traditionally, the two options for medical therapy for these secretory tumors have been DA agonists and somatostatin analogs. DA agonists provide symptomatic relief in the majority of patients but normalize IGF-1 levels only in approximately 20% to 40% of cases.

Somatostatin analogs (octreotide, Sandostatin LAR, lanreotide, and lanreotide SR) can normalize IGF-1 levels in up to 60% of patients and have a more favorable side-effect profile compared with DA agonists [9]. The recently introduced GH receptor antagonist, pegvisomant, has normalized IGF-1 levels in 90% to 100% of patients who have refractory disease, although reported experience with its administration for greater than 2 years remains limited [46,48].

*Adjuvant treatments*

Radiation therapy historically was the adjuvant treatment of choice for recurrent or residual pituitary adenomas; however, its use has waned because of its slow rate of hormone normalization and increased incidence of early and late complications. Contrary to fractionation schemes, the goal of radiosurgery is to deliver a highly effective dose of radiation to a tumor in a single session. Using image guidance and steep fall-off, radiosurgery largely spares the surrounding tissues from the harmful effects of radiation. Devices that administer radiosurgery include the Gamma Knife, a linear accelerator-based system, or proton beams.

For patients who have pituitary adenomas, radiosurgery is intended to inactivate the tumor cells, thereby preventing tumor growth and, for functioning adenomas, to normalize hormone production. Published series have demonstrated adenoma growth control in up to 95% of patients (Table 4) [4,41]. Ideally, these goals are met without damage to the adjacent pituitary gland or surrounding vascular and neural structures. It is important to differentiate a radiosurgical response from the natural history of a slow growing lesion; thus, long-term radiologic follow-up must indicate adenoma growth cessation or shrinkage over a prolonged time period [49,50]. Reported rates of endocrinologic remission after radiosurgery for functional pituitary adenomas vary greatly. This variance likely is a function of

Table 4
Gamma Knife radiosurgery for clinically nonfunctioning pituitary adenomas (minimum of 20 patients)

| Authors | Patients (n) | Mean follow-up | Margin dose (Gy) | Growth control (%) |
|---------|-------------|----------------|------------------|--------------------|
| Lim [59] | 22 | 26 | 25 | 92 |
| Witt et al [50] | 24 | 32 | 19 | 94 |
| Mokry [60] | 31 | 21 | 14 | 98 |
| Izawa et al [55] | 23 | 28 | 22 | 94 |
| Feigl [61] | 61 | 55 | 15 | 94 |
| Sheehan [62] | 42 | 31 | 16 | 98 |
| Muracevic (2003) | 60 | 21.7 | 16.5 | 95 |
| Iwai (2005) | 34 | 36 | 14 | 93 |
| Picozzi (2005) | 51 | 60 | 16.5 | NR[a] |

[a] NR, better than control.

methodology, study population size, length of follow-up, and remission criteria. Initial hormonal normalization followed by hypersecretory recurrences is observed after radiosurgery as with open surgery [51].

Many neuroendocrine centers have reported their results in patients who have CD treated with radiosurgery, with endocrinologic remission rates ranging from 17% to 83% [4,49,50,52]. At the University of Virginia, after treatment and long-term observation of 113 patients who had CD, the authors have observed a remission rate of 54% (Table 5) [4,52].

Just as the endocrinologic criteria for CD remain a subject of debate, the criteria for remission of acromegaly also are inconsistent. The most widely accepted guideline for a remission in acromegaly consists of a GH level less than 1 ng/mL in response to a glucose challenge and a normal serum IGF-1 when matched for age and gender [9]. Twenty-five studies detail the results of radiosurgical treatment for 420 patients who had acromegaly with remission rates after radiosurgery ranging from 0 to 100% (Table 6) [3,27,53–56].

In patients who had prolactinomas, the defining criteria for endocrinologic remission consistently is defined as normalization of serum PRL levels for gender. Twenty-two radiosurgical studies have been performed on patients who had prolactinomas receiving a mean dose to tumor margin of 13.3 to 33 Gy with remission rates varying from 0 to 84% [20,57,58].

Stereotactic radiosurgery also has become an important tool in the treatment of craniopharyngiomas, which generally are radiosensitive tumors. Radiation therapy could represent an important adjuvant option, allowing surgeons the opportunity to safely remove easily resectable tumors but spare patients unnecessary risk by radiating residual.

Because up to 60% of craniopharyngiomas are both solid and cystic, a variety of additional adjuvant treatments, including aspiration of the cyst or stereotactic Ommaya reservoir, are possible. This allows for intracavitary brachitherapy with the antibiotic, bleomycin, radioactive phosphorus (32P), or the alpha-emitting 90Yt. The squamous epithelial cells that are

Table 5
Radiosurgery for CD (minimum of 20 patients)

| Authors | Patients | Mean follow-up (months) | Margin dose (Gy) | Endocrine control (%) | Growth control |
|---------|----------|-------------------------|------------------|-----------------------|----------------|
| Witt et al [50] | 25 | 32 | 19 | 28 | 92 |
| Sheehan (1999) | 43 | 44 | 20 | 63 | 100 |
| Feigl [61] | 20 | 64 | 29 | 35 | 100 |
| Devin [63][a] | 35 | 35 | 22 | 49 | 91 |
| Jagannathan [64] | 70 | 42 | 24 | 52 | 95 |
| Castinetti [65] | 40 | 54 | 29.5 | 42.5 | Not reported |

[a] Linear accelerator; the rest are Gamma Knife.

Table 6
Gamma knife radiosurgery for acromegaly (minimum of 20 patients)

| Authors | Patients | Mean follow-up (months) | Margin dose (Gy) | Endocrine control (%) | Growth control |
|---|---|---|---|---|---|
| Lim (1992) | 20 | 26 | 25 | 38 | 92 |
| Hayashi [66] | 22 | 16 | 24 | 41 | 92 |
| Laws (1999) | 56 | Not reported | Not reported | 25 | Not reported |
| Izawa et al [55] | 29 | 28 | 22 | 41 | 94 |
| Pollock [67] | 26 | 42 | 20 | 42 | 100 |
| Attanaiso [68] | 30 | 46 | 20 | 37 | 100 |
| Castinetti (2005) | 82 | 49.5 | Not reported | 23 | Not reported |
| Jezkova [69] | 96 | 54 | 15 | 50 | 62.3 |

present in craniopharyngiomas are highly sensitive to these antineoplastic agents. Thus, if the solid part of the tumor is small, surgery can be avoided and patients can be treated with radiosurgery directly.

## Follow-up

Prognosis for patients who have sellar tumors is dependent on patient status, comorbid conditions, tumor size, extension, and functional histotype. Serial clinical, ophthalmologic, endocrinologic, and radiologic evaluations are required for patients who have nonfunctioning tumors. Children and adolescents should have careful monitoring of height, weight, and pubertal status. A qualified neuroendocrine team should screen patients for hypothyroidism, adrenal insufficiency, diabetes insipidus, and other endocrinopathies at regular intervals, and hormone replacement should be administered if needed. A postoperative MRI should be performed within 3 months of treatment and yearly thereafter to evaluate for tumor recurrence or for residual tumor.

For hormonally active tumors, surveillance measures should include the steps outlined previously and specific attention to ensure that the hormonal hypersecretion remains normalized.

## References

[1] Thapar K, Laws ER Jr. Pituitary tumors. In: AHK, Laws ER Jr, editors. Brain tumors. London: Churchill Livingstone; 2001. p. 803–54.

[2] Jagannathan J, Dumont AS, Jane JA Jr, et al. Pediatric sellar tumors: diagnostic procedures and management. Neurosurg Focus 2005;18:E6.

[3] Davis JR, Farrell WE, Clayton RN. Pituitary tumours. Reproduction 2001;121:363–71.

[4] Sheehan JP, Jagannathan J, Pouratian N, et al. Stereotactic radiosurgery for pituitary adenomas: a review of the literature and our experience. Front Horm Res 2006;34:185–205.

[5] Colao A, Loche S, Cappa M, et al. Prolactinomas in children and adolescents. Clinical presentation and long-term follow-up. J Clin Endocrinol Metab 1998;83:2777–80.

[6] Molitch ME. Pathologic hyperprolactinemia. Endocrinol Metab Clin North Am 1992;21: 877–901.

[7] Randall RV, Scheithauer BW, Laws ER Jr, et al. Pituitary adenomas associated with hyper-prolactinemia: a clinical and immunohistochemical study of 97 patients operated on trans-sphenoidally. Mayo Clin Proc 1985;60:753–62.

[8] Laws ER Jr. Acromegaly and gigantism. In: Wilkins RHRS, editor. Neurosurgery. New York: McGraw Hill; 1985. p. 864–7.

[9] Vance ML. Endocrinological evaluation of acromegaly. J Neurosurg 1998;89:499–500.

[10] Kanter AS, Diallo AO, Jane JA Jr, et al. Single-center experience with pediatric Cushing's disease. J Neurosurg 2005;103:413–20.

[11] Nieman LK. Medical therapy of Cushing's disease. Pituitary 2002;5:77–82.

[12] Dickerman RD, Oldfield EH. Basis of persistent and recurrent Cushing disease: an analysis of findings at repeated pituitary surgery. J Neurosurg 2002;97:1343–9.

[13] Abe T, Ludecke DK, Saeger W. Clinically nonsecreting pituitary adenomas in childhood and adolescence. Neurosurgery 1998;42:744–50, [discussion: 750–1].

[14] Lindholm J. Cushing's syndrome: historical aspects. Pituitary 2000;3:97–104.

[15] Arnaldi G, Angeli A, Atkinson AB, et al. Diagnosis and complications of Cushing's syndrome: a consensus statement. J Clin Endocrinol Metab 2003;88:5593–602.

[16] Oldfield EH, Chrousos GP, Schulte HM, et al. Preoperative lateralization of ACTH-secret-ing pituitary microadenomas by bilateral and simultaneous inferior petrosal venous sinus sampling. N Engl J Med 1985;312:100–3.

[17] Jagannathan J, Dumont AS, Prevedello DM, et al. Genetics of pituitary adenomas: current theories and future implications. Neurosurg Focus 2005;19:E4.

[18] Colao A, Di Sarno A, Landi ML, et al. Macroprolactinoma shrinkage during cabergo-line treatment is greater in naive patients than in patients pretreated with other dopa-mine agonists: a prospective study in 110 patients. J Clin Endocrinol Metab 2000;85: 2247–52.

[19] Corsello SM, Ubertini G, Altomare M, et al. Giant prolactinomas in men: efficacy of caber-goline treatment. Clin Endocrinol (Oxf) 2003;58:662–70.

[20] Shrivastava RK, Arginteanu MS, King WA, et al. Giant prolactinomas: clinical manage-ment and long-term follow up. J Neurosurg 2002;97:299–306.

[21] Jane JA Jr, Laws ER Jr. The surgical management of pituitary adenomas in a series of 3,093 patients. J Am Coll Surg 2001;193:651–9.

[22] Ciric I, Ragin A, Baumgartner C, et al. Complications of transsphenoidal surgery: results of a national survey, review of the literature, and personal experience. Neurosurgery 1997;40: 225–36, [discussion: 236–7].

[23] Kelly DF, Laws ER Jr, Fossett D. Delayed hyponatremia after transsphenoidal surgery for pituitary adenoma. Report of nine cases. J Neurosurg 1995;83:363–7.

[24] Friedman RB, Oldfield EH, Nieman LK, et al. Repeat transsphenoidal surgery for Cushing's disease. J Neurosurg 1989;71:520–7.

[25] Laws ER Jr, Fode NC, Redmond MJ. Transsphenoidal surgery following unsuccessful prior therapy. An assessment of benefits and risks in 158 patients. J Neurosurg 1985;63: 823–9.

[26] Laws ER Jr. Recurrent pituitary adenomas. In: Landolt AM, Vance ML, Reilly PL, editors. Pituitary adenomas. Edinburgh (Scotland): Churchill-Livingstone; 1996. p. 385–94.

[27] Nicola G, Tonnarelli G, Griner A. Surgery for recurrence of pituitary adenomas. In: GF, Beck-Peccoz P, BA, editors. Pituitary adenomas: new trends in basic and clinical research. Amsterdam: Excerpta Medica; 1991. p. 329–38.

[28] Cappabianca P. "Boom boom" surgery. Surg Neurol 2007;67:106.

[29] Jane JA Jr, Han J, Prevedello DM, et al. Perspectives on endoscopic transsphenoidal surgery. Neurosurg Focus 2005;19:E2.

[30] Cappabianca P, Alfieri A, Colao A, et al. Endoscopic endonasal transsphenoidal surgery in recurrent and residual pituitary adenomas: technical note. Minim Invasive Neurosurg 2000; 43:38–43.

[31] Webster J. Clinical management of prolactinomas. Baillieres Best Pract Res Clin Endocrinol Metab 1999;13:395–408.

[32] McKeage K, Cheer S, Wagstaff AJ. Octreotide long-acting release (LAR): a review of its use in the management of acromegaly. Drugs 2003;63:2473–99.

[33] Colao A, di Sarno A, Pivonello R, et al. Dopamine receptor agonists for treating prolactinomas. Expert Opin Investig Drugs 2002;11:787–800.

[34] Ferrari CI, Abs R, Bevan JS, et al. Treatment of macroprolactinoma with cabergoline: a study of 85 patients. Clin Endocrinol (Oxf) 1997;46:409–13.

[35] Inoue HK, Kohga H, Hirato M, et al. Pituitary adenomas treated by microsurgery with or without Gamma Knife surgery: experience in 122 cases. Stereotact Funct Neurosurg 1999; 72(Suppl 1):125–31.

[36] Laws ER Jr, Ebersold GP. The results of transsphenoidal surgery in specific clinical entities. In: Laws ER Jr, Randall R, EBK, editors. Management of pituitary adenomas and related lesions with emphasis on transsphenoidal microsurgery. New York: Appleton-Century-Crofts; 1982. p. 277–305.

[37] Mampalam TJ, Tyrrell JB, Wilson CB. Transsphenoidal microsurgery for Cushing disease. A report of 216 cases. Ann Intern Med 1988;109:487–93.

[38] Shimon I, Ram Z, Cohen ZR, et al. Transsphenoidal surgery for Cushing's disease: endocrinological follow-up monitoring of 82 patients. Neurosurgery 2002;51:57–61 [discussion: 61–2].

[39] Chandler WF, Schteingart DE, Lloyd RV, et al. Surgical treatment of Cushing's disease. J Neurosurg 1987;66:204–12.

[40] Martinez R, Bravo G, Burzaco J, et al. Pituitary tumors and gamma knife surgery. Clinical experience with more than two years of follow-up. Stereotact Funct Neurosurg 1998; 70(Suppl 1):110–8.

[41] Pan L, Zhang N, Wang E, et al. Pituitary adenomas: the effect of gamma knife radiosurgery on tumor growth and endocrinopathies. Stereotact Funct Neurosurg 1998;70(Suppl 1): 119–26.

[42] Shamisa A, Bance M, Nag S, et al. Glioblastoma multiforme occurring in a patient treated with gamma knife surgery. Case report and review of the literature. J Neurosurg 2001;94: 816–21.

[43] Yu JS, Yong WH, Wilson D, et al. Glioblastoma induction after radiosurgery for meningioma. Lancet 2000;356:1576–7.

[44] Zhang N, Pan L, Wang EM, et al. Radiosurgery for growth hormone-producing pituitary adenomas. J Neurosurg 2000;93(Suppl 3):6–9.

[45] Freda PU. How effective are current therapies for acromegaly? Growth Horm IGF Res 2003; 13(Suppl A):S144–51.

[46] Melmed S, Casanueva FF, Cavagnini F, et al. Guidelines for acromegaly management. J Clin Endocrinol Metab 2002;87:4054–8.

[47] Abe T, Tara LA, Ludecke DK. Growth hormone-secreting pituitary adenomas in childhood and adolescence: features and results of transnasal surgery. Neurosurgery 1999;45:1–10.

[48] Melmed S, Vance ML, Barkan AL, et al. Current status and future opportunities for controlling acromegaly. Pituitary 2002;5:185–96.

[49] Witt TC. Stereotactic radiosurgery for pituitary tumors. Neurosurg Focus 2003;14:e10.

[50] Witt TC, Kondziolka D, Flickinger JC, et al. Gamma Knife radiosurgery for pituitary tumors. In: Lunsford LD, Kondziolka D, Flickinger J, editors. Gamma Knife brain surgery. Progress in neurological surgery. Basel (Switzerland): Karger; 1998. p. 114–27.

[51] Giustina A, Barkan A, Casanueva FF, et al. Criteria for cure of acromegaly: a consensus statement. J Clin Endocrinol Metab 2000;85:526–9.

[52] Sheehan JM, Vance ML, Sheehan JP, et al. Radiosurgery for Cushing's disease after failed transsphenoidal surgery. J Neurosurg 2000;93:738–42.

[53] Cozzi R, Barausse M, Asnaghi D, et al. Failure of radiotherapy in acromegaly. Eur J Endocrinol 2001;145:717–26.

[54] Fukuoka S, Ito T, Takanashi M, et al. Gamma knife radiosurgery for growth hormone-secreting pituitary adenomas invading the cavernous sinus. Stereotact Funct Neurosurg 2001;76:213–7.

[55] Izawa M, Hayashi M, Nakaya K, et al. Gamma knife radiosurgery for pituitary adenomas. J Neurosurg 2000;93(Suppl 3):19–22.

[56] Jackson IM, Noren G. Gamma knife radiosurgery for pituitary tumours. Baillieres Best Pract Res Clin Endocrinol Metab 1999;13:461–9.

[57] Pouratian N, Sheehan J, Jagannathan J, et al. Gamma knife radiosurgery for medically and surgically refractory prolactinomas. Neurosurgery 2006;59:255–66 [discussion: 255–66].

[58] Thorsen FA, Ganz JC. Dose planning with the Leksell Gamma Knife: the effect on dose volume of more than one shot at the same target point. Stereotact Funct Neurosurg 1993; 61(Suppl 1):151–63.

[59] Lim YL, Leem W, Kim TS, et al. Four years experience in the treatment of pituitary adenomas with gamma knife radiosurgery. Stereotact Funct Neurosurg 1998;70(Suppl 1):95–109.

[60] Mokry M, Ramschak-Schwarzer S, Simbrunner J, et al. A six-year experience with the postoperative radiosurgical management of pituitary adenomas. Stereotact Funct Neurosurg 1999;72(Suppl 1):88–100.

[61] Feigl GC, Bonelli CM, Berghold A, et al. Effects of gamma knife radiosurgery of pituitary adenomas on pituitary function. J Neurosurg 2002;97:415–21.

[62] Sheehan JP, Kondziolka D, Flickinger J, et al. Radiosurgery for residual or recurrent nonfunctioning pituitary adenoma. J Neurosurg 2002;97:408–14.

[63] Devin JK, Allen GS, Cmelak A, et al. The efficacy of linear accelerator radiosurgery in the management of patients with Cushing's disease. Stereotact Funct Neurosurg 2004;82: 254–62.

[64] Jagannathan J, Sheehan P, Pouratian N, et al. Gamma knife surgery for Cushing's disease. J Neurosurg 2007;106:980–7.

[65] Castinetti F, Nagai M, Dufour H, et al. Gamma knife radiosurgery is a successful adjunctive treatment in Cushing's disease. Eur J Endocrinol 2007;156:91–8.

[66] Hayashi M, Izawa M, Hiyama H, et al. Gamma knife radiosurgery for pituitary adenomas. Stereotact Funct Neurosurg 1999;72(Suppl 1):111–8.

[67] Pollock BE, Nippoldt TB, Stafford SL, et al. Results of stereotactic radiosurgery in patients with hormone-producing pituitary adenomas: factors associated with endocrine normalization. J Neurosurg 2002;97:525–30.

[68] Attanasio R, Epaminonda P, Motti E, et al. Gamma knife radiosurgery in acromegaly: a 4-year follow-up study. J Clin Endocrinol Metab 2003;88:3105–12.

[69] Jezkova J, Marek J, Hana V, et al. Gamma knife radiosurgery for acromegaly—long-term experience. Clin Endocrinol (Oxf) 2006;64:588–95.

ELSEVIER
SAUNDERS

Neurol Clin 25 (2007) 1251–1258

NEUROLOGIC
CLINICS

# Index

*Note:* Page numbers of article titles are in **boldface** type.

0733-8619/07/$ - see front matter © 2007 Elsevier Inc. All rights reserved.
doi:10.1016/S0733-8619(07)00112-0

*neurologic.theclinics.com*

| 1. Publication Title | 2. Publication Number | | | | | | | | 3. Filing Date |
|---|---|---|---|---|---|---|---|---|---|
| Neurologic Clinics | 0 | 0 | 0 | - | 7 | 1 | 1 | 2 | 9/14/07 |

| 4. Issue Frequency | 5. Number of Issues Published Annually | 6. Annual Subscription Price |
|---|---|---|
| Feb, May, Aug, Nov | 4 | $198.00 |

7. Complete Mailing Address of Known Office of Publication (Not printer) (Street, city, county, state, and ZIP+4)

Elsevier Inc.
360 Park Avenue South
New York, NY 10010-1710

Contact Person: Stephen Bushing

Telephone (Include area code): 215-239-3688

8. Complete Mailing Address of Headquarters or General Business Office of Publisher (Not printer)

Elsevier Inc., 360 Park Avenue South, New York, NY 10010-1710

9. Full Names and Complete Mailing Addresses of Publisher, Editor, and Managing Editor (Do not leave blank)

Publisher (Name and complete mailing address)

John Schrefer, Elsevier, Inc., 1600 John F. Kennedy Blvd. Suite 1800, Philadelphia, PA 19103-2899

Editor (Name and complete mailing address)

Donald Mumford, Elsevier, Inc., 1600 John F. Kennedy Blvd. Suite 1800, Philadelphia, PA 19103-2899

Managing Editor (Name and complete mailing address)

Catherine Bewick, Elsevier, Inc., 1600 John F. Kennedy Blvd. Suite 1800, Philadelphia, PA 19103-2899

10. Owner (Do not leave blank. If the publication is owned by a corporation, give the name and address of the corporation immediately followed by the names and addresses of all stockholders owning or holding 1 percent or more of the total amount of stock. If not owned by a corporation, give the names and addresses of the individual owners. If owned by a partnership or other unincorporated firm, give its name and address as well as those of each individual owner. If the publication is published by a nonprofit organization, give its name and address.)

| Full Name | Complete Mailing Address |
|---|---|
| Wholly owned subsidiary of | 4520 East-West Highway |
| Reed/Elsevier, US holdings | Bethesda, MD 20814 |

11. Known Bondholders, Mortgagees, and Other Security Holders Owning or Holding 1 Percent or More of Total Amount of Bonds, Mortgages, or Other Securities. If none, check box. ☐ None

| Full Name | Complete Mailing Address |
|---|---|
| N/A | |

12. Tax Status (For completion by nonprofit organizations authorized to mail at nonprofit rates) (Check one)
The purpose, function, and nonprofit status of this organization and the exempt status for federal income tax purposes:
☐ Has Not Changed During Preceding 12 Months
☐ Has Changed During Preceding 12 Months (Publisher must submit explanation of change with this statement)

PS Form 3526, September 2006 (Page 1 of 3 (Instructions Page 3)) PSN 7530-01-000-9931 **PRIVACY NOTICE**: See our Privacy policy in www.usps.com

| 13. Publication Title | | 14. Issue Date for Circulation Data Below |
|---|---|---|
| Neurologic Clinics | | August 2007 |

| 15. Extent and Nature of Circulation | | | Average No. Copies Each Issue During Preceding 12 Months | No. Copies of Single Issue Published Nearest to Filing Date |
|---|---|---|---|---|
| a. Total Number of Copies (Net press run) | | | 2650 | 2400 |
| b. Paid Circulation (By Mail and Outside the Mail) | (1) | Mailed Outside-County Paid Subscriptions Stated on PS Form 3541. (Include paid distribution above nominal rate, advertiser's proof copies, and exchange copies) | 1237 | 1147 |
| | (2) | Mailed In-County Paid Subscriptions Stated on PS Form 3541 (Include paid distribution above nominal rate, advertiser's proof copies, and exchange copies) | | |
| | (3) | Paid Distribution Outside the Mails Including Sales Through Dealers and Carriers, Street Vendors, Counter Sales, and Other Paid Distribution Outside USPS® | 657 | 647 |
| | (4) | Paid Distribution by Other Classes Mailed Through the USPS (e.g. First-Class Mail®) | | |
| c. Total Paid Distribution (Sum of 15b (1), (2), (3), and (4)) | | ► | 1894 | 1794 |
| d. Free or Nominal Rate Distribution (By Mail and Outside the Mail) | (1) | Free or Nominal Rate Outside-County Copies Included on PS Form 3541 | 73 | 60 |
| | (2) | Free or Nominal Rate In-County Copies Included on PS Form 3541 | | |
| | (3) | Free or Nominal Rate Copies Mailed at Other Classes Mailed Through the USPS (e.g. First-Class Mail) | | |
| | (4) | Free or Nominal Rate Distribution Outside the Mail (Carriers or other means) | | |
| e. Total Free or Nominal Rate Distribution (Sum of 15d (1), (2), (3) and (4)) | | ► | 73 | 60 |
| f. Total Distribution (Sum of 15c and 15e) | | ► | 1967 | 1854 |
| g. Copies not Distributed (See instructions to publishers #4 (page #3)) | | ► | 683 | 546 |
| h. Total (Sum of 15f and g) | | ► | 2650 | 2400 |
| i. Percent Paid (15c divided by 15f times 100) | | | 96.29% | 96.76% |

16. Publication of Statement of Ownership

☐ If the publication is a general publication, publication of this statement is required. Will be printed in the November 2007 issue of this publication.

☐ Publication not required

17. Signature and Title of Editor, Publisher, Business Manager, or Owner

*[signature]* Date: September 14, 2007

Joel Fanucci – Executive Director of Subscription Services

I certify that all information furnished on this form is true and complete. I understand that anyone who furnishes false or misleading information on this form or who omits material or information requested on the form may be subject to criminal sanctions (including fines and imprisonment) and/or civil sanctions (including civil penalties).

PS Form 3526, September 2006 (Page 2 of 3)

# Moving?

## Make sure your subscription moves with you!

To notify us of your new address, find your **Clinics Account Number** (located on your mailing label above your name), and contact customer service at:

**E-mail: elspcs@elsevier.com**

**800-654-2452 (subscribers in the U.S. & Canada)**
**407-345-4000 (subscribers outside of the U.S. & Canada)**

**Fax number: 407-363-9661**

**Elsevier Periodicals Customer Service**
6277 Sea Harbor Drive
Orlando, FL 32887-4800

*To ensure uninterrupted delivery of your subscription, please notify us at least 4 weeks in advance of move.